Date Due

FEB 3 1994		
2-26-04		
DISCARD		

Oakton Community College
Morton Grove, Illinois

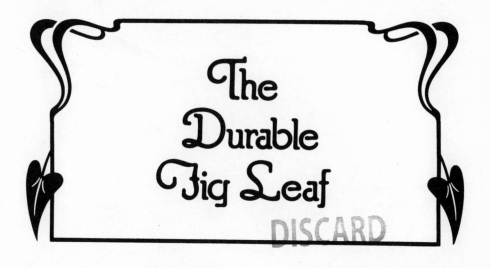

The Durable Fig Leaf

BY MARK STRAGE

The Durable Fig Leaf

Women of Power:
The Life and Times of Catherine de' Medici

Cape to Cairo: Rape of a Continent

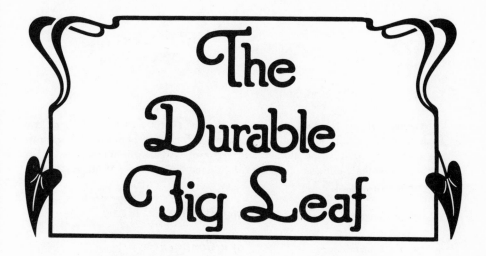

The Durable Fig Leaf

A Historical, Cultural, Medical,
Social, Literary, and Iconographic
Account of Man's Relations with
His Penis

by Mark Strage

51426

WILLIAM MORROW AND COMPANY, INC.
New York   1980

Library of Congress Cataloging in Publication Data

Strage, Mark.
    The durable fig leaf.

    Includes bibliographical references and index.
    1. Penis. 2. Masculinity. 3. Men—Sexual behavior. I. Title.
GT495.S86   301.41   79-20722
ISBN 0-688-03582-5
ISBN 0-688-08582-2 pbk.

Book Design by Michael Mauceri

Printed in the United States of America.

First Edition

1 2 3 4 5 6 7 8 9 10

This one is for Michael

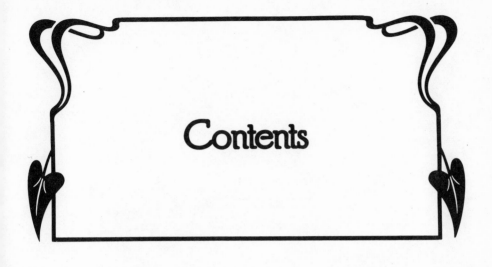

Contents

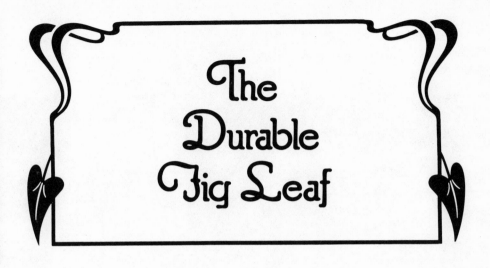

The
Durable
Fig Leaf

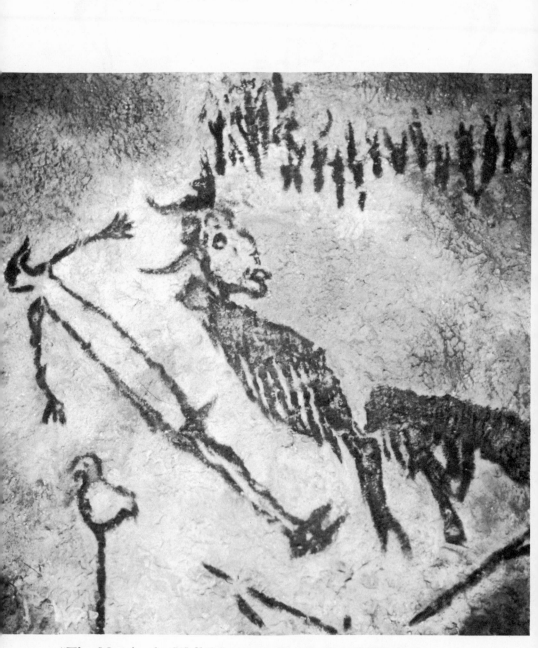

"The Man in the Well." Lascaux, France (*ca.* 13,000 B.C.)
Editorial Photocolor Archives

Introduction

On September 12, 1940, four village youths from Montignac, in the Dordogne region of France, were out hunting rabbits on a wooded crest overlooking the Vézère River when their dog vanished into the bramble-screened root hole of a fallen tree. In the course of retrieving it, two of the boys lowered themselves into the hole, slid down a slope of slippery clay, and came to rest on the cool, dry floor of a wide gallery. They struck some matches which one of them was carrying in his pocket, looked around, and rushed back to tell their schoolmaster what they had seen.[1]

They had accidentally discovered the great painted cave of Lascaux, perhaps the noblest, most astonishing monument of prehistory. Here, preserved by a layer of calcite crystals and so fresh that they could have been finished yesterday rather than 15,000 years ago, are murals of hundreds of animals: lines of trotting ponies, aurochs grazing and tossing their heads, gravid mares, a herd of reindeer swimming a river, bulls and stags pawing the ground, lions, ibexes, boars—all drawn with such attention to form and detail that zoologists have no difficulty identifying species which they previously knew only through skeletal remains.

More careful investigation revealed that the cave is on two levels, and on the lower of them, at the bottom of a twenty-foot well, was found the most extraordinary painting of all. It shows a badly wounded bison, his entrails spilling out in great loops, his legs quivering under him, and his tail furiously whipping the air. His head is turned, and his horns are leveled toward a man who appears to be falling backward. In contrast with the animal, which is startlingly lifelike, the man has been sketched with a few simple lines, as if by a child. At his feet lie his spear and a hooked stick; near his side,

11

also sketched, is the figure of a bird perched on a pole. To the left, facing away from the scene, is the figure of a retreating rhinoceros.

It is an arresting composition which has received more attention than any other cave painting. One reason is that it is one of the earliest representations of a human figure. Another is its obvious narrative intent. A third, which leaps to the eye on a closer look, is that the human figure, so economically drawn, displays a conspicuous erection.

Millions of words have been written about prehistoric painting. Almost a dozen books have been devoted to the Lascaux cave alone.[2] The scene of the man and the bison has been the subject of numerous interpretations. But to the knowledge of this writer, no one has ever explained the meaning of that odd anatomical detail. This omission is about to be rectified, but first, something should be said about the artist who drew the picture.

Obviously we don't know his name, but we do know a great deal about him. In appearance, he was taller, stronger, and probably more handsome than we are, with a well-proportioned body, a high forehead, and cleanly formed cheekbones. In comparison to his predecessors, he possessed highly developed skills. He could strike and shape flint into scrapers, chisels, and blades so keen that they can still cut flesh at a touch. Moreover, he had learned to use them to fashion still other implements. From markings left on the joints of animals, we know that he skinned his game, and from ivory objects that could have served only as needles or punches, we know that he, or his women, sewed the hides into clothing. He had artificial light—crudely scooped-out stones with the marks of calcined wicks around their lip could have served no other purpose—and probably artificial heat as well. Pebbles and gravel have been found carefully piled on the remains of live coals; they would have served to store and slowly to release heat, as they still do in stoves used in the cold parts of Europe.

He also used his tools to shape animal bones and teeth, shells, fish vertebrae and then to thread them into pendants and necklaces. That he would take the time for such activity is profoundly significant because it proves that he had at last reached a milestone in his long evolutionary voyage—a voyage that had begun with the capacity for objectification and led in turn to articulated speech, to the notion of symbols, to abstract thought, to the concept of persons and of values, and finally to the acquisition, for the first time, of an awareness of himself. Then, as now, a necklace or pendant is not necessary to satisfy any immediate material need. But self-awareness arouses needs of its own. Whatever they may have been, they could be satisfied only by wearing, or giving, a decoration which nature had withheld from him.

Self-awareness, a condition we associate uniquely with man, brought with it another equally exclusive human attribute—anxiety. Ritual burial, which is a response to the realization that death may not be the final end, was one of the manifestations of this anxiety. The painted caves are another.

Shortly after its discovery in 1879, the great painted cave at Altamira was inspected by a delegation of eminent scholars. They looked at the vast ceiling fresco of prancing, rearing bulls and pronounced it a fake. Time, and the discovery of more than 100 other sites forced a reversal of this judgment, but posed another problem. Why did early man, heretofore considered an unfeeling, incoherent brute hardly distinguishable from the animals he hunted, decorate the insides of his caves with such splendor?

The suggestion was made that the paintings were the spontaneous expression of a creative urge, supported by an emerging aesthetic sensibility—Art for Art's sake. But most of the paintings were found in remote, inaccessible caves, guarded by narrow tunnels and uncertain escarpments. Many of them were placed in such hidden crannies that it has been necessary to use mirrors in order to photograph them adequately. "No one," the British scholar R. R. Marett points out, "would dream of hedging round a mere picture-gallery with such trying turnstiles." [3]

Commentators then turned to Sir James G. Frazer's *The Golden Bough* and reinterpreted the paintings as examples of homeopathic or sympathetic magic—the belief that an effect resembles its cause and that objects which have once been in contact continue to act on each other at a distance. The animals that man hunted were the source of both his food and the materials of his technology. They were central to his survival and thus to his anxiety. Was it not possible, therefore, that he painted representations of them in order to celebrate them or even to help hunt them down? Scholars took another look at the paintings and noticed details they had not seen before, or had seen but not understood. Many of the animals appeared to be wounded by javelins or about to be pierced with flying darts. Squarish or oval geometric designs found in many of the paintings and previously inexplicable now became traps or nets.

When they were thus viewed as "wishful paintings," the very inaccessibility which had militated against the Art-for-Art's sake explanation became a potent supporting argument. The painted caves were not dwellings at all, but sanctuaries inside which magic rites were performed. A few imprints of what may have been human heels in the floor of one cave were accepted as evidence of ceremonial dances. Moreover, because the prints were small enough to have been left by children, some prehistorians even inferred the existence of initiation or puberty rites. The fact that paintings and drawings were frequently found superimposed over each other, while nearby stretches of wall had been left untouched, was taken to signify some ritual intent.[4]

But even this assumption did not help explain the scene of the falling man and the bison. The first to try was Henri Breuil, the French cleric-anthropologist who, by virtue of seventy years of exploration, writing, and lecturing, was until his death in 1961 the world's recognized authority on prehistoric art. Abbé Breuil, who had been called in to authenticate Lascaux upon its discovery, proposed that the scene "commemorated some fatal accident that occurred during the course of a hunt." The man has been mortally wounded by the bison, he explained, but the spear could not have inflicted the wound through which the bison's entrails are spilling. This was done by the rhinoceros, seen by Breuil as "stalking off with a contented air, having just destroyed what annoyed it before."[5] As for "the pole surmounted by a conventional bird without feet and almost without tail," Breuil pointed out that it was reminiscent of funeral posts used by the Alaskan Eskimos and Vancouver Indians. To support this interpretation of the painting as a commemorative monument, he also suggested that it might well have marked the actual grave of the fallen hunter.

Such was the weight of Breuil's prestige that the painting is still occasionally referred to as "The Prehistoric Tragedy," even though excavation of the cave floor revealed no skeleton or other signs of burial. A more serious objection to his interpretation, however, is that it raises the question of why the artist would have chosen to perpetuate a tragic, undesirable event in a context of magic and ritual.

Subsequent explanations have proposed that the rhinoceros was painted by a different hand and therefore not a part of the scene at all. The bird on the stick has been described as a hunting decoy, a special spear thrower, or a totemic emblem. It has been suggested that the bison is caught in a trap and therefore could not have attacked the man, and that to judge from the position of his head, he could not even see him. One interpretation holds that the scene depicts a confrontation between the bird clan and the bison clan. Still another sees significance in the shape of the bison's entrails.

All these versions start with the assumption that the man is dead or dying, but this is not necessarily true. Frazer has also observed:

> The explanation of life by the theory of an indwelling and practically immortal soul is one which the savage does not confine to human beings but extends to the animate creation in general. . . . Thus to the savage, who regards all living creatures as practically on a footing of quality with man, the act of killing and eating an animal must wear a very different aspect from that which the same act presents to us.[6]

The hunter *must* kill, and the act of murder which is necessary to his existence comes to weigh upon him, if not in moral, then in practical terms. To resolve this conflict and the fundamental anxiety it generates, he conceives an intermediate who can by appropriate means communicate with the animals, intercede on the hunter's behalf, and persuade them to return. Horst Kirchner, a German historian, proposed that the man in the well is precisely that intermediate —a shaman—and that he is therefore not dead or dying, but in a deep trance.[7]

This interpretation explains both the bird mask and the bird on the pole. If the spirit of the shaman is to leave his body and visit those of departed animals, it is logical to suppose that it would assume the form of life which the artist associated with free-ranging, effortless flight. Bird images are indeed found among Eskimos and other northern hunting cultures, but more specifically as attributes of shamans than as funerary decorations. That the human figure is rendered not only crudely but as a minimal representation is explained by the fact that the artist was attempting to portray a human being in a supernatural state, a concept beyond his powers of expression. But he did manage to convey a most impelling characteristic which he had himself undoubtedly observed: the rigidity of a subject undergoing extreme psychic stress.

Finally, the assumption that the painting portrays a shamanistic exercise has the additional virtue of accounting for a key aspect of the composition which all previous explanations, including Kirchner's, decorously ignored. The fallen figure is drawn with such economy of line that a single dot serves to represent its facial features. Why then did the artist take pains to indicate the penis and, more specifically, an ithyphallic—erect—penis?

The reason, quite possibly, is that he was drawing exactly what he had seen—that the shaman, in the performance of his ritual, had roused himself into a state of erection. Physiologically, erection is one of the manifestations of extreme masculine tension. Under the weight of culturally induced repression, we now tend to associate it exclusively with a single aspect of virile behavior. But there is evidence that this need not always be the case nor in fact *is* always the case.

Furthermore, just as the bird is the symbol of flight, the falling man's erection can also be interpreted as the visible attribute of power or domination. This idea is clearly expressed in another context: a Bronze Age rock carving found in southern Rhodesia. The scene depicts a rain-invoking ceremony. All the personages, the supplicants and the victim about to be sacrificed, are drawn normally. Only the central figure, the rain bringer, displays a conspicuous erection. Even more explicit is another early rock carving, this time of a hunting scene, in Tiut, Algeria. The hunter is shown kneeling as he aims an arrow at a passing animal. To his side is a larger human figure, its arms raised in a protective gesture. The two figures are connected by a continuous line drawn between their sexual organs, as if to provide a path for the flow of power.

Carved on huge boulders along the southern Scandinavian shore there exists an entire body of art—thousands of drawings which together give a comprehensive view of daily life some 3,500 years ago. Animals still appear, but they no longer predominate. Some of them have been domesticated. We know this from other evidence, but we could tell as well from the slope of their shoulders and the set of their feet. Many symbols appear, but unlike those in the caves, they are easy to interpret. Plain circles, circles with dots, circles quartered, and circles with spokes, they all represent the sun. Taken for granted in southern France and Spain, the sun would assume greater significance in these latitudes, especially to people who had begun to plant crops.

We see, for instance, a drawing of a man tilling the land, and we note that he is using a plow made of a forked tree branch shaped very much like the plow blades that were still used until recently in Sweden and Denmark. We note, too, that the artist has endowed him with an erection which, although too generous, points at the correct anatomic angle. Perhaps the intention, as some scholars maintain, was to invoke the concept of fertility—in the same way that, until not long ago, peasants in various parts of Europe would go out and copulate in the fields they had just sown. Looking further, however, we see men sailing on ships, men jumping, men blowing horns, men wielding enormous battle-axes, men playing some kind of game with a ball, men on skis. All of them have huge erections. We even see a jaunty little man doing nothing except walk along empty-handed but with an air of such obvious delight at the stiff penis which precedes him that the full implication of the word "cocky" pops into mind. The promotion of fertility cannot explain these exaggerated, eternally ready organs.

Additional examples of prehistoric art could be cited—in the Sahara, on the icy shores of the White Sea, in a hidden Alpine valley, in the American Southwest. From the moment he first achieved self-awareness, man has been preoccupied with his penis. He saw and drew it as the badge of his power and dominance—and as will be shown, he has used it as an instrument to achieve these ends. He recognized and appreciated that it was, as nature had intended, the agent of his keenest pleasure. And he very early discovered, as will also be shown, that it could be the cause for crushing, unremitting anxiety.

This preoccupation has not abated. On the contrary, the constellation of his conflicting emotions regarding the organ of his malehood has profoundly affected the manner in which man has organized his civilization, ordered his institutions, treated women and his fellow men, and even expressed the creations of his own imagination.

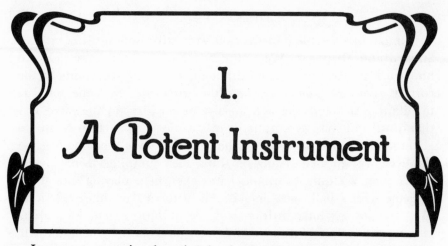

1.
A Potent Instrument

It appears certain that, in the beginning, God was a she. The earliest-known cult objects, dating back some 20,000 to 30,000 years, are statuettes of women. More than 130 have been found, in places scattered across Europe from France and the Apennines to the Don Valley and the shores of Lake Baikal in Siberia. Although they are made of ivory, bone, stone, coal, and even baked clay—the entire range of materials available to the artist—virtually all of them embody the same stylistic conventions: The breasts are large and pendulous, the loins and hips broad, the buttocks ample, the pubic triangles prominent, and the vulvas clearly incised. By contrast, the arms are so short as to be almost vestigial, and the legs are often unfinished and dwindle to a footless point.

Because of this emphasis on sexual characteristics, the most famous of these statuettes was christened the Venus of Willendorf, after the small Austrian village where it was found in 1908, and initiated speculation which still remains unresolved. The earliest published description of the statuette sounded an equivocal note: "The artist who modeled this figure showed great skill, and a daring realism pushed to a horrible extreme." [1] But the author went on to forgive the artist, because he was trying to invoke the concept of fecundity. This interpretation was probably inspired by Sir James Frazer, whose *Golden Bough*, first published in 1890, had noted, "To live and to cause to live, to beget children, these were the primary wants of man in the past, and they will be the primary wants of man in the future so long as the world lasts." [2]

These may indeed have been the primary wants of a dynastically minded late Victorian gentleman, but they were not necessarily shared by paleolithic man. The economic advantage of having chil-

18

dren is manifest in crop-planting societies in which additional hands can multiply the food supply, but it does not apply to hunting cultures in which food is dearly won and many years must pass before the young cease being a liability. It is always risky to draw analogies between early man and existing societies which happen to display equivalent technological skills, but it is significant that many of the surviving hunter cultures, scattered as far apart as the Kalahari Desert and the circumpolar North, practice population control through means ranging from sexual continence to infanticide. There is no evidence that early man availed himself of such controls, but neither is there evidence that he sought to promote fruitfulness of his own kind. The "erotic" explanation, which prompted the British historian Grahame Clarke to describe the figurines as "characteristic products of unregenerated male imagination," [3] is equally unsupported. The statuettes are small; the Venus of Willendorf is just 11.5 centimeters tall. Some are worn so smooth as to suggest extended manipulation. But even if they were intended for such use, the motivation need not have been exclusively erotic—not any more than the worn toe of the bronze Saint Peter in Rome attests to the foot fetishism of generations of worshipers. To make such an assumption is to see the reflection of what we deem to be sexual only in terms of our repertory of images and habits.

A more intriguing explanation, drawing upon the setting in which some of the statuettes were found, has been proposed by Franz Hancar. In Gagarino, in the Ukraine, six figurines carved out of mammoth ivory were discovered near the sunken walls of a dwelling. Elsewhere in Russia, another figurine was found inside the foundation itself, buried in a squarish hole which bore traces of fire. At other sites the statuettes were associated with burned animal bones and, in one instance, with animal skulls arranged in the form of a circle. Hancar points out that human figurines—invariably female—are still carved by present-day Siberian reindeer hunters as representations of their ancestral origin and as guardians of the hearth which they placate into benevolence with offerings of food. He describes paleolithic home life during the long winter months: The men, unable to hunt, work on their weapons or sit idle while the women carry on their tasks of sewing hides and curing meat. It is they who, by the division of labor, are charged with all the household industries which provide whatever comforts exist. From this role, it is an easy step to that of symbol for the family or kinship group. The statuettes, Hancar suggests, were the central object of a cult and, as such, "the earliest detectable expression of that undying idea which recognizes woman as the center and source of an effective magical force, and sees in her the embodiment of the beginning and continuance of life." [4] Not Venuses at all, but Junos.

The goddess, still steatopygous, reappears among the earliest vestiges of human presence in Asia Minor and the Near East. In *The Cult of the Goddess*, published in 1959, E. O. James notes that numerous headless clay female statuettes, all with pendulous breasts, prominent navels, and highly developed buttocks, were found in the neolithic village of Tell Arpachiyah, which dates back to before 4000 B.C. Subsequent digging has unearthed still earlier settlements such as Catal Huyuk in what is now Anatolia, where James Mellaart found no fewer than forty-nine shrines or sanctuaries dating back to 6000 B.C. "The principal deity," he writes, "was a goddess who is shown in three aspects, as a young woman, a mother giving birth, or as an old woman, in one case accompanied by a bird of prey, probably a vulture." [5] Still more recent diggings at Ganj Dareh, in Iran, dated at 7300 B.C., have turned up what one author chooses to call "pottery toys in the form of sexually explicit female statuettes." [6]

One of the astonishing aspects of the goddess is her ubiquity. She has been found in the Tigris Valley, in Egypt, on Crete and other Aegean islands, in Turkestan, in the Indus Valley, in Greece, and, as late as 1949, in an ancient flint mine in Grimes Graves in Norfolk, England. With time and the increased sophistication of her creators, her form changed. She became the slender, bare-breasted snake goddess of Knossos, the stately, regal Isis, the life-giving Ishtar, the all-powerful Cybele, flanked by her lions. She has come down to us in thousands of representations, in figurines, on bas-reliefs, cylinder seals, and signals, as decoration on clay vessels and sarcophagi. At various times and places she appears as the Mistress of the Trees, the Lady of the Beasts, the Great Spinstress weaving the web of life. But always, she is the all-supporting, all-including goddess: her two hands offering her breasts, or her left pointing to her genitals and the right to her left breast; nursing or fondling a male child; standing upright among animals; arms extended, holding tokens of her specific role.

In time she acquired a consort, but whether he is identifiable as her young lover, her servant, or even her son, he is clearly subservient to her. The divine qualities—to bring life, to sustain and enrich it, and eventually to take it away—all are vested exclusively in her. She causes the crops to grow, the flocks to multiply, the sun to rise, and the stars to move. In only one respect—a significant one, as will be seen—does she fail to exert her divine power. She hands down no laws.

Arguing in part from such archaeological finds and in part from interpretations of myth and legend, a few scholars and amateur historians have postulated an extended period during which mankind thrived under matriarchal rule, benignly administered by wise, gentle queens and enforced, to the extent that recidivist males made force necessary, by bands of amazons.[7] There is not a shred of direct evidence that such a system ever existed, and save for a few feminist polemicists, no serious writer of either sex now gives it more credence than such other happy inventions as Cockaigne and the Land of Oz. There is no question, however, that during the millennia which correspond to the age of the goddess, the position of women was different from what it became after she was eased from her throne.

With the retreat of the glaciers some 12,000 years ago, the protracted age of the Great Hunt came to an end. Fortunately, however, man learned to plant crops and domesticate animals. In consequence of the acquisition of these two useful skills, he was able to abandon his uncertain, nomadic existence and eventually to settle down in permanent communities, where he gradually perfected the other tools and talents that enabled him to create the civilization which we, in turn, have inherited.

The details and precise sequence of this process are still being worked out by archaeologists and anthropologists, but certain assumptions seem safe. Hunting, especially the hunt for large, dangerous animals, required strength and stamina, if no conspicuous degree of superior intelligence, and therefore almost certainly was a masculine occupation. In a period when the requirements of subsistence permitted no idle hands, the gathering of additional food— nuts, berries, roots, grains—was therefore relegated to women and children. During the excruciatingly gradual transition from hunting to agriculture—one can hardly imagine one Cro-Magnon saying to another after an unsuccessful hunt, "Hey, the mammoth are getting scarce, let's plant some corn"—this division of labor almost certainly prevailed.

It is also possible that while transporting grain, a woman may have

spilled some of it and subsequently noticed that it had sprouted.*
Whatever the actual mechanism—accident or inspired deduction—
that set it into motion, agriculture became women's work. Women
marked out the fields because they, better than the men, knew where
grain grew best. They prepared and planted them, probably with
the same pointed, fire-hardened sticks that they had used for digging
up edible roots. With the help of the children, they harvested the
crops, stored them, and prepared them for eating. When, in time,
there were sheep or goats to take care of, the women did that, too,
collecting the milk and turning it into cheese.

It also seems likely, since it was the women who tended the fires,
that one of them noticed one day that if ordinary clay is subjected
to heat, it hardens into permanent form. From that observation to
the first crude piece of pottery was a step which should not require
thousands of years. Pottery making became women's work and still
is in virtually every preliterate society from Australia to the Congo.
Weaving was women's work, too. Did not the goddess herself weave?
As the noted Harvard anthropologist Irven de Vore writes, "It was
woman, the gatherer, not man the hunter who fed the primitive
family. As still happens, man's activities got the publicity and made
the bigger outward impression, but it was woman's work which kept
things going." [8]

And what did the men do all this time? Apparently not a whole
lot. They continued to hunt, probably well past the point of useful,
profitable return. They helped with the heavy work of clearing fields
and of construction, although the bulk of building was done by
women. A group of recent studies by the UN Economic Commission
for Africa has shed light on the relative work inputs of women and
men in contemporary agricultural societies. The findings were that
women account for 100 percent of the rearing and education of children, of cooking, cleaning, washing, and food processing. They also
account for 90 percent of providing the community's water supply
and 80 percent of its fuel supply. They contribute 70 percent of the
effort required for food production, 50 percent for animal husbandry,
domestic food storage, and house repairs. In addition, they do 90
percent of the work connected with brewing and 70 percent of what
the studies lump together under the heading of "community self-

---

* Using grains of einkorn, a cereal plant known to have existed in neolithic
times, modern scholars have replicated such a serendipitous event.

help projects." [9] The men, when they are not consuming the products of the brewing activity, account for the rest.

Sheltering, protecting, nurturing, giving, and sustaining life, the women of the neolithic emulated their goddess in one additional respect. They, too, handed down no laws. As best as can be reconstructed, early neolithic society was egalitarian. If the goddess was served by priestesses or even by priests, they had not yet succeeded in arrogating a favored position for themselves as an attribute of their calling. Eynan, one of the earliest villages yet uncovered, consisted of some fifty circular, domed one-room huts 7 meters in diameter, each containing its own hearth and collectively enclosing a circular courtyard measuring some 2,000 square meters. During this early period of the neolithic—10,000 to 8000 B.C.—the men were still away hunting for extended periods of time, and the settlement served them as a permanent base. The huts were occupied by the women and children—traces of infant and child burial have been found under some of the hut floors—and, presumably, by the males of the households when they were home. There were, at this early stage, no craft shops, no public or communal buildings, no indications of social caste or differentiation.

Possibly it was the innate, biological nature of women which caused them to reject, or not even to consider, a social organization based on hierarchy and dominance. Possibly, and more likely, the social system simply did not require any such structure. One can easily imagine all the necessary decisions being taken by the women in concert as they gathered in the courtyard to plan out and assign the day's activities and then their going about their work, collective or individual, without any need to exert authority. Within the home, the primary bond was between mother and children. As Elise Boulding writes in *The Underside of History*:

> One very distinctive feature of the women's culture is the omnipresence of children and the continuing nature of responsibility for infants and very small children. There is no moment of the day or night when this responsibility wholly lapses. . . . Additionally, pregnancy is a twenty-four-hour-day "activity" since it requires energy and resources from the mother's body. Pregnancy merges imperceptibly into the continuing responsibility for infants after birth, a responsibility that really stretches from the moment of conception until the age of three or four.

The breastfeeding that begins after birth merges imperceptibly into the activity of preparing and serving food to children that extends for women to the activity of feeding all adult males in her household.[10]

Because the woman was literally the keeper of the homesite, it is logical that society should arrange itself along what anthropologists now call matrilocal and matrilineal lines. Under such a system, Boulding proposes:

When a new household was to be formed, a young woman would build her home, and a young man would come to live there somewhat on sufferance, bringing gifts. He could easily be sent away if he didn't please his wife, or his wife's mother. Older men (and sometimes young men) would have a thin time if their wives sent them away and they could not persuade any other woman to take them in.[11] *

Undisturbed by external forces, such a social system in which descent is reckoned on the mother's side and in which the groom literally moves into his bride's family could have sustained itself almost indefinitely, as it has among not only the Tongans but also the Ashanti, the Trobrianders, and the Nayat. But obviously something happened to change matters radically.

In fact, a whole set of factors combined to challenge and eventually to topple the existing order, but it is tempting to single out just one decisive event: the invention of the plow. Even though it made its appearance after change had already begun, the temptation is especially attractive, in the light of subsequent developments, because the plow is so obviously phallic, in form as well as function.†

* Describing divorce among the contemporary matrilocal Plateau Tongans, Elizabeth Colson writes: "Old women chuckle happily at their independence; old men try desperately to find wives through whom they can once more establish a household unit catering to their wishes and giving them prestige and ritual potency." [12]

† As Sophocles notes in *Oedipus the King*: "O Oedipus . . . How, Oh how have the furrows ploughed by your father endured to bear you, poor wretch," and Shakespeare in Sonnet III:

For where is she so fair whose unear'd womb
Disdains the tillage of thy husbandry?

The immediate effect of the plow, which first appeared in the Near East around 4,000 B.C., was to multiply food yields and thus set the stage for the accumulation of wealth. Wealth—in movable form—in turn created the basis for trade, and with it the beginnings of occupational specialization. Salt, sulfur, and bitumen from the Dead Sea, obsidian from Anatolia, turquoise from Sinai, cowrie shells from the Red Sea—all these had been well known to the hunters on the track: well known and worthless beyond their purpose for personal use. Now, however, they acquired a value far in excess of even the animals which had been the object of the hunt. How quickly and with what decisive effect this lesson was learned were revealed during the excavation of Beidha, where successive settlements were found superimposed on the same site. Level VI, dating to 7000 B.C., consisted of the familiar, crude circular huts. But above them, on Level IV, separated by fewer than 500 years, archaeologists found:

> Three large rectangular houses measuring 16 by 20 feet displayed interiors finely finished in plaster, equipped with hearths bordered by plastered sills. Set into the sills were stone bowls; food could have been boiled by filling them with water and then dropping hot stones into them. These houses faced a large open space, like the central plaza of a Latin American town. Around them and across the plaza were much smaller rectangular houses.[13]

Where the opportunity to amass wealth exists, the class system does not lag far behind.

Wealth also mandated the creation of a profession totally new to mankind—the military. As the noted historian V. Gordon Childe observes, "Positive evidence for warfare multiplies only when the importance of stock-breeding in the rural economy increases. The correlation can hardly be altogether accidental."[14] To this day, hunting people tend to live and let live.

Vast technological change—the discovery of metals—further fragmented society into new lines of occupational specialization. There was nothing inherently masculine about bronze making or bartering, any more than tending goats was inherently feminine, but women of the neolithic age tended not to participate in these new activities. Accounting for this reluctance in sociological terms, Boulding suggests:

The instability of matrilineal systems can be explained entirely in structural terms. Had women given more attention to spin-off activities with which they were not directly concerned, and adapted their communication patterns to encompass a wide range of happenings, matriliny might have adapted to a new scale of social operation. The fact that women did not do so should not be put in primarily biological terms, although their triple producer-breeder-feeder role may have put them at a disadvantage. An inspection of their daily work load compared with that of the earlier hunting-and-gathering era suggests that they were probably suffering from work overload and information overload, and did not stand back to get the larger picture.[15]

As for why women, who certainly had the power to do so, did not abandon some of their prior occupations to enter these promising new growth fields, a number of explanations are offered. One is the "traditional conservatism" of women, born of or at least conditioned by long experience. "Care of children," Boulding notes, "does not admit of much variation, particularly in feeding." [16]

Another explanation proposes that conservatism is a trait associated with occupation rather than sex. Farmers, who become conditioned to the immutable cycle of the seasons, are traditionally set in their ways whether they plant their crops in Nebraska, New Zealand, or Nyasaland. So, too, are potters. In a cross-cultural study entitled "Sociology of Pottery," George M. Foster investigates pottery villages in Mexico, Tibet, India, Tunisia, Spain, and South America and concludes that potters, whether male or female, "are more conservative in basic personality structure than are non-potter villagers . . . and as a class are more resistant to innovation of all kinds than are non-potters."[17] *

Whatever their reason, women's reluctance to involve themselves in these new activities inevitably led, in Boulding's words, to "the

* As explanation, he suggests: "The reason lies in the nature of the productive process itself which places a premium on strict adherence to tried and proven ways as a means of avoiding economic catastrophe. Pottery-making is a tricky business at best, and there are literally hundreds of points at which a slight variation in materials and processes will adversely affect the result. . . . [E]conomic security lies in duplicating to the best of the potter's ability the materials and processes he knows from experience are least likely to lead to failure. . . . [T]his breeds a basic conservatism, a caution about all new things that carries over into the potter's outlook on life itself."

progressive lessening of their participation in significant decision-making as clan-based roles receded in importance." [18] This effective abdication had many consequences, the most immediate of which was the rapid—dizzyingly rapid in contrast with the pace of change during the prior seven millennia—disappearance of egalitarianism and its supplantation by systems of political power. In theory, notably utopian or socialist theory, there is no reason why egalitarianism should not survive the development of increasingly complex social or economic organization. In fact, it does not seem to, no more in our time than it did some 6,000 years ago. Two sociologists have made a painstaking review of seventy-one different contemporary cultures which have been sufficiently studied by anthropologists to permit graded scoring on certain traits such as level of technology, caste system, codified laws, sex dominance, and polygyny. Correlating fifty-seven such traits, they find a consistent positive relationship between the level of technology and an autocratic pattern of social organization. As one rose, so did the other. And as they both rose, the position of women within the society edged downward into stricter subjection.[19]

This last finding was confirmed by another cross-cultural study, this time of the family unit. The study was able to trace a connection between the development of civilization and the growth of autocratic political states. It also demonstrated that autocratic power structure usually entails the greater subjection of women, particularly in the realm of sexual restrictiveness.[20] *

Obviously, the power in these autocratic societies, as it does in all societies, rests firmly in the hands of men. The question is, why should male rule automatically entail the subjection, if not the subjugation, of women? Or, to paraphrase Professor Henry Higgins, why can't a man be more like a woman?

In a sense, this entire book is an attempt to answer the question. And perhaps, since we began our inquiry with her, the proper way to start is by considering what happened to the goddess.

Myth serves many functions, not the least of which are to explain, vindicate, and justify. Bronislaw Malinowski writes:

---

* Hitler's Germany was not one of the societies considered in the study, but the well-remembered Nazi triple exhortation of *Kinder, Küche, Kirche* fits the pattern.

> Myth . . . is a story which is told in order to establish a
> belief, to serve as a precedent in ceremony or ritual, or to rank as
> a pattern of moral or religious conduct. Mythology, therefore,
> or the sacred traditions of a society, is a body of narrative woven
> into their culture, dictating their belief, defining their ritual,
> acting as the chart of their social order and the pattern of their
> moral behavior.[21]

The winds of political and economic change which swept across
the Near East during the fourth, third, and second millennia before
Christ did not immediately topple the goddess from her throne.
Rather, they began by inflating the importance of her consort. In
Egypt he was Horus, the son whom Isis had once been shown, in an
early statuette, solicitously nursing. There had been no question of
Isis's position then. She was "the natural mother of all things, mistress
and governess of all the elements, the initial progeny of worlds, chief
of the powers divine, queen of all that are in hell, the principal of all
that dwell in heaven, manifested alone and under one form of all
the gods and goddesses." [22] But Horus proved to be a less than dutiful
son, for in later elaborations on the myth we learn that "thereupon
Horus, the son of Isis, was angry with his mother, and he went forth
and his face was savage like a panther of Upper Egypt. And he removed the head of his mother, Isis, and he put it on his bosom and
he ascended into the mountains." [23]

The Sumerians had once worshiped Inanna as their principal goddess, but later tales describe how she wandered incautiously into
the underworld and was released only through the intercession of the
shepherd, Dumuzi, who later married her and himself became the
god of everything that grows. The Canaanites, who in the second
millennium B.C. came out of the deserts of southern Mesopotamia
to settle in Palestine, had at one time worshiped Astarte, but the god
they brought with them and imposed over their growing empire was
Baal, who could assume many forms but most commonly was portrayed as a bull.*

In Babylon, where the mother goddess, Tiamat, "had fashioned
all things," it was her very fecundity which led to her downfall. According to the *Enuma Elish*, the Babylonian account of the Creation,

---

* A bull is a powerful, frequently ferocious animal, but equally significant is
his ability, hardly lost on a tribe of herd tenders, to take care of the sexual needs
of a large number of cows.

Tiamat sought revenge over a slight to her majesty by letting loose
a fearful horde of monsters: "She set up the viper, the dragon, and
the Lahamu, the great lion, the mad dog, and the scorpion man,
mighty storm demons, the dragonfly and the bison, bearing relentless
weapons, unafraid of battle." [24] Frightened, the lesser gods chose one
of their own, Marduk, as their defender. He destroyed the demons
and, for good measure, their creator: "The lord trod upon the legs
of Tiamat, and with his relentless club he split her skull. He cut
open the arteries of her blood, causing the north wind to carry it to
far places; like a mussel he split her into two parts." [25] As reward, he
was made king of the gods and also patron of Babylon itself.

The new, masculine divine *dramatis personae* reflected a harsher
attitude toward the world itself. Joseph Campbell writes in *The
Masks of God*:

> It is now perfectly clear that before the violent entry of the
> late Bronze and early Iron Age Aryan cattle-herders from the
> north and Semitic sheep-and-goat herders from the south into
> the old cult sites of the ancient world, there had prevailed in
> that world an essentially organic, vegetal, non-heroic view of
> the nature and necessities of life that was completely repugnant
> to those lion hearts for whom not patient toil of earth but the
> battle spear and its plunder were the sources of both wealth and
> joy. In the older mother myths and rites the light and dark
> aspects of the mixed thing that is life had been honored equally
> and together, whereas in the later, male-oriented, patriarchal
> myths, all that is good and noble was attributed to the new,
> heroic master gods, leaving to the native nature powers the
> character only of darkness—to which, also, a negative moral
> judgment was now attached. . . . Where the goddess had been
> venerated as the giver and supporter of life as well as consumer
> of the dead, women as her representative had been accorded a
> paramount position in society as well as in cult. . . . Opposed
> to such without quarter is the order of the Patriarchy, with an
> ardor of righteous eloquence and a fury of fire and sword.[26]

The changes, both in the mythic heavens and on earth, came
gradually and at different times in different places, but in retrospect
they reveal both a pattern and a purpose. To cite Campbell again:

> It is an effect of the conquest of local matriarchal order by

invading patriarchal nomads, and their reshaping of the local lore of the productive earth to their own ends. It is an example, also, of the employment of a priestly device of mythological deformation, which has been in constant use (chiefly, but not solely, by Western theologians) ever since. It consists simply in terming the gods of other people demons. . . . It is used in the present case to validate in mythological terms not only a new social order but also a new psychology.[27]

Furthermore, to dramatize the fact of change, to attest to the superior power of the new gods, and to impress upon the faithful the permanence of the new order, the process of mythical deformation was frequently dramatized by an epic struggle which pitted the Great Mother and her dark brood on one side and the younger, fairer gods on the other. The most familiar example of this struggle, in Western tradition, occurs in Greek mythology: the victory of Zeus over the Titans, the offspring of Gaea, the goddess Earth.*

A similar epic combat and victory preceded the ascendancy of another of the patriarchal gods—a god who was not above boasting of his triumph. "Canst thou draw out leviathan with a hook? or his tongue with a cord?" Yahweh asks Job. "Canst thou fill his skin with barbed irons? or his head with fish spears? Lay thine hand upon him, remember the battle, do no more. Behold, the hope of him is in vain: shall not one be cast down even at the sight of him? None is so fierce that dare stir him up: who then is able to stand before me? Who hath prevented me, that I should repay him? whatsoever is under the whole heaven is mine." [28]

Once the new male gods were established on their thrones, the next step was predictable. Sargon of Agade, who around 2350 B.C. became one of history's first documented despots, left this autobiographical note for posterity:

> My lowly mother conceived and bore me in secrecy; placed me in a basket of rushes; sealed it with bitumen, and set me in the river, which, however, did not engulf me. The river bore me up. And it carried me to Akku, the irrigator, who took me from the river, raised me as his son, made of me a gardner: and

---

* The account of how Indra, the king of the Vedic pantheon, gained supremacy over Vritra, the cosmic serpent, bears strong resemblances to the Greek myth.

while I was a gardner, the goddess Ishtar loved me. Then I ruled the kingdom. . . .[29] *

A few short centuries after Sargon, a better-remembered king was even more explicit about the legitimacy of his power:

> When exalted Anu, king of the Angels and Baal, who is the lord of heaven and earth . . . made Marduk great among the great gods, when they proclaimed his name to Babylon. . . . At that time, Anu and Baal called to me, Hammurabi, the pious prince, worshipper of the gods, summoning me by name to bring about the rule of righteousness in the land, to wipe out the wicked and evil, to prevent the strong from oppressing the weak, to go forth like the sun over the human race to illuminate the land, to further the welfare of mankind.[31]

Hammurabi, it will be recalled, was a bloodthirsty conqueror who is chiefly remembered as the author of the earliest-known code of law, of which the words quoted above form the prelude.

We do not know for certain what the status of women was in the Babylon of 1750 B.C., but we can make certain assumptions based on the Hammurabic code itself, which stipulates that "if a married lady who is dwelling in a man's house persists in behaving foolishly and belittling her husband . . . they shall convict her and her husband may marry another woman" and that "if a man takes himself off and there is the necessary maintenance in his house, his wife shall not enter another man's house."

We can make safer assumptions about woman's lot in a country lying not far from Babylon. One of the documents which has come down to us from that country reads in part:

> And God said, Let us make man in our image, after our likeness: and let him have dominion over the fish of the sea, and over the fowl of the air, and over the cattle, and over all the

---

* Otto Rank, one of the early disciples of Freud, wrote a paper on the myth of the birth of the hero, in which he analyzes some seventy accounts of similar tales, collected from Mesopotamia, Egypt, India, China, Japan and Polynesia, Greece and Rome, Iran, the Bible, Celtic and Germanic, Turkish, Finnish and Estonian lore. From them all he was able to construct was a formula which resembled that of a certain type of neurotic daydream. Its main components were: a birth shrouded in some mystery; infant exile or exposure; adoption by people humbler than himself; return to his "rightful" estate through the intercession of a higher power; final triumph and vindication.[30]

earth. . . . And the rib, which the Lord God had taken from man, made he a woman, and brought her unto the man. . . . And the Lord God said unto the woman, What is this that thou hast done? And the woman said, The serpent beguiled me, and I did eat. . . . Unto the woman he said, I will greatly multiply thy sorrow and thy conception; in sorrow thou shalt bring forth children; and thy desire shall be to thy husband, and he shall rule over thee." [32]

The story of the garden of Eden is hardly original to this document. It had already been graphically told, complete with serpent, tree of knowledge, and eternal life, on a series of three Syrian-Hittite clay seals which are on display at the Louvre. The significant difference, however, is that in this earlier version no one is cast out of Eden. There is no theme of human guilt or of divine wrath and retribution. All this is a latter-day addition, fashioned to demonstrate the jealous new god's power to mete out punishment for disobedience and to establish once and for all woman's guilt for all the ills of the world.

Denigration of woman is not unique to the Bible. Campbell notes that "throughout all patriarchal mythologies, the function of the female has been systematically devalued, not only in a symbolic cosmological sense, but also in a personal, psychological one." [33]

The classical scholar Jane Ellen Harrison points out that the whole constellation of glories and tragedies of the Trojan Wars derives from a "trivial and even vulgar . . . opera-bouffe" [34] incident in which three goddesses decide on the spur of the moment to participate in a beauty contest, a frivolous impulse more feminine than divine. But still, the gods of Olympus consorted with women, married them, and were born of them. Not so this new god, so jealous that He shared his power with no one, much less a mother or wife, and so awesome that men were enjoined against using His name in their prayers. This, then, was the final fate of the goddess: to be supplanted by a deity who required His male worshipers to thank Him as follows: "Blessed art Thou, O Lord our God, King of the Universe, that I was not born a woman."

Through the millennia of the goddess's rule, her presence had frequently been indicated by synecdochic symbols. The great paleolithic caves contain hundreds of drawings and carvings of downward-facing triangles with vertical clefts bisecting their bottom angle. In the earlier, more prudish days of prehistoric scholarship, several interpretations were advanced for this design, but none could obscure its simple, obvious allusion to female anatomy.

Of the endless different seashells that exist, one in particular—the cowrie—has been prized for tens of thousands of years. It has been found, thousands of miles from its native habitat, in Cro-Magnon tombs, in predynastic Egyptian crypts, in Anglo-Saxon graves. As the *concha veneris*, it was perforated and worn as an amulet by the Romans. One author has documented its use throughout Europe;[35] another has suggested that it was the original inspiration for the Turkish crescent.[36] It was, well into the nineteenth century, a standard medium of exchange in large areas of Africa.

Again, interpretations of the meaning of the cowrie shell vary, but it is sufficient to pick one up and observe its underside with its deeply involuted pinkish mouth to understand the reason for its special fascination. For primitive man in particular, as G. Elliot Smith notes, "If the loss of blood was the first only recognizable cause of death, the act of birth was clearly the only process of life giving. The portal by which a child entered the world was regarded, therefore, not only as the channel of birth but the actual giver of life."[37]

Representations of breasts, too, occur repeatedly throughout the paleolithic and neolithic periods, first as crude cup-shaped indentations and later in explicit detail. On the island of Malta an entire neolithic civilization which lasted for some fifteen centuries occupied itself by erecting fantastic stone temples the basic floor plans of which faithfully reproduce the form of a woman's body.

Symbols or actual representations of male genitals appear far more rarely, especially if one discounts the predilection of some scholars to ascribe phallic significance to any object of elongated or roughly cylindrical shape.* The later deification of the bull and the ram, and the proliferation of the horn as their symbol, are

---

* A conspicuous and mystifying exception is the large quantity of bones and antlers which had obviously been selected because of their similarity in shape to the erect penis and then incised or carved to heighten that similarity. Because they seem to have a vaguely martial air, and because of their general shape, a French archaeologist named them *batons de commandement*—swagger sticks. Barring their use as double-headed dildos, which they uncannily resemble, no one has yet advanced an even remotely plausible explanation of their function.

clearly intended to assert the rising power of the male principle. Just as the vulva and the breast had betokened nurturance, the horn-penis came to stand for procreative potency and, on occasion, sexual passion.

But the new patriarchs, determined to assert their supremacy, endowed the male sexual organ with an additional attribute. We are told that when Abraham asked his servant to make a promise to him, he said, "Put, I pray thee, thy hand under my thigh: And I will make you swear by the Lord, the God of Heaven, and the God of earth. . . ." [38] And later, when Jacob is dying: ". . . and he called his son Joseph, and said unto him, If now I have found grace in thy sight, put, I pray thee, thy hand under my thigh, and deal kindly and truly with me. . . ." [39]

The Authorized King James Version of the Bible contains numerous euphemisms, including, in these two instances, the substitution of the word "thigh" for "genitals." As the *Encyclopaedia Biblica* notes: "With regard to the practise of putting the hand under another's thigh, it seems plain that it grew out of the special sacredness attaching to the generative organ; fruitfulness being of specially divine origin, the organ of it in man could by the primitive Semites be taken as symbolizing the Deity." [40]

The notion of fruitfulness, as was pointed out, is itself a recurring euphemism, invoked by earlier generations of commentators to render any sexual activity respectable. In this instance, moreover, the euphemism seems to be the result of purely reflex action because there is no context of sexuality to explain away. The penis is not being used for procreation or for passion. Rather, it serves as the emblem of power and as such is intended to establish a relationship of dominance and submission—in one instance between master and servant and in the other between father and son.

To the patriarchs, this elevation of the penis to the rank of status symbol may have been merely an observance of natural law. What they could not know is that they were not the first to do so. The establishment of a similar relationship, expressed in similar fashion, is, in fact, common among many other primate species. Studying the habits of a large colony of hamadryas baboons at London's Regent's Park Zoo some years ago, a young South African biologist named Solly Zuckerman * noticed certain peculiar but recurring

---

* Now Sir Solly Zuckerman. The book which reported his observations, *The Social Life of Monkeys and Apes* (London: 1932) has become one of the early classics of ethology.

patterns of behavior. When a male baboon felt threatened by a stronger male, he would ward off danger by assuming the attitude of a female in heat, turning around with lifted tail and arched back to expose his hind parts to the superior male. The latter would then cease to harass and would mount the submissive one, imitating the act of mating.

Similar behavior has since been observed on the part of other monkeys and apes and of other animal species that live in bands or flocks structured by a fixed hierarchy. Indeed, the pattern was first noted by Buffon in 1766, when he described a baboon he had seen as "insolently lascivious in satisfying its strong desires in public. It seemed to make a parade of its nakedness, presenting its posteriors oftener to the spectators than its head." [41]

For once the great French naturalist misunderstood completely because sexual desires had nothing whatever to do with the animal's performance. It was simply frightened and seeking to appease the onlookers. As Claire and W. M. S. Russell note in *Violence, Monkeys and Men*: "A male engaged in true sexual mounting would be, so to speak, swept off his feet: he would grasp the female's hocks with his own hind-legs, bringing himself into position for complete intercourse." [42] By contrast, a monkey seeking to establish dominance almost always kept his feet on the ground and was thus often actually incapable of penetration.*

The psychologist A. H. Maslow defines this kind of dominance-subordination behavior as "pseudosex." That it occurs among human beings, he notes, is obvious to any clinician and is illustrated by language itself—in phrases such as "Kiss my ass." [44] Especially in social situations which, by imposing a strict hierarchical order, most nearly resemble baboon life—the military, for instance, or corporate

* Earlier in the same book, the authors, clearly meaning no slur, depict hamadryas baboon society as follows: "The resulting patriarchal democracy is strikingly like that of certain human societies, such as the ancient Hebrews, with their polygamous families moving about independently, their two-family teams (Abraham and Lot) and their combination of equal status (for the patriarchs) and respect for experience. Kummer observed that food was relatively scarce in Ethiopia, and that the baboons had to scatter widely in the day-time to get enough to eat. Dispersal into small family units is evidently necessary in these conditions, and each patriarch has to develop the independence and initiative shown in the cynocephalus baboons by a few males of the establishment. Leadership is thus spread among all the males. The Hebrew patriarchs, traveling far and wide to find grass and water for their flocks, were in a rather similar position. In both cases, the status of the female appears extremely low." [43]

life—a subordinate who attempts to appease a superior or curry favor with him is likely to be categorized as a "brown-noser," an "ass-licker," or a "corn-holer." (The phrase "curry favor" may itself refer back to the primate practice of grooming, which is another form of demonstrating a dominant-subordinate relationship.)

Another genital mode of demonstrating dominance was described by Drs. Detlev Ploog and Paul MacLean after observing a captive colony of six spider monkeys for a full year. As expected, the monkeys—Bert, Casper, Dwight, Edgar, Frances, and Gertrude—quickly established themselves into a hierarchy of dominance which could be confirmed by their feeding and grooming habits, as well as by their general behavior. The surest indication of rank, however, proved to be order of precedence in displaying penile erections:

> In this display, the male approaches a female or another male head-on, places one or both hands on its back and thrusts the erect penis toward the face. . . . The animal receiving the display sits in a cowering position while ducking its head as though dodging a blow. . . . If it does not remain quiet during the display, it may be viciously attacked.[45]

Casper turned out to be the dominant member of the group. He displayed to the other males, but none dared display to him. Moreover, "on a number of occasions single males were introduced into the colony for short periods. Casper was the only male of the established group that persisted in tracking the new animal and displaying. If the newcomer did not remain passive and quiet during the display, it was viciously attacked." The lowest member of the group was Edgar. He displayed to none of the other males, but all displayed to him. Edgar, the authors note, displayed only to humans.

The ethologists Wolfgang Wickler and Irenaus Eibl-Eibesfeldt have independently observed that many species of primates use penile presentation as both a territorial threat and as a demonstration of dominance. "When a group of vervet monkeys is feeding, several males always sit and keep watch with their backs to the group and display their vividly colored genitals. If an unknown member of the species approaches, the 'guards' have an erection." [46] This action, Eibl-Eibesfeldt observes, is generally accompanied by a threatening facial expression.

Citing other examples of penile threat, Wickler notes that "the genitals of African monkeys of the genus *Cercopithecus* have become extremely colorful for this signal function: the penis can turn bright red, the scrotum a luminous blue. The color combination can vary from species to species and is one of the brightest body colors found among mammals." [47] He then points out that contemporary inhabitants of the Sunda Islands, comprising the western part of the Malay Archipelago, still carve and erect life-sized ithyphallic wooden figures. "These figures," he explains, "are guards. They stand at the entrance of villages, houses and temples, as well as on graves and property boundaries. They always stand with their back to the guarded object and display their genitals to the outside." Furthermore, he adds, "often the phallus is painted in conspicuous colors, for instance red." [48] He concludes:

> Even psychoanalysts are in danger of overlooking the fact that the phallus has two meanings—which are biologically related but can be separated: primarily, the phallus is a symbol of power; it only became a symbol of fertility secondarily, on the roundabout route of its possible associations in the human mind. So it would be one-sided to relate the phallus only to the sexual realm.[49]

Many phallic symbols, customs, and usages make sense only when understood as expressions of dominance or aggression. The Kiwai hunter in New Guinea who presses his penis against the trunk of the tree he has selected to make into a harpoon shaft is not concerned that the tree he is about to cut down should reproduce itself. He wants his harpoon to be straight, strong, and capable of deep penetration and is thus attempting to imbue it with those qualities. A Maori warrior, fearful of being bewitched before going into battle, crawls between the legs of a great chief whose penis will shed its strength upon him. Galla tribesmen in southern Ethiopia still wear simple phallic ornaments made of light shining metal on their brows as a sign of rank and valor. Indonesians who believe that wind and waterspouts are provoked by evil spirits take their bared penises in their hands and point them in the appropriate directions. In the essay accompanying his translation of *The Arabian Nights*, Sir Richard Burton relates a common punishment for strangers caught in the harem was to "strip them and expose them to the embraces of the grooms and Negro slaves." Surely the administration of such a sentence relied upon the satisfaction of aggression and the pleasure of humiliating another human being as much as upon simple erotic arousal.

Nor is the practice limited to superstitious, preliterate savages. In classical Greece the sight of protective herma stones—four-sided columns topped by a man's head and decorated with an erect, protruding phallus—was so commonplace that Aristophanes alludes to them in *Lysistrata* when describing the Spartan envoys who arrive in Athens to negotiate peace.* The hundreds of Roman amulets depicting flying penises or rampant penises or penises riding in chariots which now fill the closed cases of numerous museums were intended to repel evil or misfortune and therefore to protect their wearer, rather than to promote fecundity or potency. (A similar purpose is served by the gesture, originally Mediterranean but now largely universal, of clenching the fist with the thumb protruding between the index and middle fingers.) Among the trinkets which knowledgeable visitors to Japan seek out are the small, round amulets which can be purchased in certain temples. On the outside, they display only a stylized, threatening face, but if one opens a little panel on the back, one discovers a meticulously realistic erect penis set into a little shrine.†

In the West, public display or explicit representation of the penis is still not generally accepted. Nevertheless, the concept of phallic power has found forceful modes of expression. For instance, one of the antique artillery pieces displayed in the courtyard of the Musée de l'Armée in Paris is a sixteenth-century bronze cannon which is decorated, among other traceries, with the figure of a naked woman so positioned that her legs straddle the touchhole. Charles Ferguson notes in *The Male Attitude* that "under Henry VIII, a man's man, cannon took on a symbolic as well as a military value. Cannon were exhibited with pride in public places. Founders made barrels in long shapes. They pointed erect at all times. Craftsmen were encouraged to display artistry that would carry over the sentiments of chivalry into the new weapons." [51]

The advent of functional design has eliminated this kind of ex-

---

* The unfortunate Spartans, it will be remembered, were suffering the effects of their women's prolonged withholding of sexual favors.

† Although amulets of this kind have a long history, they have been adapted to cope with twentieth-century exigencies. Eibl-Eibesfeldt writes that "orderly as the Japanese are, they write on the back what the amulet offers protection against—for example, against car accidents!" [50]

plicit identification, but the United States Marine Corps, which prides itself on how it trains men, has taken pains to revive it. No one who has ever gone through boot camp can forget the drill-ground litany, shouted out and accompanied by appropriate gestures:

This is my rifle, this is my gun.
This is for business, this is for fun.

All guns big and small are phallic, not only because of their form but also because of their function. They discharge; they pierce; they penetrate. The first definition of "ejaculate" in the *Oxford English Dictionary* is to "shoot forth." In the vernacular we shoot our load or our wad. A rod, a joint, a piece are commonplace slang expressions for a gun and also for a penis. We can use either one of them to bang a broad or to drill her. Even women, who could be expected to resent the double identification, fall into it naturally. How many, in orgasmic ardor, have yelled out, "Shoot"?

But among all guns and things that shoot, the pistol occupies a special place. Ian Fleming, who owes at least part of his spectacular success to James Bond's inexhaustible armory of phallic weapons and gimmicks, disingenuously has one of his characters say: "It is a Freudian thesis, with which I am inclined to agree, that the pistol, whether in the hands of an amateur or a professional gunman, has significance for the owner as a symbol of virility, an extension of the male organ, and that excessive interest in guns is a form of fetishism." [52]

Indeed, one of the earliest issues of the *Internationale Zeitschrift für Ärztliche Psychoanalyse*, which Freud himself edited—with Ferenczi, Rank, Jones, Abraham, Brill, Jung, and Hanns Sachs as co-editors—contains a note on *Pistolensymbolik*.[53] It deals with a young man who proudly shows a newly acquired pistol to a lady friend, commenting on how handsome it is and how well it performs. Her reply is that she finds it not handsome at all, but rather disgusting and unappetizing.

A pistol fits comfortingly—reassuringly—into the palm of the hand. If it is an automatic, it has a powerful, tireless mechanism that can be made to slide back and forth. If it is a revolver, it has a round protuberance at the base of the shaft, and it can be cocked. Whichever it is, it can be lovingly oiled and rubbed, stripped down, and put together again as good as or better than new. It can shoot, and when it shoots, it has enormous, decisive impact on the intended target. Furthermore, it can be depended upon to work even when its flesh-and-blood equivalent fails. In Mickey Spillane's *I, the Jury*, the heroine absorbs all of Mike Hammer's sexual attention but still persists in betraying him. So, in the book's closing scene, Mike permits her to finish stripping for him and then shoots her lovingly in the lower abdomen—the fuck she'll never forget.

This scene, or another undistinguishable from it, has become the obligatory trademark of all the Mike Hammer books and of their hundreds of imitations. It has been adapted to the screen, in films which are invariably advertised with posters showing the hero brandishing a huge gun while, in the background, several women enact various stages of arousal. Usually the weapon is a pistol, but sometimes a shotgun or submachine gun is used instead. Always, however, the barrel is absurdly long, and the weapon, held high against the upper thigh, is pointed upward at a suitably virile angle.

There are, by conservative estimate, somewhere over 100 million guns in civilian hands in the United States, approximately as many as there are penises. The astonishing success of the National Rifle Association in blocking even the most innocuous regulations of those guns suggests that their owners would as soon give up one as the other. The only legal uses to which guns can be put in the United States are hunting, marksmanship, and self-protection. Handguns, which constitute the large majority of the 100 million, are hardly ever used by hunters, and only a few very expensive models are accurate enough for target shooting. As for protecting one's home and loved ones, it has been estimated by the National Commission on the Causes and Prevention of Violence that householders succeed in shooting burglars less than once in 500 instances—thus accounting for only a negligible proportion of the 20,000 people in the United States who are annually killed with guns.[54] Perhaps we would all do better to resume erecting *herma* stones and wearing amulets.

That the automobile satisfies needs other than transportation was understood very early by psychoanalysts. In an article which appeared in the *International Journal of Psychoanalysis*, one author offers, among many others, the following insights:

> I need not describe in detail the ways in which Oedipus impulses find expression in driving; in the urge to overtake and

resentment in being overtaken, in the wish to keep the road to oneself. . . . A boy reports that he was afraid of being run over by a small gray car; he associates the colour of the car to the shade of his father's suit. . . . Fast driving symbolizes genital, anal or urethral potency, but also oral greed. . . . The fear of losing control over the car stimulates earlier anxieties about losing control over the excretory system. The noisy smelly car is also conceived of as excrement. . . . Masturbation anxieties may be expressed in fear of having damaged the engine by faulty handling. . . . Anxiety-dreams of being chased by motor cars usually express sadistic intercourse, but may have a paranoid character. . . .[55]

Those who have reservations about psychoanalytic interpretations may be skeptical about some or all of these conclusions, but their basic implication has clearly not been lost on the practical men who earn their living designing and selling automobiles. Why else did they decide in near unanimity that an automobile, which functionally is no more than a container on wheels, should look like a chromed bat-winged self-propelled penis, erect and straining to thrust?

For all the attention it has received, the phallic significance of the automobile has generally been treated with tolerant, boys-will-be-boys amusement. If a grown man can derive psychosexual wish fulfillment or allay his fears of impotence by sitting behind the wheel of a ludicrously designed fuel-guzzling monster, more power to him. If he lavishes time and money on his automobile, cleaning and polishing it and loading it down with inane gadgets, his behavior is deemed no more aberrant than that of his wife when she decides that what the house needs is a good top-to-bottom cleaning and a few more appliances. Some years ago Theodor Reik proposed the notion that women make an unconscious identification between their homes and their own bodies and that the compulsion which some of them feel regarding scrubbing, dusting, and polishing is in effect the acting out of purification and atonement for early forbidden erotic activities. A man's compulsive care of his automobile-penis, it is argued, is merely the male equivalent of such *Hausfrauen-neurosis*.[56]

But it is not only grown men who drive cars. On the contrary, our society has made the granting of the right to drive a car into the nearest thing we have to an initiation rite—the formal, socially sanctioned mark of passage from adolescence to adulthood. Unfortunately for the recipients, we have chosen to grant them this right at the exact time when they are least equipped to cope with it. As Joseph D. Noshpitz writes in "The Meaning of the Car":

> The youth who is going through the body growth of puberty, who is enormously conscious of his own body, who is becoming increasingly aware of girls' bodies—to such a boy, the endless tinkering, the putting together, taking apart, looking into the insides of, looking up under the bottom of, having, in short, complete control over this object of his attention is an attempt to master the fact that he has no control to speak of about his own body growth. He has fears about the control of his erections, and although he is vitally interested in the body growth of the females about him, he has absolutely no control over them. He is often subject to intense fantasies of undressing girls, or entering into sexual interaction with them in one way or another and not infrequently he is very inhibited in the attempts to enact these fantasies in the real world—what a wonderful chance to have total control of a body: to look anywhere one wants to, to handle whatever he may wish to, make something, somebody respond exactly as one orders it to.[57]

And having looked and handled and controlled to his heart's content, he will call the fruits of his labors a hot rod, leaving no doubt that, just like Dad, he knows what anatomical part it is intended to represent.

For teenagers, and for many adults as well, a car frequently serves as the powerful reinforcement for an insecure body image—a machine body which is far superior to their own because it does not tire and because it is obedient to their will, responding to command at the touch of a finger or toe. A reassuring boon at any time, this new body is likely to be invoked in stressful situations: An adolescent who has just had an argument with his parents—or a grown man with his wife—will storm out of the house, get into his car, and go for an aimless ride, just to "cool off." It is especially necessary in circumstances which test or challenge an adolescent's uncertain masculinity. A teenager asking to borrow the family car, or, better yet, to have one of his own, will, when pressed, argue that girls will not go out with boys who don't have "wheels." What he is really saying was verbalized by one of the subjects in an in-depth study of accident-prone motorcyclists: "There is a strength and power in it. It's masculine and makes me feel strong. I approach a girl on a cycle and I feel confident. Things open up and I am much more at ease." [58]

Fast and reckless driving, which accounts for the appalling accident rate of drivers under twenty-five, may simply be the result of carelessness or irresponsibility, but there is growing evidence that much of it is motivated by unconscious counterphobic action.[59] Indeed, in an investigation of drivers who were involved in collisions, Dr. James W. Hamilton has suggested that it is not only teenagers who are prone to this dangerous acting out. Discussing the widespread negative response to mandatory safety features on automobiles, he writes:

> If the car were regarded by the buyer as primarily a narcissistic adornment, then any factors which would detract from the styling of the car, as some safety additions do, could create a certain reluctance to buy the product. But more importantly, there may be a greater resistance related to the counterphobic quality of driving seen not infrequently in this country where the emphasis is upon acceleration, speed and taking chances or courting disaster. By such behavior one exposes oneself to the feared situation, be it of death, castration, etc., only to recover magically each time. Hence, opposition to safety features or to the use of already installed items such as belts, creates a greater risk, maintains a higher level of excitement, omnipotence, and subsequent elation, and supports denial and repression in maintaining the conflict on an unconscious level.[60]

In December 1977, a survey conducted by the National Highway Traffic Safety Administration among 84,682 drivers in fourteen United States cities determined that only 18.5 percent used the safety belts provided in their cars. In an additional insight, the survey notes that use of the belts was three times more common among owners of Volvos, Toyotas, and Volkswagens—all generally considered "sensible" cars—than among owners of Cadillacs, Lincoln Continentals, and sports cars.

Redolent with phallic appeals, automobile advertising also strives to energize the aggressive tendencies of prospective buyers by giving their products such names as Fury, Panther, Wildcat, Dart, Sabre, Charger, and Cougar. In so doing, they are tacitly endorsing a theory which has been advanced independently by such disparate observers as Sigmund Freud and Eldridge Cleaver: that there is a close link in the masculine makeup between the sexual and aggressive drives.

Freud was never comfortable with his successive formulations of aggression. In *Three Essays on the Theory of Sexuality*, which was published in 1905, he took an essentially Darwinian position: "The sexuality of most male human beings contains an element of *aggressiveness*—a desire to subjugate; the biological significance of it seems to lie in the need for overcoming the resistance of the sexual object by means other than the process of wooing." [61] Aggression, thus, was evolutionarily adaptive to the extent that those males who were best able to subdue females into mating ended up making the largest proportionate contribution to the gene pool. Later, in 1915, he changed his mind and described aggression as a primary drive, distinct from sexuality. Still later, and presumably at least in part as a result of pondering the dreadful carnage of World War I, he elaborated this notion into the theory of the death instinct. In *Beyond the Pleasure Principle* (1920) he proposed that the aggressive instinct was primarily self-destructive rather than directed toward mastering the external world. Man's aggression was a secondary phenomenon, a diversion of the energy of the "death instinct" away from the self against which it was originally directed. Finally, in 1937, he arrived at the conclusion that there were two groups of instincts: "Erotic instincts which are always trying to collect living substances together into even larger unities, and the death instincts, which act against that tendency and try to bring living matter back into an inorganic condition." [62]

Psychoanalysis is still struggling its way out of this maze erected by its founder.* Meanwhile, physiological investigation into the functioning of the brain has provided tantalizing hints that he may have come closest to the truth with his original notion. In the course

* One of the most widely held current views, first stated by Heinz Hartmann and colleagues, is that aggression is a separate instinctual drive which bears the same relation to pleasure and to unpleasure as does libido: Discharge of aggression, generally speaking, gives rise to pleasure; accumulation and lack of discharge, generally speaking, give rise to unpleasure.[63]

of experiments intended to map neural pathways in the brain of squirrel monkeys, Paul MacLean has discovered that electrical stimulation of the structures within the limbic lobe—in evolutionary terms, the "old" brain of premammalian species—could cause immediate penile erection. Then, by moving the electrode less than a millimeter, he was able to elicit a rage response from the animal— "an angry or fearful type of vocalization, with showing of fangs." [64] This intimate neural proximity prompted MacLean to cite another passage from the early Freud's *Three Essays on the Theory of Sexuality*: "A number of persons report that they experienced the first signs of excitement in their genitals during fighting or wrestling with playmates. . . . The infantile connection between fighting and sexual excitement acts in many persons as a determinant for the future preferred course of their sexual impulse"—a conclusion which anyone who has experienced the embarrassment of telltale bite marks on the side of the neck would probably endorse.

That aggressive behavior is associated with sexual responses even in newborn babies was first noted forty years ago and would be common knowledge among mothers were it not for the circumstance that babies tend to wear diapers while they are being fed. Studying the nursing habits of one- to forty-three-week-old babies, H. M. Halverson was able to distinguish a pattern of behavior which recurred when feeding was interrupted by the removal of the breast or by the substitution of a difficult nipple: "As the infant begins to make strong and rhythmic sucking movements the legs contract stiffly so that the knees are raised high over the abdomen with the toes sharply flexed. The hands are fisted near the shoulders. The scrotum tightens and the testicles retract toward the inguinal rings." In thirty-four out of forty-four instances observed, these actions were accompanied by penile erection, which invariably subsided when normal feeding was resumed. [65]

The connection between male sex hormones and aggression has been known, if not understood, ever since the first Egyptian or Sumerian farmer discovered a simple method for reducing a savage bull into a plodding ox. Medieval texts accurately describe changes brought on by the removal of the testicles, and it has been more than a century since testicular implants were first successfully performed on animals under laboratory conditions. But it was only with the isolation and identification of testosterone as the principal male sex hormone in 1934 that scientists have been able to demonstrate its explosive potential as a trigger of aggression. Prepubescent rats, which are normally meek and peaceful, will start fighting with each other after being injected with testosterone.[66] Male ring doves, given the same treatment, will tend to enlarge the territory they lay claim to.[67] In experiments with a flock of hens it was shown that the lowest bird on the pecking order would, after treatment with testosterone, fight its way to the top.[68]

Because of ethical considerations, experiments involving intentional attempts to heighten aggression in human males are difficult to construct. Nevertheless, two recent studies strongly suggest that there is a direct, positive correlation between aggressive behavior and blood levels of testosterone. In the first of them, performed in 1971, two groups of men, aged twenty-one to twenty-eight and thirty-one to thirty-six respectively, were given batteries of standard psychological tests designed to measure aggressive and hostile characteristics. Measurements were also taken of their testosterone output. In the case of the older men there was no consistent relationship between the two, but among the younger subjects it was found that individuals who described themselves as more aggressive—more likely to get into fights or lose their tempers—also had higher levels of plasma testosterone.[69] The second study involved the observation of twelve psychiatric inpatients over an eight-week period. Levels of plasma testosterone were taken weekly and correlated with behavioral data and interviews. The results showed a wide variance in testosterone levels from one subject to another. However, within eight of them, the changes in testosterone level correlated well with observations of change in aggression over the eight-week period of the experiment. The conclusion to be drawn, it seems, is that what may be a high level of testosterone for one man may not be high for another, but whatever that level may be, its increase either causes or coincides with increased aggression.[70]

Other investigators have tried to determine whether a causal relationship exists between aggressive and sexual arousal: whether by increasing someone's hostility and anger, one also simultaneously stimulates them sexually. One of the most revealing experiments of this kind, carried out while its principal author was himself an undergraduate, used a group of 124 students, male and female, at the University of Connecticut. As part of the test, one-half of the group was subjected to a form of aggression arousal:

The subjects were expected to receive back their midterm examinations. Their instructor told them that their exams were terrible and that he had graded them more harshly than was his custom. He then put a fictitious grading curve on the board showing nearly all failing grades. He went on to say that he was keenly annoyed with the work of the class in general and that he could not understand why they had not worked harder. He told the class that he would hand the tests back after a demonstration which had been arranged through the auspices of Yale University. The experimenter was then introduced as a Yale Ph.D., and the class was turned over to him. He greeted the students in a cold, formal manner and proceeded to give them a short introduction in which . . . he stated that the work was part of a research program at Yale and that he was interested in determining the imaginatory capacity of college students on the basis of their ability to make up stories on short notice. He delivered the instructions in an arrogant and authoritative manner that was designed to focus the aggression already aroused and to create more.[71]

The students were then handed sets of four cards, each of which depicted a man and a woman in a commonplace situation—a boss giving dictation to a secretary; two people playing chess; a teacher and a student; a couple sitting on a couch—and were asked to write out a description of what they imagined was actually happening.

The other half of the group, acting as a control, was given the same set of cards but was not subjected to the disparaging charade about failing grades or to the insulting behavior of the visiting Yale Ph.D. All the descriptions were then evaluated on the basis of standard scoring systems by two judges who had not been told which group had composed them.

The first finding was that there was significantly more aggressive imagery in the stories of the group which had been aroused to anger, a finding which in effect validated the construction of the experiment. At the same time, however, the aroused group also produced a considerably greater volume of sexual imagery, indicating a strong linkage between the two motivations. Furthermore, although male subjects produced more sexual imagery, female subjects also showed evidence of dual arousal. "It appears," the authors conclude, "that women respond with sexual arousal to an angry man who in fantasy they see as making a sexual rather than hostile advance. Thus, from a female's point of view, aggression is an important aspect of a male's sexual appeal."

Several follow-up studies have confirmed these findings. In one of them, the connection between aggression and sexual arousal was demonstrated in reverse: Subjects who had been given a pornographic story to read, and were then offered the opportunity to administer punishment by means of an electric shock machine did so in far greater degree than a control group which had read some innocuous science fiction.[72] In another, designed to test the thesis that the raising of *any* drive in an organism tends to energize *all* drives, it was shown that the aggression provoked by sexual arousal could not be duplicated, under identical circumstances, by the arousal of either anxiety or laughter.[73] In still a third, the investigators experimentally reduced anger and aggression in the laboratory and found a parallel decline in the arousing qualities of erotic stimuli—in effect coming full circle back to the ancient farmer and his gelding knife.[74]

One of the serious shortcomings of the research just described is that the two categories which investigators customarily draw upon for their subjects—college students and prison inmates—can hardly be considered as representative of our society as a whole. Nevertheless, anyone attempting to draw generalizations about that society on the basis of what it seems to prefer in films, books, television programs, even the kinds of events reported in its newspapers would have to conclude that sexual arousal and aggression not only are related but are often treated and perceived as the two sides of the same coin. Indeed, the association between sexual behavior and violence is so natural and automatic as to have permeated our language centuries ago.

In the course of preparing a paper on the relationship between slang and dream symbolism, Calvin Hall had occasion to go through Eric Partridge's *Dictionary of Slang and Unconventional English* word by word, extract every expression for sexual intercourse—212 in all—and classify them into categories.[75]

The largest group, forty-eight terms (23 percent), consists of expressions which are primarily aggressive in meaning—words such as "ram, "stab," "impale," "thump," "invade," "push," "prod," "poke," "switch," "prong." The next most frequent class of words (forty-five terms, or 21 percent) describe the purely mechanical aspects of the act: those of entering, joining, lying under or over, moving back and forth. The third class consists of expressions related to physical work and manual activity. Examples include: "night-work," "post a letter," "grind one's tool," "thread the needle," "grease the wheel," "wind up the clock," and, of course, "screw." In all, there are thirty-four such expressions, or 16 percent.

The fourth category—sixteen terms, or 8 percent—consists of terms which, in one fashion or another, allude to the pleasurable aspects of sexual intercourse: "merry bout," "four-legged frolic," "jig." *

Hall sums up:

> The principal conceptions of sexual intercourse as they are revealed by slang are (1) a sadistic or aggressive attack by a man upon a woman, (2) a mechanical action which consists of a man getting on a woman, entering her, joining bodies, and bouncing around, and (3) a form of physical or manual work performed by a man upon a woman. The conception of coitus as an activity which gives pleasure is a poor fourth.

There is hope for the future, however. One of the newest slang expressions for sexual intercourse, recent enough not to be included in Partridge's *Dictionary*, is "to ball." Brought into the language through the youth culture, the expression has not only pleasurable but even festive connotations. Furthermore, its usage denies the compulsory notion of male aggression in sexual encounters. A woman cannot readily ram, impale, thump, prod, poke, or prong a man, but a chick can ball a guy just as well as a guy can ball a chick.

The ultimate amalgam of aggression and sexuality would appear to be rape—the intrusion into a woman's body without her consent.

* The most common slang expression for coitus has given rise to considerable etymological speculation. It has been connected to the German *ficken*, which mean "to strike," to the Latin *futueo*, the French *foutre*, the Italian *fottere*, the Greek *phutueo*, and, prior to all that, to the Indo-European roots "BHU" and "BHUG." If experts cannot agree on the etymology of the principal four-letter word in the English language, it is not likely that ordinary persons know what they are expressing when they use it. However, for every time that the word is used to describe a sexual act, it is used a dozen times to express aggression or hostility, as in "I got fucked," "I'll fuck the bastard," or the simple "Fuck you!"

Feminist writers have adopted the position that rape is a symptom —an inevitable consequence—of our social order. In an article entitled "Rape: The All-American Game" which appeared in *Ramparts* magazine in 1971, Susan Griffin concludes: ". . . rape is not an isolated act that can be rooted out from patriarchy without ending patriarchy itself." [76] Four years later, in a well-publicized book, Susan Brownmiller fleshed out this thought and projected it backward into time: "From prehistoric times to the present, I believe, rape has played a critical function. It is nothing more or less than a conscious process of intimidation by which *all* men keep *all* women in a state of fear." [77] And in *Sexual Assault: Confronting Rape in America*, Nancy Gager and Cathleen Schurr provided an additional economic dimension: "Rape is not an isolated phenomenon of 'sick' males, but rather an inevitable part of the entire social matrix which denigrates women—psychologically, physically, economically, and politically—and which still tends to regard females as male 'property.' " [78]

One can hardly believe that the authors of these statements intended them to be taken in any spirit other than polemical. * If so, they have succeeded at least to the extent of directing fresh attention to rape and to rapists. To support her contention of male indifference to rape, Brownmiller charged: "Articles on rape in psychology journals have been sparse to the point of nonexistence." [81] Whether or not the statement was true in 1975—and its accuracy, like that of so many others, depends on the author's definitions—it is no longer so. In particular, psychologists have taken advantage of a Massachusetts statute which requires diagnostic evaluation of anyone convicted of sexual assault to look more closely at the motivation of rapists.

What they are learning—work is still in progress—gives support to feminists' basic contention about the nature of rape, while at the same time rejecting their monolithic, conspirational view of it:

* Reviewing Brownmiller's book *Against Our Will: Men, Women and Rape,* Edmund Fuller points out that her view of rape is "as grotesquely exaggerated as to say that because some men murder, it keeps all mankind in a constant state of intimidation and that the murderer is the tacit agent of all those who slay." [79] In a sympathetic treatment of *Against Our Will*, Gilbert Geis chides its author for "a violation of fundamental rules of fairness and logic, rules which insist that a person should not be accused of meretricious actions only on the basis that he possesses the potentiality for engaging in them." [80]

One of the most basic observations one can make about rapists is that they are not all alike. Similar acts are performed for different reasons, or different acts serve similar purposes. Our clinical experience with convicted offenders and with victims of reported sexual assault has shown that in all cases of forcible rape three components are present: power, anger, and sexuality.[82]

The sample used in the study consisted of 133 convicted rapists and 92 adult rape victims. The principal conclusion which emerged from interviews with members of both groups is as follows:

> We have found that either power or anger dominates and that rape, rather than being primarily an expression of sexual desire, is, in fact, the use of sexuality to express issues of power and anger. Rape, then, is a pseudo-sexual act, a pattern of sexual behavior that is concerned much more with status, aggression, control, and dominance than with sexual pleasure or sexual satisfaction. It is sexual behavior in the service of non-sexual needs.*

One of the objectives of the study was to see whether rapists could be differentiated according to any discernible personality patterns. Again on the basis of interviews with both offenders and victims, the authors hazard the following four categories:

> The *power-assertive rapist* regards rape as an expression of his virility and mastery and dominance. He feels entitled to "take it," or sees sexual domination as a way of keeping "his" women in line. . . . The *power-reassurance rapist* commits the offense in an effort to resolve disturbing doubts about his sexual adequacy and masculinity. He wants to place a woman in a helpless, controlled position in which she cannot refuse or reject him, thereby shoring up his failing sense of worth and adequacy. . . . The *anger-excitation rapist* finds pleasure, thrills and excitation in the suffering of his victim. He is sadistic, and his aim is to punish, hurt, and torture his victim. . . .

---

* A companion study, important if only because medical evidence in cases of rape often focuses on the presence or absence of semen in the victim, showed that, of 170 men convicted of sexual assault, 55 had experienced sexual dysfunction which prevented ejaculation. Moreover, half of 23 victims who had been subjected to gang rapes had negative laboratory tests for sperms.[83]

The *anger-retaliation rapist* commits rape as an expression of his hostility and his rage toward women.

Of the four, the last category was numerically the most common, followed by the first. Together, they accounted for 103 of the 133 cases. But why rage and hostility? Why the need to assert mastery and dominance?

Let us grant, despite extreme feminist views, that convicted rapists do not as yet represent a fair cross section of male humanity. Nevertheless, these same drives and emotions, checked or repressed below the threshold of pathology, often intrude upon males' relations to women. The reason this should be so may be something as simple as fear.

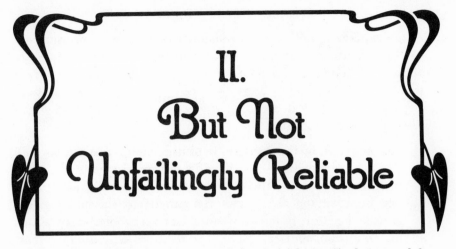

II.
But Not
Unfailingly Reliable

The correspondence columns of the *British Medical Journal* for March 9, 1968, carried a letter from Singapore describing an unusual epidemic. "Those affected with the disease," writes Dr. Chong Tong Mun, "experienced a sudden feeling of retraction of the penis into the abdomen with great fear that, should the retraction be permitted to proceed, and if help was not forthcoming, the penis would disappear into the abdomen with fatal outcome." [1]

The letter goes on to note: "In their fear and anxiety to prevent such a mishap, they held on to the penis either by their hands or with instrumental aids, such as rubber bands, strings, clamps, chopsticks, clothes-pegs, etc. sometimes with severe injury to the penis."

The outbreak, during which some 4,500 cases were reported over a two-month period, was more severe than most, but it was hardly the first recorded instance of the disease. Koro, or *suk yeong* to give it its Chinese name, was first described in the medical literature in 1895 [2] and has since been sporadically noted in Borneo, South China, the Celebes, Hong Kong, and the Sudan.[3-6] Typically, the afflicted are sixteen to forty-five years old, although in Singapore a young mother was seen rushing into a clinic, clutching her four-month-old baby's penis, and they are almost always Chinese.

In the most comprehensive review of koro yet made,[7] Dr. P. M. Yap describes it as "a state of acute anxiety leading to the conviction of penis shrinkage and to fears of dissolution" and notes that most of the cases he investigated exhibited immature, dependent personalities and sexual histories of conflict and maladjustment. As for the Chinese's particular susceptibility to koro, Yap proposes that it is somehow related to the theory of harmonious equilibrium between the yang and yin principles.

This explanation may be farfetched, but because koro does appear to be culture-bound, and because there is something inescapably funny about the notion of a man's using chopsticks to prevent his penis from shrinking away, a note of condescension tends to creep into the clinical accounts of its incidence. One American writer, for instance, states:

> Any assertion by the doctor . . . that the penis is quite normal, that it does not show any signs of diminishing in size or disintegration, and that there is no danger whatever present, does not improve the anxiety of the patient to the slightest degree. . . . He is usually able to alarm the whole family about his condition, and several of his relatives will usually stand around his bed and join the patient in his urgent appeals to the medical staff for immediate help.[8]

The spectacle of conflict-ridden, maladusted Chinamen running around and frantically clutching at themselves may have its comic side, but it is far from being the most absurd or damaging manifestation of a fundamental male fear. One of man's earliest, most dismaying discoveries about himself was that his penis, for all its desirable attributes, was an unreliable, capricious instrument with a will of its own. Because he could not control it, because he could not understand how it worked, because it could fail him at the most crucial time, the penis became a cause for anxiety. In this chapter, we shall trace some of the manifestations of this anxiety—how, because of it, men have attempted to segregate women, to impute them with sinister intentions, and to persecute and punish them. We shall then show that the level of this male anxiety rises as women, through no action or fault of their own, are perceived in a context of increased femaleness or sexuality. Finally, we shall look at some of the ways men have devised to resolve, or at least attenuate, their anxiety—thereby inflicting harm on women, on the world, and, perhaps most grievously, on themselves.

But first, a note on nomenclature. The most persuasive evidence for the existence and intensity of male anxiety regarding the penis may be that like superstitious natives, we cannot even bring ourselves to utter its correct name. Textbooks and articles speak of castration anxiety, castration complexes, castration fears. In conversation, we complain about women who are ball-breakers or who glory in cutting a man's balls off. Dictionaries, however, define castration as the removal of the testicles, which is not at all the fate that castration anxiety is all about. Laymen may perhaps be excused their anatomical inaccuracy, but psychiatrists ought to know better. Indeed, to borrow another term from their vocabulary, their choice of words constitutes a collective case of displacement so colossal in scale so as to border on the conspiratorial.[9] *

The central irony of male penile anxiety is that woman lies irreducibly at its root. It has, for instance, been observed that only very rarely do men experience impotence while engaging in homosexual relations or while masturbating. Thus, because anxiety is a basic drive in the formation of social institutions and because men have, for the past four or five millennia at least, been essentially unchallenged by women in how they chose to design and administer their world, they elected to do it by attempting wherever possible to exclude them from it. To this aspiration we owe—or until very recently owed—the near-undiluted masculine nature of our political, professional, religious, military, and economic organizations, as well as the division of labor which has marked virtually all societies and even the pattern of leisure and recreational activities they have observed.

Men have constructed elaborate pretexts to justify this segregation, but one of the earliest and in some respects the most satisfactory was simply that women were the carriers of a peculiar kind of communicable disease. It was this—the fear of contagion—which Ernest Crawley proposes as the explanation for the almost universal practice of separation of the sexes which he found among what were then called savage societies. In his two-volume *The Mystic Rose*, first published in 1902, he cites the practice, common in all parts of the world, of building separate men's living quarters which women were forbidden to enter and notes all kinds of additional proscriptions:

> Every inhabited island in the Torres Straits has a certain area set apart for men into which the women may not go. . . .
> In the Pelew Islands, men and women hardly live together and family life is impossible. . . . In Cambodia, a wife may

---

* As evidence that they do know their anatomy, they were careful in another context—this one not only nonthreatening but rather flattering to men—to use the proper term. Not one of them has ever charged women with suffering from testicle envy.

never use the pillows or mattress of her husband because she would hurt his happiness thereby. . . . Among the Karens of Burma, going under a house where there are females within is avoided. . . . Amongst the Samoyeds and Ostyaks a wife may not tread in any part of the tent except her own corner.

Segregation was further enforced by custom: "Husband and wife among the Kaffa in Africa see each other only at night, never meeting during the day. . . . In Fiji, women apparently are considered even more dangerous than dogs, for, while these are kept out of some temples, women are excluded from all of them." [10]

Language was enlisted to perpetuate this exclusion of women:

Among the Arawak, men and women have different words for even common objects. . . . The Karaya have a special women's dialect, which, it has been suggested, is an older form of the tribal speech. . . . In Japan, female writing has quite a different syntax and many peculiar idioms; the Japanese alphabet possessed two sets of characters, for the use of men and women.* . . . In Madagascar, there are terms proper for a woman to use to her own sex, others for women to men, and for men to women.

The act of eating—"commensal relations," as Crawley calls it— was considered fraught with particular dangers. "Biologically, the sexual impulse is a development from the nutritive, and the primary close connection of the two functions is continued in thought, subconscious and physiological, and appears sometimes above the threshold of consciousness." He enumerates scores of societies where men and women ate apart and notes additional taboos such as:

Amongst the Narriyeri, boys during the progress of their initiation are forbidden to eat any food which belongs to women, "lest they grow ugly or grey." . . . The Indians of Guiana believe that, if a pregnant woman eats of game caught by hounds they will never be able to hunt again. . . . Algonkin priests may not even eat food prepared by a married woman.

It all sounds quaint, but what will future anthropologists make of the practice of twentieth-century American businessmen to gather daily at luncheon clubs where sexual segregation, de facto, if not

* It still does.

de jure, is purchased at the price of exorbitant dues and preserved from pollution by so much as a waitress or hatcheck attendant? As far as language is concerned, English-speaking women are not required to use a separate idiom, but certain words and phrases have become exclusively their property. "I could just scream," "I nearly fainted," "I died laughing," "I let my hair down"—a man would no more think of using any of these expressions than he would of wearing a dress in public.*

Crawley makes the point that if contact between the sexes is always hazardous, "it is expected that the danger of contagion should be multiplied and deepened when the contact is of the most intimate kind possible." To support this hypothesis, he notes: "In South Africa a man must not, when in bed, touch his wife with his right hand, for if he did so, he would have no strength in war, and would surely be slain"; "the North American Indians dared to go to their wives' cabin only at night"; and "In Fiji, *rendezvous* between husband and wife are arranged in the depths of the forest" [11]—presumably out of sight not of others, which could be more conveniently arranged, but of each other.

One of the stray tidbits in the cornucopia of information served up by Dr. Alfred Kinsey is the revelation that among American men whose education did not go beyond grade school, more than half (57 percent) regularly engaged in sexual intercourse while clothed.† In commenting on this practice, Kinsey notes: "This intercourse with clothing is not a product of the inconveniences of the lower level home, nor is it dependent upon the difficulties of securing privacy in a small home, as too many sociologists have gratuitously assumed. It is primarily the product of the lower level's conviction that nudity is obscene." And he adds:

> There are some cases of lower level males who have been highly promiscuous, who have had intercourse with several hundred females, and who emphasize the fact that they have never turned down an opportunity to have intercourse except "on one occasion when the girl started to remove her clothing before coitus. She was too indecent to have intercourse with." [12]

---

* Except, of course, if he were mimicking a "faggot."

† With increased education, pajamas—and possibly underwear—tended to come off. The corresponding figures are 34 percent for men who went to high school and 10 percent for those who attended college.

Why a woman's naked body should be "obscene" or "indecent" will be considered in due course, but the unwillingness to look at it during copulation—whether in Fiji or the United States—appears to be the limit of where segregation can be carried.

When one surveys the mass of anthropological lore, as well as the extensive literature of misogyny and the depressing evidence of history itself, the conclusion is hard to escape that, as H. R. Hays writes in *The Dangerous Sex*, "one half of the human race regards the other at best with condescension and suspicion, at worst with hatred." [13] Seldom, in our culture, has this hatred been expressed more virulently than in the teachings of the early Church Fathers. The Bible records that women were among the first converts—and remained among the most faithful—that they devoted themselves to charity, supported their men in adversity, labored to spread the Gospel, and, in one instance, even "expounded . . . the way of God more perfectly" than men.[14] Nevertheless, Paul urged Timothy: "Let the woman learn in silence with all subjection. But I suffer not a woman to teach, nor to usurp authority over the man, but to be in silence." [15]

Clement of Alexandria held: "Every woman should blush at the thought of what she is." Saint John Chrysostom argued: "Among all savage beasts, none is found as harmful as woman" and called her a "whited sepulchre." [16] * A church council in the sixth century even prohibited women, because of their impurity, from receiving the Eucharist into their naked hands.[17]

Underneath the virulence of the hatred, and surely at least in part responsible for it, there can be discerned an insistent, audible harmonic of fear. Woman is not only inherently impure and evil but inherently dangerous. And when Tertullian accuses woman of being "the devil's gateway" or describes her as "a temple built over a sewer," his metaphors leave little doubt regarding which specific aspect of her is fraught with peril. As for the nature of the danger, the anonymous author of the Apocrypha is explicit: "Give not thyself to a woman, so as to let her trample down your manhood." [18]

---

* The full passage reads: ". . . if you consider what is stored up inside those beautiful eyes, and that straight nose, and the mouth and the cheeks, you will affirm the well-shaped body to be nothing else than a whited sepulchre; the parts within are full of so much uncleanliness."

This fear—that women can cost a man not only his soul but also more palpable corporeal loss—runs through all the misogynistic ravings of the Jeromes, Ambroses, Origens, Hilarions, Odos of Cluny, Augustines, and even tinges the gentle Aquinas, who described woman as a "failed man." As Wayland Young notes in *Eros Denied*, their anxiety can be summed up in one sentence from Cardinal Hughes de Saint Cher: "Woman pollutes the body, drains the resources, kills the soul, uproots the strength, blinds the eye and embitters the voice." [19]

Human beings capable of inflicting such harm could not be permitted to run loose. At the same time, however, it was unacceptable for men to concede that mere women could hold such power over them. The solution to this dilemma was man's invention of the witch. She had already appeared in the person of Lilith, Lamia, and Circe, but it required Christian zeal to define her, describe her mode of operation, and prescribe appropriate punishment for her. In response to a request from Pope Innocent VIII, two Dominican monks named Jacob Sprenger and Heinrich Kramer in 1486 put together the first comprehensive guide to witchcraft. Entitled *Malleus Maleficarum*—"The Hammer of Witches"—their compilation was endorsed by the faculty of the University of Cologne, ran through nineteen editions, and became one of the basic, approved texts of the Inquisition.[20]

The authors list the old charges: "What is woman but a foe to friendship, an unescapable punishment, a necessary evil, a natural temptation, a desirable calamity, a domestic danger, a delectable detriment, an evil of nature, painted with fair colors." But then they quickly get to the point. Why is "this kind of perfidy [witchcraft] found more in so fragile a sex than in men"? The natural reason, they propose, "is that she is more carnal than a man, as is clear from her many carnal abominations." In fact, states the *Malleus*, "All witchcraft comes from carnal lust, which is in women insatiable." And the text supports the points by paraphrasing the Bible: "There are three things that are never satisfied, yea a fourth thing which says not: It is enough, that is, the mouth of the womb."

Although they intended to deal with all aspects of their subject, most of the fifty-nine "Questions" in the *Malleus* betray the authors' preoccupation with problems of sex—and rather peculiar problems at that. Question VIII asks "Whether witches can hebetate the powers of generation or obstruct the venereal act," * and Question IX examines "Whether witches may work some prestidigitatory illusion so that the male organ appears to be entirely removed and separated from the body." Not only is this answered in the affirmative, but it is illustrated with examples:

> And what, then, is to be thought of those witches who in this way sometimes collect male organs in great numbers, as many as twenty or thirty members together, and put them in a bird's nest, or shut them up in a box, where they move themselves like living members, and eat oats and corn, as has been seen by many and is a matter of common report? . . . For a certain man tells that, when he had lost his member, he approached a known witch to ask her to restore it to him. She told the afflicted man to climb a certain tree, and that he might take which he liked out of a nest in which there were several members. And when he tried to take a big one, the witch said: "You must not take that one"; adding, "because it belonged to a parish priest."

In a recent commentary on the *Malleus*—a book which, although it now elicits amusement, in its own time not only legitimized but prescribed the killing, after protracted torture, of tens of thousands of women †—the British psychiatrist W. H. Trethowan has written: "What the demonologist appears to have ascribed to possession or bewitchment, the psychoanalyst recognizes as an instinctual impulse derived from the 'id.' " And he adds with understatement: "The *Malleus Maleficarum* contains much that a psychoanalyst would at once interpret as castration anxiety." [21]

If women, merely by their existence, can occasion male anxiety, how much more so when they are exhibiting evidence of their femininity. Among the physiological manifestations peculiar to women, none has provoked keener male apprehension, usually expressed in terms of revulsion, than their periodic discharge of some

---

* The answer is: "The truth is sufficiently evident . . . although the method of obstruction has not yet been specifically declared."

† It is not appropriate here to describe, as the *Malleus* did, the techniques to be used in interrogating suspected witches, but in intensity of sexual sadism, they lack only the intervening invention of electricity to match the practices perfected by the French for dealing with female guerrillas in Algeria.

four to six ounces of blood and mucous matter. Menstruation may, in fact, as some anthropologists believe, have been responsible for the original institution of the concept of taboo. Around the world and through history, menstruating women have been locked into suspended cages, fumigated and roasted, buried in the ground up to their waists. It is probably impossible to enumerate the full range of disasters—ruined crops, soured wine, scarce game, ailing flocks, hailstorms, floods, lost battles, sudden sickness, and unexplained accidents—which men have blamed on menstruating women or the indignities and cruelties they have devised to punish them. Robert Briffault, whose monumental *The Mothers* contains twenty-five pages of examples,[22] conceded that his list is far from exhaustive.

The Bible warns: "And if a man shall lie with a woman having her sickness, and shall uncover her nakedness . . . both of them shall be cut off from among their people." [23] According to the Talmud, if a menstruating woman were to walk between two men, one of them would die. Even today an Orthodox Jewish woman may not, while she is menstruating, hand any object to a man, not even her own husband.[24] Preoccupied as they were with spiritual matters, the early Church Fathers took note of the phenomenon. In the canonical writings he handed down as Archbishop of York in 729, Saint Egbert required that women, including nuns, who attended divine services while menstruating should atone for their sin with 20 days of fasting.

Several writers have cited a letter which appeared in the March 2, 1878, *British Medical Journal* and posed this question:

> It is a very prevalent belief amongst females (both rich and poor) that in curing hams, women should not rub the legs of pork with the brine pickle at the time they are menstruating, or the hams will go bad. I shall be glad if any of your readers can tell me if this be mere imagination, or if such be really the case. . . .

The ensuing correspondence, published over several issues of the *Journal,* indicates that as of the time, medical opinion in Britain was divided on the question.

That menstruation is still a source of acute unease is perhaps best illustrated by the odd position it occupies among one small, aberrant subgroup of our society. In the words of one of their own members, the Hell's Angels are ". . . complete social outcasts—outsiders against society. And that's the way we want to be. Anything good we laugh at. We're bastards to the world and they're bastards to us." [25] Hell's Angels' costumes and accessories are carefully chosen to complement this image: filthy, grease-caked Levi's, peaked Prussian helmets, Iron Crosses, swastikas, and variously colored pilot's wings—red to indicate that the wearer has performed cunnilingus on a menstruating woman, and black for the same act on a Negress.

If the intent is to shock, it succeeds. At the height of the Angels' activity in California during the early sixties, the state's attorney general compiled a report of their depredations. Notable among them is:

> Early on the morning of October 25, 1962, it was reported that three Hell's Angels had seized a 19-year-old woman in a small bar in the northern part of Sacramento and while two of them held her down on a barroom floor, the third removed her outer clothing. The victim was menstruating at the time, her sanitary napkin was removed and the third individual committed cunnilingus upon her. . . .[26]

One of the ways some women try to discourage a rapist is to tell him they are menstruating. Long before science had identified the process of ovulation,* the primitive's common and not illogical explanation for vaginal bleeding was that it was the consequence of a wound. Various legends relate how snakes, lizards, birds, or supernatural creatures inflicted this wound. The Carib Indians believed that their own ancestors had no women until, one day, they caught some strange creatures that had fallen out of a tree. They bound them, tied woodpeckers to them in the proper place, and that was that.[27] Until recently New Guinea tribesmen carved intricate figurines illustrating their particular legends. They showed reclining women with a crocodile attacking their vulva or a hornbill plunging its beak into it.

But what is there about a wound which is repulsive? Or, for that matter, about blood? On the contrary, blood as often connotes life-sustaining attributes. It has been used in numberless sacred cere-

---

* The distinction of doing so belongs to Dr. Eduard Pfluger, whose demonstration was published in 1873. Fourteen years earlier, an alternative explanation had been offered by the historian Jules Michelet: "Woman is forever suffering from the cicatrization of an interior wound which is the cause of a whole drama. She suffers incessantly the eternal wound of love." Only a Frenchman could have thought of that.

monies, by the Masai and presumably by the Mafia. Germaine Greer writes in *The Female Eunuch*: ". . . I must confess to a thrill of shock when one of the ladies to whom this book is dedicated told me that she had tasted her own menstrual blood on the penis of her lover. There are no horrors present in that blood, no poisons; I would suck a bleeding finger, I would not scruple to kiss a bleeding lip, and yet. . . ." [28]

Revulsion is the manifestation of anxiety, but perhaps its cause is not just the blood itself but where it came from, not just the wound but where it was inflicted. A man sees, or imagines, that particular blood and that particular wound, and they remind him of what could happen to him. If he is an Australian aborigine, he in fact does believe that there was once something where the wound now is. If he is a normally adjusted civilized male with perhaps only a trifle less than perfect confidence in the infallibility of his manhood, he knows that the wound is not really a wound, and yet. . . .

If woman is seen as revolting, how much more so that specific part of her which makes her a woman. Consider for a moment the historic fate of the cunt. We have seen that prehistoric artists, out of superstition, respect, or awe, drew representations of it on the walls of the caves. If we accept the interpretation of archaeologists, it was the central object of worship in elaborate religions. Today it is still drawn on walls, but mostly in the stalls of men's public toilets, and one measure of the reverence it commands is that if we wish to find it in most dictionaries, we must look under "pudendum," which is also defined as "that of which one ought to be ashamed"—or, as the common French phrase for the female sexual apparatus puts it, *les parties honteuses*. In one of his treatises on nature, Linnaeus characterized the female genitals as "abominable" and refused to describe them. The French physician Des Laurens asked, "How can this divine animal, full of reason and judgement, which we call man, be attracted by those obscene parts of women, defiled with juices and located shamefully at the lowest part of the trunk?" [29]

Again, the manifestation is disgust. A possible cause for the underlying anxiety was suggested by Karen Horney in an extraordinary paper entitled "The Dread of Women." She says:

> This dread of the vagina appears unmistakably not only in homosexuals and perverts, but also in the dreams of every male

analysand . . . e.g., a motorcar is rushing along and suddenly falls into a pit and is dashed to pieces; a boat is sailing in a narrow channel and is suddenly sucked into a whirlpool; there is a cellar with uncanny, blood-stained plants and animals; one is climbing a chimney and is in danger of falling and being killed.[30]

Horney explains the dreams in terms of one of the basic psychic mechanisms: "Everywhere, the man strives to rid himself of his dream of women by objectifying it. 'It is not,' he says, 'that I dread her; it is that she herself is malignant, capable of any crime, a beast of prey, a vampire, a witch, insatiable in her desires. She is the very personification of what is sinister.' " *

One of the most vivid manifestations of this malevolence, lurking beneath the surface of male consciousness, is the ubiquitous myth of the vagina dentata. In its classic form, it runs like this:

A Brahmin and wife went to live in a Baiga's house. Every day the Brahmin went out to beg and the wife stayed at home flirting with the two fine sons of the Baiga. . . . At last she called the elder boy to live with her. In her vagina were teeth and these cut off the boy's penis. The woman laughed at him, saying, "You're very quiet today, go to it with more vigour." But he had lost his penis and went away. Then the woman called the younger boy and cut off his penis also.

The boys sat by the roadside and when the Brahmin came home they told him what had happened. . . . He entered his wife's room and made her lie down. He had secretly brought a pair of tongs from the smithy. He began to play with his wife's vagina with one hand, telling her how beautiful she was, while with the other hand he inserted the tongs and removed the teeth. . . . Neither said a word about what was happening. But then when the teeth were gone the woman could get no pleasure, her vagina was so large. She called many men to her but there was no joy in it. At last she went to the Brahmin's horse, but it went into her with such violence that it killed her.[31]

This story, and twenty-one others very much like it, were collected by the ethnographer Verrier Elwin in central India, but similar tales

* And she adds this intriguing insight: "May not this be one of the principal roots of the whole masculine impulse to creative work—the never-ending conflict between the man's longings for the woman and his dread of her?"

were related by North American Indians,[32] by Siberian Eskimos, and by otherwise completely dissimilar tribes in Africa, South America, and the Pacific.[33] Wolfgang Lederer, in *The Fear of Women*, records that the New Mexico Jicarilla Apache have a tale about a murderous old man named Kicking Monster, whose four daughters were at one time the only women in the world who possessed vaginas:

> They were "vagina girls," and they lived in a house that was full of vaginas. Other vaginas were hanging on the walls, but these four were in the form of girls with legs and all body parts and were walking around. As may be imagined, the rumor of these girls brought many men around; but they would be met by Kicking Monster, kicked into the house, and never returned. And so Killer-of-Enemies, a marvelous boy hero, took it upon himself to correct this situation.

As soon as Killer-of-Enemies enters the house, the four girls approach him, craving intercourse. But he asks: "Where have all the men gone who have been kicked into this place?" "We ate them up," they reply, "because we like to do that." Killer-of-Enemies promises to do what they wanted but tells them that first they must all eat some medicine made of berries which he had brought along. They agree, but the berries pucker first their mouths and then their vaginas, so that finally they cannot chew at all, but only swallow.[34] Thus, the vagina was put to its proper use.

By and large, our culture is too well organized—indeed, culture is in itself a wholesale exercise in objectification—to let the vagina dentata survive, although it continues to linger in unexpected contexts. What, for instance, are we to make of children's stories about witches who live deep in the heart of dark forests, who lure their victims with promises of unbounded pleasure (such as a whole house made of candy), and who then proceed to eat them? Or of the tale of Briar Rose—the Grimm version of Sleeping Beauty—in which all suitors for the young girl's hand are pierced by the thorns of a hedge and die horribly, until the prince comes along and discovers: "The hedge was nothing but large and beautiful flowers, which parted from each other of their own accord to let him pass unhurt." *

---

* The vagina dentata may also, to those who recall the peculiar shape of its front grille, have contributed to the near-instant demise of the Edsel. One of the jokes current at the time dealt with the distraught Edsel dealer who came home, asked his wife to remove her panties and sit tailor-fashion on a table. "My God, he said after a moment's study, "they're right!"

The vagina dentata did, however, recently make a rare public appearance in, of all places, the *New York Times Magazine* of April 21, 1974. The article describes the manner in which the publishing industry tries to create a made-to-order best-seller and uses the saga of *Jaws* as its example. It relates the agonies through which the editors put author Peter Benchley, the careful planning which went into each step of the book's creation, and its unveiling before the marketing staff. "The sales managers loved the book and the title," the *Times* reports, "but there was considerable resistance to the jacket. It made them think of Freud's classic dream of castration, the vagina dentata." The jacket was redesigned, but not so radically as to lose its predatory character. And the reason, perhaps, is that on second thought the sales managers remembered that in the United States far more women than men buy books.

Jean-Paul Sartre writes in *Existential Psychoanalysis*: "The obscenity of the feminine sex is that of everything which 'gapes open.' It is a summons to being, as all holes are. In herself, woman appeals to a strange flesh which is to transform her into a fullness of being by penetration and dissolution. . . . Beyond any doubt, her sex is a mouth and a voracious mouth which devours the penis." [35] Or, as a clay-daubed Arunta aborigine once explained more simply to psychoanalyst-anthropologist Geza Roheim, "The vagina is very hot, it is fire and every time the penis goes in it dies." [36]

Both notions are concisely expressed by the Gallic notion of *la petite morte* and given exegesis by Freud himself:

> . . . Man fears that his strength will be taken from him by woman, dreads becoming infected with her femininity, and then proving himself a weakling. The effect of coitus in discharging tensions and inducing flaccidity may be a prototype of what these fears represent; and realization of the influence gained by the woman over a man as a result of sexual relations, and the favor she extorts by this means, may all conduce to justify the growth of these fears. There is nothing in all this which is extinct, which is not still alive in the heart of man today.[37]

That it is even more alive today than when Freud wrote these words in 1918, we will see presently. What is most remarkable, however, is not that men should voice these sentiments, but that they should have communicated them, intact, to women—and especially to women more than commonly aware of their femininity.

This is Simone de Beauvoir, on the subject of sexual organs:

> The sex organ of a man is simple and neat as a finger; it is readily visible and often exhibited to comrades with proud rivalry; but the feminine sex organ is mysterious even to woman herself, concealed, mucous, and humid as it is. . . . Man "gets stiff," but woman "gets wet"; in the very word there are childhood memories of bedwetting, of guilty and involuntary yielding to the need to urinate. Man feels the same disgust at involuntary nocturnal emissions; to eject a fluid, urine or semen, does not humiliate; it is an active operation; but it is humiliating if the liquid flows out passively, for then the body is . . . a vessel, a container, composed of inert matter and but the plaything of capricious forces.[38]

And this is Germaine Greer:

> The worst name anyone can be called is _cunt_. The best thing a cunt can be is small and unobtrusive: the anxiety about the bigness of the penis is equalled only by the anxiety about the smallness of the cunt. No woman wants to find out that she has a twat like a horse-collar.[39]

But why should a woman be concerned about the size of her cunt? As recently as a generation ago, she might have worried that bigness would betray excessive or indiscriminate use, but Masters and Johnson, among others, have by now certified that the vagina is "infinitely distensible from a clinical point of view" [40] and that in any case virtually all the neural sensors serving the vaginal barrel are concentrated in its outer third.

If women worry about the size of their cunts, it may be because they know that men worry about it.* And the reason men worry about it, quite simply, is their anxiety about being able to fill it adequately. It is not by accident that Horney begins her paper on the dread of women with two poetic passages dealing with water. From Homer onward, the image of woman-as-water has been one

---

* One indication of the prevalence of this worry among men is the enormous number of variety of "big cunt" jokes. As G. Legman has demonstrated exhaustively in _The Rationale of the Dirty Joke_, humor, especially sexual humor, is usually an attempt to relieve the fear or uneasiness which the teller feels, partly by verbalizing it and partly by exposing the listener to the same anxiety.

of the abiding metaphors of our culture. Both are primal elements; both evoke a nurturing, amniotic security, a gentle, hospitable presence.

But those are not the only characteristics which give the metaphor its force. One of the poems Horney selected is "The Song of the Fisherboy," from Schiller's *Wilhelm Tell*:

> The clean smiling lake woo'd to bathe in its deep,
> A boy on its green shore had lain him to sleep;
> Then heard he a melody
> Flowing and soft,
> And sweet as when angels are singing aloft.
> And as thrilling with pleasure he wakes from his rest,
> The waters are murmuring over his breast;
> And a voice from the deep cries,
> "With me thou must go, I charm the young shepherd,
> I lure him below." *

The operative analogies, clearly, are that woman is alluring, deep, and dangerous—that she is, in the last analysis, a bottomless pit which man can try to plumb only at the risk of his life. Mythology is peopled with beautiful, sexually aggressive damsels—undines, naiads, nymphs—who lure men to watery graves. Ulysses, when approaching the sirens' rocks, orders his men to stop their ears with wax and has himself tied to the mast of his ship. Heine's Lorelei, combing her golden hair on the bank of the Rhine, enraptures passing boatmen to their death. More recently the psychiatrist James Leuba has advanced the speculation that a great many deaths by drowning may actually be precipitated by sudden panic over being pulled down by some aquatic creature, getting entangled in water plants or seaweed, or being attacked by a fish—all expressions of castration anxiety.

Not only is the pit dangerous, but because it is bottomless, men can never hope to fill it. Erik Erikson incurred the fury of feminist polemicists for at least alluding to this corollary in his "Inner and Outer Space: Reflections of Womanhood." [41] Perhaps, in so singling

---

* The other poem, the same author's "The Diver," is a more melodramatic expression of the same idea which ends: "Salamander-snake-dragon-vast reptiles that dwell/In the deep, coil'd about the grim jaws of their hell."

him out, they have overlooked the prior, and more explicit, formulation of the same idea by Carl Jung:

> . . . it should be remarked that *emptiness* is a great femi-
> nine secret. It is something absolutely alien to man; the
> chasm, the unplumbed depths, the *yin* . . . A man may say
> what he likes about it; be for it or against it, or both at once;
> in the end he falls, absurdly happy, into this pit, or, if he
> doesn't, he has missed and bungled his only chance of making
> a man of himself. In the first case one cannot disprove his
> foolish good luck to him, and in the second one cannot make
> his misfortune seem plausible.[42]

Horney writes in *The Dread of Women*: "Male homosexuality
has for its basis . . . the desire to escape from the female genital,
or to deny its very existence. . . . Only anxiety is a strong enough
motive to hold back from his goal a man whose libido is assuredly
urging him on to union with the woman." [43]

That anxiety, expressed by denial and the desire to escape, is
one of the factors which lead men to make the homosexual choice
seems a reasonable supposition. One of the most startling findings
of the first Kinsey study—more startling even than the proportion
of males who had experienced homosexual contact*—was the sheer
volume of these contacts which homosexuals managed to generate
in the pursuit of their sexual activity. Many homosexual men reported having had hundreds of partners, and some placed the number in the thousands. A more recent study by the Institute for Sex
Research, conducted in San Francisco and published in 1978, found
that among 572 white male homosexuals more than one-half had
had more than 500 different partners during the course of their
sexual careers and that 28 percent had had more than 50 partners
during the past year alone.[44]

Several reasons for this transitory nature of male homosexual
relationships have been proposed: the tendency to fetishize sex
as the central component of a relationship, confusion over which

---

* The figure was originally reported as 37 percent, but Dr. Wardell Pomeroy,
one of the coauthors of the study, subsequently noted that it may have been
overstated. "Probably," he corrected, "33 percent would have been closer to the
mark."

partner is to assume the dominant social role, and even the economic circumstance that "the gay relationship does not receive the
financial subsidies that the heterosexual marriage enjoys, in the
form of reduced taxes and discounts given to married couples by
many private associations and businesses." [45] A more persuasive
explanation is given by Donald Webster Cory, himself a homosexual and one of the first to write intelligently on the subject:

> . . . because for many of these people homosexuality is not
> a search for but a flight from something unknown, something
> that holds them in constant terror and fear. Their imperious
> desires for male-male relationships are actually vicarious and
> substitutive diversions from other desires, and therefore leave
> unanswered and unresolved the basic need of the individual. It
> is for this reason that the astonishingly frequent partner-chang-
> ing and the short-lived character of homosexual relations must
> be viewed not as healthy varietism and freedom from puri-
> tanical codes of artificial fidelity, but as a revolt against the
> partner with whom sex has been consummated. . . .[46]

Anxiety's involvement being granted the answer to the deeper
question of why certain males should be more susceptible to this
anxiety than others has thus far eluded psychiatrists. Their difficulty, starting with Freud, has at least in part been due to their
assumption that humanity comes in one of two sexual models and
to the complementary conclusion that any individual who does not
see it that way is, ipso facto, psychotic and a potential subject for
cure. Clearly, male homosexuals have chosen to reject certain
aspects of the masculine role. At the same time, however, it is an
observable fact that, as one pair of writers notes, ". . . if most gay
men were interested in playing a feminine role in sexual activities,
a set of masculine players was also needed." [47] There had, therefore, to be at least two kinds of male homosexuals, each with its
own set of psychosexual symptoms. And since such symptoms do
not arise spontaneously, there also had to be at least two sets of
psychosexual etiologies. This, in turn, led to some fairly involuted
formulations, even by psychoanalytic standards. One practitioner,
for instance, concludes:

> All the available evidence points to the fact that homo-
> sexuality is a psychological disease. . . . The writer has found

it in young men where there has been (1) hostility to the mother; (2) excessive affection for the mother; (3) hostility to the father; (4) both (2) and (3), i.e. the Oedipus complex; and (5) affection for an insufficiently masculine father.

And just in case he has omitted a permutation, he adds: "No doubt there are many other possible factors." [48]

Because attacking the problem from a masculine-feminine orientation did not shed much light, a psychiatrist named Irving Bieber proposed in 1962 an alternative means of classification. Having studied many hundreds of male homosexuals and their sexual habits, he divided them into two classes: inserters and insertees.[49] Not especially romantic, the categories at least had the virtue of being physiologically descriptive. Unfortunately, given the force of sexual stereotypes, they carried unmistakable judgment over active-passive, dominant-submissive roles.* The implication is clear that even between two homosexual men, the more manly would choose to be the inserter. But in fact, is the act of sucking a penis passive? Is the placement of one's penis in another man's mouth active? If so, why do we speak of the resulting activity—"being blown"—in the passive voice?

More to the point, the new classification did not improve the very low rate of success which psychiatrists had enjoyed in "curing" homosexuals. Indeed, so far did this rate eventually drop that to account for it, the profession came to the belated conclusion that its patients had not been sick in the first place. In December 1973 the Board of Trustees of the American Psychiatric Association voted to reclassify homosexuality as a "sexual orientation disturbance" rather than as a "mental disorder."

As early as 1965 Evelyn Hooker, whose perceptive studies of homosexuals began in the 1950s, had written: "I propose that, in the context of their subcultures in relation to the larger society, homosexuals develop working solutions to problems of sexual performance and psychological gender which cannot be understood in the perspective of the two-sexed heterosexual world." [50] This

---

* The same stereotypes underlie a well-known modern riddle: A father and his son are walking along a road when they are hit by a passing car. The father is killed, but the son is only injured and rushed to a hospital. There the attending surgeon takes a look at him and says, "I can't operate on this child because he is my son." How is this possible? Because, of course, the surgeon is a woman.

view now appears to be gaining ground in psychiatric circles. It has, to judge by their writings, long been considered an axiom among most homosexuals.

Additional research has shed further question on the inserter-insertee distinction. The Institute for Sex Research study contained a series of questions dealing with sexual techniques, which for ease of tabulation were divided into seven categories—"masturbating a partner," "being masturbated by a partner," "reaching orgasm by rubbing their body against the body of a partner," as well as the four inserter-insertee combinations. Of the 676 respondents, some 95 percent had, during the past year, performed or received fellatio. Some 80 percent had performed anal intercourse, and some 70 percent had received it.[51] There are, to be sure, such categories as inserters and insertees, but the roles are freely interchangeable. Because the study included both black and white subjects and was coded to distinguish between their responses, it was possible to isolate one interesting finding: The favorite sexual activity of black homosexual males, selected by 44 percent of the 108 respondents, was performing anal intercourse. No other sexual technique scored nearly as high among blacks, and the favorite among whites—being fellated—received only 27 percent. In the absence of other evidence, one may hazard the guess that this preference among blacks has less to do with erotic taste than with the acting out of a culturally conditioned sense of status.[52] *

Another recent study, this time in Detroit, sought to discover, among other things, whether there is any pattern to the personal sexual preferences of homosexuals. Did men who preferred the inserter role in oral-genital contacts also prefer to be the inserter in anal-genital contacts? Was there a corresponding insertee type? Their findings, based on 243 subjects, were that not only was there no consistency, but the combinations of preference ranged across the full spectrum of statistical possibilities. "The most common set of sexual preferences among gay males," the authors conclude, "is for all roles, both oral and anal and active and passive." In other words, homosexuals are into sex.[53]

In 1970 a mild stir was caused in sociological circles by the appear-

---

* Interestingly, the study also found that among female homosexuals, black women chose the receiving of cunnilingus as their favorite activity (29 percent), while none of them preferred performing the same act. The corresponding findings among white female homosexuals were 20 percent and 6 percent.

ance of a study entitled *Tearoom Trade*. It was not so much the subject of the study—male homosexual practices—which was unusual as the fact that a "tearoom" is, in the vernacular of the homosexual subculture, a public rest room, usually in a park, movie house, hotel, or bus station, where sex is freely available and the further fact that the study's author, Laud Humphreys, had collected his material by personally observing over a two-year period the encounters which occurred in several "tearooms" of a large city.

As a sociologist Humphreys was not as much interested in the psychological drives of homosexuals as he was in the "rules and roles" which governed their behavior. What he discovered was that in the environment he was studying, the first are as strict as the second are flexible:

> The homosexual games of cruising for the one-night stand exhibit the universal and protective nature of rules, which are standard for all situations: 1. Avoid the exchange of biographical data. 2. Watch out for chicken (teenagers)—they're dangerous game. 3. Never force your intentions on anyone. 4. Don't knock [criticize] a trick [sex partner]. 5. Never back down on trade agreements.[54]

As for roles, he notes that the psychiatric preconceptions did not apply in practice:

> Of fifty-three acts of fellatio that I observed systematically, later analysis indicated that the insertee was the "aggressor" in twenty, the insertor was the "aggressor" in twenty-seven, the two seemed equally aggressive in two cases, and the data was [*sic*] insufficient for determination in four of the acts. The "aggressor" was defined as the player who first made an irrevocable commitment, an unmistakable overture.[55]

If anything, he further notes, it is age which determines the choice of roles: "In most cases, fellatio is a service performed by an older man upon a younger." For the rest, he concludes: "This study of restroom sex indicates that sexual roles within these encounters are far from stable. They are apt to change within an encounter, from one encounter to another, with age, and with the amount of exposure to influences from a sexual deviant culture."[56]

Within this shifting pattern of roles, Humphreys did observe the presence of one constant, which has been noted by almost all writers on male homosexuality: The vast majority of gay men prefer a sexual partner who is quite masculine; few desire one who is effeminate. This preference is evident from a cursory look at the ads which appear in male homosexual publications. The May 3, 1979, issue of the *Advocate*, for instance, announced the availability of "Talk of the Nation!!! 6'1" Ex-Col Boxer. EN-DOWED LIKE A HORSE!!! 9AM-Midnight-$50" and "Want it Huge? Rugged!! Handsome! Giant Tool!!! Call Blue Anytime." If there are any limp-wristed "nellies" out there, they are not spending their money on advertising.

Analyzing the contents of 359 ads placed in the *Advocate*—a bi-weekly newspaper with a circulation of approximately 60,000, published in California but distributed nationally—two researchers found that more than half claimed or sought explicit masculine attributes, ranging from "rugged" and "husky" to "junior executive" to "Ivy League type."[57] A more detailed study of the same publication noted that fully one-third of the ads in the "Models, Masseurs, and Escorts" section contained references to the advertisers' penises:

> Of these, 108 (74 percent) described themselves as "ample," "real (very) well endowed," or "hung nicely." Another 32 (22 percent) used extravagant terms to characterize their endowments as "exceptional," "huge," "super," or "thick and meaty." Two (1 percent) listed actual sizes, such as 8" or 10", and 5 (3 percent) identified themselves as "cut" (circumcised) or "uncut" (uncircumcised).[58]

A number of writers have ascribed this male homosexual preoccupation with masculinity and its most distinctive attribute to purely social factors:

> . . . an interest in masculine men need not be explained by involuted theories of Oedipal conflict. Masculinity and dominance are a standard part of the male gender role and are considered erotic and desirable when desired by women. Since dominating behavior, or its appearance, is considered erotic in men in our culture, a desire for that behavior among gay men need not be explained in terms of psychopathology. They

seem to have simply internalized their culture's conceptions of what is desirable in men. Hence one need not resort to Oedipal explanations of psychopathology to understand the sexual tastes of gay men.[59]

Martin Hoffman, whose *The Gay World* is one of the most perceptive books on male homosexuality, has also noted this sexual taste and penile preoccupation, but his explanation for their existence touches on different ground. Citing the behavior of some homosexuals, he asks:

> What is the reason for this compulsive desire for fellatio? It seems that this . . . is very much like what the Biblical historian W. Robertson Smith referred to as a sacramental feast, in which the participant eats the flesh and drinks the blood of the divine animal during a primitive religious ceremony, in order to get the *mana* or vital power which is present within the animal. . . . The compulsive fellator is unwittingly re-enacting an ancient religious rite. By sucking the penis of what he believes to be an especially masculine male, he feels he is incorporating some of this masculinity and vitality into his own person. . . .
>
> This explanation fits in very well with the well-known emphasis on penis size among male homosexuals. Any student of gay life can attest to the fact that very many male homosexuals are particularly fetishized on the size of the penis, and that this forms a recurrent topic of discussion among them. While this can partly be attributed to reasons no more pathological than the heterosexual male's interest in his partner's breast size, such an interest on the part of the homosexual male very often results in his going to great lengths to secure a partner with the largest possible penis.[60]

The same sentiment is voiced, with some poignancy, by "Mark Rosen," one of the anonymous subjects interviewed in depth by Alan Ebert in his interesting collection *The Homosexuals*:

> The plot is to keep us cock-happy. Give the gays their meat— a chicken in every bed—and they'll never focus on the real issues. And that's what's happening. Think of the energy we are wasting in baths and sex bars that could be put to use in gaining real freedom and acceptance. But, until the gay community

looks up from the cock it's sucking and gets its head together, we won't move one inch politically. But the day we give up those six to eight inches that fascinate us for the one inch that is more vital to our daily lives is the day we become a power to be reckoned with.[61]

The wish to "move politically" and to "become a power to be reckoned with" are unusual concepts to associate with what is, after all, nothing more than the exercise of a sexual preference. But in the United States at least, male homosexuality is viewed as something more threatening. Whatever level of anxiety is implicated in a man's choosing to become a homosexual, it is almost benign in comparison to the level of anxiety which the existence of male homosexuality seems to generate among the majority of American heterosexual men.

Kinsey was evidently aware of this phenomenon because in revealing his findings regarding the incidence of homosexuality among American men, he made the point of observing: "There are practically no other European groups, unless it be in England, and few if any cultures elsewhere in the world, which have been as disturbed over male homosexuality as we have here in the United States." [62]

"Disturbed" is, in keeping with Kinsey's style when venturing into editorial comment, a mild term. Geoffrey Gorer, who has earned a place among foreign observers of the United States, writes: "Among the generality of Americans, homosexuality is regarded not with distaste, disgust, or abhorrence, but with panic; it is seen as an immediate and personal threat." [63] In other words, the very fact that someone else may be a homosexual is sufficient cause for anxiety.

It should be noted, however, that it is not the aberration of sexual relations between two members of the same sex which is the cause of the panic. The fact that Gorer does not bother to qualify the term underscores the tacit agreement that the other form of homosexuality is socially, morally, and legally acceptable. To the extent that they have paid attention to it at all, men's attitude toward female homosexuality has generally ranged from indifference to mild amusement. The Mosaic laws, which had something to say—generally negative—about every possible kind of sexual permutation, do not even mention it. Ronald Pearsall, writing about lesbianism in *The Worm in the Bud*, says:

> Allusions to male homosexuality in Victorian England resulted almost entirely from court cases, and men without homosexual tendencies became acquainted, much to their surprise, with this other side of the heterosexual coin solely through reading newspaper reports of the various unsavory cases that were sure-fire circulation raisers for the Sundays. Many of them remained in the dark about the precise activities. . . . If the man on the street was oblivious to homosexuality in men, how much more was he in respect of homosexuality in women.[64]

The reason that the Criminal Law Amendment Act of 1885, which made it a crime to commit homosexual acts in private, refers only to men is that Queen Victoria had no idea that women could enjoy sex together, and no one could think of an appropriate way to describe to her how they would go about it.[65] Searching though the hundreds of legal opinions on "unnatural" sexual behavior handed down during the 256 years prior to 1952, the Kinsey researchers could not find a single case sustaining the conviction of a female for homosexual activity.

The explanation for this exceptional tolerance may well be, as Catherine Stimpson has suggested, that "Men regard the Lesbian choice as that of a lesser for a lesser." There seems to be more to it, however, judging by the kind of interest which the current coming out of lesbianism is evoking in men. It is possible that many recent films such as *The Vixen* and *The Killing of Sister George*, as well as the dozens of paperback glosses on D. H. Lawrence and Pierre Louÿs, are directed to female audiences. But *Playboy* and *Penthouse*, when locked in circulation combat, have both resorted to long, hard, breathing photographic essays of women making love, and almost every pornographic film has its obligatory Lesbian scene.

In *Group Sex*, the nearest approach to a scientific study on the subject yet published, Gilbert Bartell notes: "Ninety-two percent of the women at large [sex] parties become involved in sexual activity with one another."[66] And he adds: "We found not one exception to the rule that the husband approves and enjoys watching. Most swinging husbands admit that this turns them on."[67]

By contrast, in describing, however ungrammatically, the unwritten etiquette of present-day orgies, he observes: "One rule that immediately removes the transgressor from everyone's guest list is that no male should attempt any homosexual activity. . . . Even for men to touch each other accidentally in group action scenes is considered poor form by most male participants." [68]

A woman can deck herself out like a stevedore or a truck driver and not attract a second glance, but a man who wears a dress in public still runs the risk of being arrested in many communities. Male transvestism is acceptable only when it is clearly nonthreatening, and even then it requires the accompanying reassurance of laughter: the life-of-the-party guest who puts a lampshade on his head; the chorus girls in prison-camp movies, with their hairy legs and grapefruit breasts; Milton Berle's grotesqueries; Charley's Aunt with her cigar and her provenance—"Brazil, where the nuts come from." * To cite pornographic films, if only as a certified male-to-male medium of communication, with the exception of those films which are made expressly for them, male homosexuals do not appear in dirty movies except as the rare and clearly labeled butt of humor.

In *Deep Throat*, for instance, one of the male participants in the film's inaugural orgy looks around and, in a high-pitched voice, exclaims, "What am *I* doing here?" †

Lesbianism, then, is a lark which men not only tolerate but can vicariously enjoy. Male homosexuality, however, is another matter. As Wainwright Churchill has noted, "It may be justly claimed that a person of known homosexual persuasion or even a person merely suspected of homosexual inclination is likely to suffer common abuse as well as abridgment of his human rights in the United States more often and in more ways than a member of any other minority." [69]

This was written in 1967. Since then some superficial attitudes have moderated, but the underlying hostility has not abated—and has in fact received additional judicial sanction. Commenting on the fact that during World War II the United States was alone among the warring nations in automatically rejecting all recognizable

* By contrast, when T. C. Jones appeared on Broadway in *Almanac* a few years ago, the shocked gasp with which audiences invariably greeted his removal of his wig was not exclusively a tribute to his skill at female impersonation.

† The one-line role is played, with nicely scaled restraint, by Gerard Damiano, the film's creator.

male homosexuals from its armed forces, Gorer notes: "This selection was not made through any belief that the homosexuals would
be less efficient soldiers; it was a necessary protection for the rest." [70]
In discharging Sergeant Leonard Matlovich, the Air Force conceded
that, as of 1975, this protection was still necessary.

Until recently studies of attitudes toward male homosexuality
were hampered by the difficulty of measuring the subject's responses
with any degree of accuracy. The new development of instrumenta-
tion and techniques to measure changes in penile volume have,
however, permitted the shedding of some interesting light.* Using
as his subjects a group of twenty-two male homosexuals and a
control group of eleven male heterosexual medical students, the
psychiatrist Nicholas McConaghy sought to determine the degree
of sexual arousal elicited by films of men and women performing
such actions as undressing, combing their hair, and drying themselves with towels.[71] Predictably, he found that members of the
homosexual group showed a positive response, in terms of tumescence, to nude males. But he also discovered that upon being shown
the same films, his control heterosexual test subjects—incipient
doctors all—experienced varying degrees of penile shrinkage. As
Dr. George Weinberg points in *Society and the Healthy Homosexual*,
the only explanation for this reaction, the only psychic stimulus
which causes penile shrinkage, is fear.[72]

But fear of what? Geoffrey Gorer says:

> The chief reason would seem to be the feminine conscience,
> the encapsulated mother. . . . Because every American man
> has a feminine component in his personality, there is always a
> deeply hidden doubt concerning his own masculinity; and any
> person or situation which might bring this into question is
> seen as a drastic threat to a man's integrity and reacted to with
> violence and panic.[73]

Geoffrey Gorer is not a psychiatrist—a circumstance which may
make his opinions more acceptable in certain quarters. But what
he describes in lay language is the near-classic prototype of reaction
formation, the mechanism of protecting oneself against an impulse
by taking a stand against it in others. Dick Leitsch, then the head

---

* The methodologies, applications, and revelations of this subscience, as well
as those of the still more recent subsubscience of vaginal volume measurement,
are reviewed in the chapter which follows.

of the New York Mattachine Society, one of the first outspoken male homosexual organizations, was lecturing at Ohio University in Athens when a male member of the audience challenged him: "But if you take the laws away, and the social stigmas, then everyone will become a homosexual."

On the face of it, May 4, 1960, should have been a red-letter day for men everywhere. After fifteen years of testing and field trials, G. D. Searle, Inc., then a small Chicago pharmaceutical company, on that day received permission from the Food and Drug Administration to market a new drug called norethynodrel-mestranol, better known under its trade name of Enovid and still better and more familiarly as the pill.

The full side effects of the pill—social, economic, psychological, and demographic as well as pharmacological—are still far from being reckoned. As an interim evaluation, one social historian has proposed that in revolutionizing the position of women, it ranks second only to the invention of the typewriter. For men, however, its benefits have been mixed. If one reasons from the position of man-as-seducer, or at least man-as-persuader, it would appear that anything which would enable millions of females to shed their inhibitions and become sexually playful was cause for rejoicing. Matters seem not, however, to have worked out that way. Rather, it appears that many of these females have used their new freedom to become, in David Riesman's phrase, "critical consumers of male performance." [74]

Approximately ten years after the introduction of oral contraceptives, the *Ladies' Home Journal* took note of the fact that sex was still a two-handed game by publishing an article entitled "What 'the Pill' Does to Husbands." [75] What it did, according to Dr. Robert W. Kistner, was nothing to write home about. He cites several case histories, including a Chekhovian vignette of a bluff, extroverted salesman who on his nights home suddenly began experiencing incapacitating headaches just before bedtime, and concludes: "The heightened receptiveness and aggressiveness of a woman on the Pill poses a problem for some men who achieve ego satisfaction from their sexual prowess and who cannot adjust to a changed sexual role for their wives."

Part of this change, possibly the most affecting part, is that the pill has caused the decision of whether or not to make a child to pass largely from the man to the woman—at least to the extent that it cannot be done unless the woman is agreeable to it. In his article, Kistner tells of a young working wife who blackmailed her husband out of buying himself a new sports car by threatening to throw away her pills. The illustration may be frivolous, but the underlying problem is posed on a more fundamental level by Karl Bednarik:

> When the woman interferes with the ovarian cycle by taking the pill, man deposits his semen in vacuum, so to speak. How does this affect him psychologically? . . . This factor deserves the utmost attention, because the very ability to procreate by his own free decision is one of the strongest characteristics of masculinity and has been regarded as such throughout history.[76]

Sexual intercourse and pregnancy have been immemorially inseparable in man's thinking. Religious and civil law, social custom, and standards of behavior all recognize this natural condition. Women recognized it, too, and viewed male potency with appropriate respect. The penis was a powerful weapon; it could knock you up.

The issue of abortion on demand is, ostensibly at least, not related to oral contraception. Certainly, the feminist demand of "control over our own bodies" appears to be reasonable and fair. But to grant it requires an abdication of power on the part of men, and it just may be that men, having inadvertently given women the means to reduce them to shooters of ineffectual cap pistols, are not prepared to be reasonable and fair when it comes to permitting women to erase at will the most irrefutable evidence of their manliness. The current retreat from a liberalized position regarding abortion—a retreat evident in legislative action and court decisions as well as in public opinion polls—may therefore be attributable less to a revival of moral resolve than to punitive animus. In the spirit, if not the words, of Mike Hammer, "You've been fucked, lady, you'll stay fucked."

The core of the male's problem, the inescapable reason for his anxiety has been described many times, but never more explicity than in the clinical phrases of Masters and Johnson:

> Over the centuries, the single constant etiological source of all forms of male sexual dysfunction has been the level of

cultural demand for effectiveness on male sexual performance. The cultural concept that the male partner must accept full responsibility for establishing successful coital connection has placed upon every man the psychological burden for the coital process and has released every woman from the suggestion of similar responsibility for its success. . . . During coition woman has only to lie still to be physically potent. While this role of physical passivity is no longer an acceptable psychological approach to sexual encounter in view of current cultural demand for active female participation, it is still an irrevocable physiological fact that woman need only lie still to be potent.[77]

All the shrillness of some feminist writers, their categorical rejection of anatomy as destiny, their insistence on eradicating all differences between the sexes cannot eradicate this difference. As Dr. Emil Gutheil has pointed out, women do not commit suicide because of frigidity, but men have committed suicide because of impotence.[78]

The magnitude of an effect tends to be scaled to the intensity of its cause. The anxiety which woman occasioned, and which was quickened by the organ of her sex, rises by another level at the actual prospect of sexual performance. That men fear sexual intercourse is not a Freudian invention; it finds expression in the oldest surviving literary utterance of man, the Babylonian Gilgamesh epic. When he is confronted with the appearance of a rival named Enkidu, Gilgamish sets out to destroy him by making him a present of a temple harlot:

> The prostitute untied her loin-cloth and opened her legs, and he took possession of her comeliness: She used no restraint but accepted his ardor. She used on him, the savage, a woman's wiles. His passion responded to her. For six days and seven nights Enkidu approached and coupled with the prostitute. After he was sated with her charms, he set his face toward his game. [But] when the gazelles saw him, Enkidu, they ran away.
>
> The game of the steppe fled from his presence. Enkidu tried to hasten after them, but his body was as if it were bound.
>
> His knees failed him who tried to run after his game.[79]

Gilgamish's discovery that sexual intercourse is debilitating was, from earliest times, given the support of medical opinion. K. C.

Wong's *History of Chinese Medicine* quotes a physician from the Golden Period (about 1000 B.C.) to the effect that women should be approached only in "strictest moderation" because "excessive contact with them produces internal heat ending in *ku* disease," an incurable and sometimes fatal affliction.[80] Aretaeus, a disciple of Galen's, taught that impotence, effeminacy, and, eventually, gonorrhea result from excessive sexual indulgence and its attendant loss of semen. Albertus Magnus, the most encyclopedic thinker of his time and the teacher of St. Thomas Aquinas, writes:

> Too much ejaculation dries out the body because the sperm has the power of humidifying and heating. But when warmth and moisture are drawn out of the body, the system is weakened and death follows. This is why men who copulate too much and too often do not live long, for bodies drained of their natural humidity dry out and the dryness causes death.[81]

And in the United States, Benjamin Rush, physician and signatory of the Declaration of Independence, warned in 1812 that sexual appetite, "when indulged in an undue or promiscuous intercourse with the female sex . . . produces seminal weakness, impotence, tabes dorsalis, pulmonary consumption, dyspepsia, dimness of sight, vertigo, epilepsy, hypochondriases, loss of memory, manalgia, fatuity and death. . . ."[82]

Writing twenty-five years later in *The Influence of Slavery upon the White Population*, abolitionist Louise J. Barker cites as one of the evils of slavery the custom of black women to lure young slaveholders into carnal attachments in order to destroy their constitution through physical indulgence.

The belief that sexual intercourse robs a man of his strength was common to nearly all primitive societies and accounted for the numberless taboos against men's indulging in sex prior to undertaking such masculine activities as fighting, hunting, and fishing. In somewhat the same spirit the London *Daily Telegraph* for June 19, 1958, reassures its readers: "The Coldstream Guards are taking strict precautions to stop men fainting at the Trooping of the Colour. . . . Men below the rank of sergeant are to be confined to barracks, and married men condemned to bachelor barrack beds on the night before big parades."

Against such unanimity of opinion, this writer has been able to find only one dissenting voice. In 1958 an investigator named W. R.

Johnson collected a sample of fourteen college athletes and, having made sure that they remained sexually continent for six days, asked them to perform a series of exercises designed to measure their strength and endurance. He then had them repeat the tests on a morning after all of them had indulged in sexual intercourse. Johnson does not explain how these arrangements were made or monitored, but his results, as published in *Journal of Sex Research,* show absolutely no difference in levels of performance.[83]

Despite this clinical evidence, the belief persists. An athlete who suffers a particularly bad day is, by common accord, understood to have "left it in the sheets." In 1974 the *New York Times* carried an ad for *Playboy* which consisted of a smiling close-up of Muhammad Ali and the headline "Does Ali or Doesn't Ali?" The copy goes on to say: *"Playboy* knows for sure. Now the most colorful, outspoken figure in boxing is back again, this time to take on the old wives' tale concerning no sex before athletics. . . ." [84] *

The first male rationalization, then, is that sexual intercourse is dangerous. The second rationalization is that woman is sexually insatiable. Therefore, not only is it impossible to satisfy her, but the failure to do so is the consequence of her defect, and not the result of any shortcoming on the man's part.

Just as they guarded against the dangers of sexual intercourse through taboos, primitive societies warned against the insatiable female in their myths. One of the tidiest—it could be the account of an orgy written by Woody Allen—was related to Malinowski by his Trobriand islanders:

> Far away beyond the open sea, you would come to a large island. . . . Only women live there. They are all beautiful. They go about naked. They don't shave their pubic hair. . . . These women are very bad, very fierce. This is because of their insatiable desire. When sailors are stranded on the beach, the women see the canoes from afar. They stand on the beach awaiting them. The beach is dark with their bodies, they stand so thick. The men arrive, the women run toward them. They throw themselves upon them at once. The pubic leaf is torn off; the women do violence to the men. . . . They never leave the men alone. There are many women there. When one has

---

* The answer, for readers who may have missed the January 1975 issue of the magazine, is that Ali does but does not recommend it for his opponents.

finished, another comes along. When they cannot have intercourse, they use the man's nose, his ears, his fingers, his toes— the man dies.[85]

In the West, the theme is sounded by Hesiod, who first told the tale of Pandora, and by Homer, whose Circe turned her suitors into swine. Juvenal was writing about Messalina, wife of Claudius, but he had in mind all Roman women when he describes how she worked in a brothel where she:

> Showed her golden tits and the parts where Britannicus came from. Took the customers on with gestures more than inviting. Asked and received her price and had a wonderful evening. Then, when the pimp let the girls go home, she sadly departed, Last of all to leave, still hot, with a woman's erection. . . .[86]

Expressed in various accents, the theme runs through the whole of literature—Montaigne, Milton, Diderot, Voltaire, Rousseau, Keats, Poe, Schopenhauer, Baudelaire.* Their attitude is fairly summed up by William Faulkner in his description of Temple Drake in *Sanctuary*:

> With hips grinding against him, her mouth gaping in straining profusion, bloodless, she began to speak. "Let's hurry. Anywhere . . . Come on. What're you waiting for?" She strained her mouth toward him, dragging his head down, making a whimpering moan . . . "Please, Please. Please. Please. I'm on fire, I tell you."

Paradoxically, it appears that this rationalization—that women are insatiable—has some justification. The Masters and Johnson studies have shown that under certain artificial conditions, women are capable of prodigious orgasmic demonstrations. Dr. Mary Jane Sherfey, who collaborated with them, goes farther to suggest: "It could well be that the 'oversexed' woman is actually exhibiting a normal sexuality—although because of it her integration into her society may leave much to be desired." Indeed, Sherfey adds:

> No doubt the most far-reaching hypothesis from these biolog-

---

* For longer lists, amply documented, the reader is directed to *The Anti-Sex* by R. E. L. Masters and Eduard Lea (New York: 1964), *The Troublesome Helpmate* by Katherine M. Rogers (Seattle: 1966), *Not in God's Image* by Julia O'Faolain and Lauro Martines (New York: 1973), and numerous others.

ical data is the existence of the universal and physically normal condition of woman's inability ever to reach complete sexual satiation in the presence of the most intense, repetitive orgasmic experiences, no matter how produced. Theoretically, a woman could go on having orgasms indefinitely if physical exhaustion did not intervene . . . I must stress that this condition does not mean a woman is always consciously unsatisfied. There is a great deal of difference between satisfaction and satiation. A woman may be emotionally satisfied to the full in the absence of *any* orgasmic expression (although such a state would rarely persist through years of frequent arousal and coitus without some kind of physical or emotional reaction formation). Satiation-in-insatiation is well-illustrated by Masters' statement, "a woman *will usually* be satisfied with 3-5 orgasms . . ." I believe it would rarely be said, "A man will usually be satisfied with 3 to 5 ejaculations." The man *is* satisfied.[87]

Having thus put down males, Sherfey slips smoothly out of her clinician's whites and into archeologist's khakis:

Many factors have been advanced to explain the rise of the patriarchal, usually polygamous, system and its concomitant ruthless subjugation of female sexuality. However, if the conclusions reached here are true, it is conceivable that the *forceful* suppression of women's inordinate sexual demands was a prerequisite to the dawn of every modern civilization and almost every living culture. . . . There are many indications from the prehistory studies in the Near East that it took perhaps 5,000 years or longer for the subjugation of women to take place. All relevant data from the 12,000 to 8000 B.C. period indicate the precivilized woman enjoyed full sexual freedom and was often totally incapable of controlling her sexual drive. Therefore I propose that one of the reasons for the long delay between the earliest development of agriculture (c. 12,000 B.C.) and the rise of urban life and the beginning of recorded knowledge (c. 8000–5000 B.C.) was the ungovernable cyclic sexual drive of women. Not until these drives were gradually brought under control by rigidly enforced social codes could family life become the stabilizing and creative crucible from which modern civilized man could emerge.[88]

Other scholars have yet to endorse Dr. Sherfey's reconstruction of prehistory, but her assertion that the rigid control of women's sexual drive is conducive to the stabilizing of family life is amply supported by the evidence of a more recent age. The Victorians hallowed woman. They crowned her with moral superiority, placed her on a pedestal, and then removed the stepladder that permitted access to her. It was their way of paying homage to her, but not accidentally it also served as still another rationalization of their fear of sexual intercourse, as ingenious in its way as any other product of that invention-minded era.

Dr. William Acton, author of *The Functions and Disorders of the Reproductive Organs* . . . and the recognized expert in the field, stated in 1857:

> I should say that the majority of women (happily for society) are not very much troubled with sexual feeling of any kind. . . . A modest woman seldom requires any sexual gratification for herself. She submits to her husband's embraces, but principally to gratify him; and were it not for the desire of maternity, would far rather be relieved from his attentions.[89]

It was as simple as that. If woman is an asexual being, devoid of all erotic desire and capacity for fulfillment, men need not worry about being able to satisfy her sexually.

Acton's reassuring dictum became one of the social and psychological underpinnings of Victorian life, in the United States as well as in Britain.* His book was endorsed by the *American Medical Record* as "a classic based on sound philosophy, science and a religious stand-point."[90] Other experts rushed to support his thesis. George Napheys held that only rarely did women experience a fraction of the sexual feelings familiar to men. "Many of them," he writes, "are entirely frigid, and not even in marriage do they ever perceive real desire." [91] One of the standard nineteenth-century college texts on physiology taught that, for the "majority of women belonging to the more luxurious classes," sexual intercourse after the age of twenty-three was "a mere nuisance." [92]

For those few women who might not share these male judgments,

---

* Learned men elsewhere were quick to agree with him. Cesare Lombroso, who as professor of forensic medicine and psychiatry at Turin was the most celebrated criminologist of his time, wrote in 1893 in *La Donna deliquente*: "Woman is naturally and organically frigid."

there were disagreeable consequences in store. "Any spasmodic con-
vulsions" during sexual intercourse, one popular marriage manual
threatened, would interfere with conception—"the primary function
of the act." [93] Another warned that "voluptuous spasms" on the part
of the woman were likely to cause a weakness and relaxation which
would leave her barren.[94] The recommended posture for the woman
during intercourse was to lie "motionless on the stalk, sheltering in
a dazzling tabernacle the reproductive organs of the plant." [95] *

Frequency of intercourse also received its share of attention.
Acton was willing to permit it every ten days or so, but his American
colleague Dr. John Cowan considered this excessive. "The man and
woman," he prescribes, "should come together . . . with the desire
for offspring: impregnation and conception follow, and from that
time until the mother has again menstruated—which occurs after the
weaning of the child, and which in duration extends to about
eighteen or twenty-one months—sexual intercourse should not be
had by husband or wife." [96]

This continence, and the woman's assigned botanical role, was not
the result of puritanical rejection of pleasure. Far more important
matters were at stake, for even as they erected another defense for
themselves, Victorians did not for a moment abandon the old argument that sexual intercourse was dangerous and debilitating. On the
contrary, their consumingly mercantile mentality led them to elaborate it into a complete economic system.

To begin with, they revived an old euphemism for the sexual act—
to spend.† But spend what? The new currency of the system was
semen. Acton called it a "life-giving substance" and claimed that, if
retained, it could revitalize and invigorate the entire system.[97] A
writer named N. Venel extolled it as "the most ethereal or subtilized
portion of the blood, a highly rectified and refined distillation from
every part of the system, particularly the brain and spinal mar-
row." [98] Possibly aware that this sounded suspiciously like the teachings of Hippocrates and Pythagoras—who had, in fact, called semen

---

* A formula which, at least, has the virtue of being more poetic than the Victorian lady's classic advice to her about-to-be married daughter: "Just shut your
eyes, my dear, and think of England."

† Readers, particularly readers of *My Secret Life,* in which it is used in-
numerable times, may suppose that the expression has pornographic connotations, but it appears in all kinds of Victorian writing and even crossed the ocean
to show up in *Moby Dick.*

the "flower of the blood"—others rushed to offer the support of more contemporary scholarship: the Lamarckian theory of the hereditability of acquired characteristics; the work of Darwin and Herbert Spencer; Helmholtz's mechanistic principles of "conservation of force."

In essence, the argument ran, man was endowed with a certain amount of semen, and he could, through clean, careful living, add to his store. He could also choose to spend it—and the American physician J. Marion Sims even helpfully told him how much each withdrawal would cost. ("I do not know that anyone has thought of measuring the quantity of semen ejected in the act of copulation . . . I was induced on several occasions to measure it . . . and I found that ordinarily there was about a drachm and ten minims.* ") [99]

The Victorian attitude toward masturbation—which can be summed up in the nanny's warning "If you don't stop playing with it, it will fall off"—was preeminently a reaction to the severe strain which the "solitary vice" placed on a young man's balance sheet. Insanity was hardly punishment enough for self-inflicted bankruptcy. But there was a danger still greater than masturbation, and more insidious because it did its damage by stealth. As C. Bigelow warns in *Sexual Pathology*:

> Of all the diseases or derangements which affect or which can affect the generative organs, there is none equal nor half so bad as Spermatorrhoea. All others together, or one after another, in a continuous round, are not capable of producing— and never have and never can produce—half so much mischief, derangement and ruined health as this one evil of Spermatorrhoea or involuntary emission of Semen! [100]

All the engineering skills which had gone into the construction of the Crystal Palace were mobilized to guard against spermatorrhoea, or, as it is called today, wet dreams. One could buy an electric alarm which sounded under the sleeper's pillow when the penis, expanded by erection, completed an electrical circuit. Another popular device was a urethral ring consisting of a sheath with four steel points which turned inward, but which would rise and press into the skin of the penis at the first appearance of an erection.

* A little more than an eighth of an ounce.

Still another, described by Frank Harris in his autobiography, consisted of a piece of leather whipcord which was wound around the penis at night. "As soon as the organ began to swell and stiffen in excitement," he writes, "the cord would grow tight and awake me with pain." One physician recommended the insertion into the rectum of a wooden object resembling, in size and shape, a pigeon's egg. Worn day and night, the device was designed not to prevent erection or ejaculation but, by pressing on the prostrate gland, to force the semen backward into the bladder.[101]

It would have been surprising if, having established such vigilance over all other expenditures of semen, Victorian experts had overlooked the risk of its depletion during normal sexual relations—especially as it was this context, and neither masturbation nor nocturnal emissions, which occasioned their male anxiety to begin with. Predictably, Acton set their minds at rest. Since the sexual act imposes such an enormous drain on his system, he writes, the male should perform it in as short a time as possible, preferably in a few minutes.[102] Physicians advised husbands and wives that it was their joint responsibility to maintain the male's sperm at the desirable level of richness. To do so, it was essential that no more sperm than was necessary for the production of a child be released during copulation and that the wife therefore make no demand which would require additional expenditure. J. H. Kellogg, whose accumulation of a fortune in the fledgling cornflake industry made him a respected voice in all matters pertaining to health, suggested the revolutionary notion that husband and wife should habitually occupy separate beds—with any migratory movement being at the husband's discretion, naturally.[103] G. Stanley Hall, the man who in other respects was sufficiently enlightened to sponsor Freud's only visit to the United States, sums up the era's attitude: "Thus the sex organs have two functions: the first is reproduction and the other is to give force and energy to all other parts and to character generally. All work involving great effort, either mental or physical, requires sexual temperance, and Delilah always robs Samson of his strength.[104]

None of the foregoing is intended to suggest that the Victorians were opposed to sexual intercourse. In 1850 there were at least 10,000 full-time prostitutes in London, many of them barely in their teens. There were at least as many, and reputedly a greater variety of them, only a Channel crossing away. There were, on sounder testimony than that of *My Secret Life*, a virtually limitless number of shopgirls, factory girls, farm girls, and domestics who were accessible for the price of a few coins. There was also a monumental amount of jiggery-pokery carried on in the stately homes and red-brick mansions. No, Victorian males were not opposed to sex. Like men before them, they were frightened at the prospect of having to perform. And as members of one of the most male-dominated societies of all time, they took good care to see that they wouldn't have to.

For the preponderance of Victorian women, the price of granting their men this psychic tranquillity was merely the abdication of their own rights to sexual gratification. In addition, a nastier lot lay in store for a number of them. Despite the overwhelming weight of expert counsel, there cropped up here and there among the "more luxurious classes" * a backsliding female who perversely appeared to enjoy sex and even, with appropriate delicacy, dared hint as much to her husband.

Having defined the absence of sexual desire in women as normal, physicians had no choice but to diagnose its presence as an indication of disease. According to Dr. Augustus Kinsley Gardner, who received his M.D. from Harvard in 1844, taught at the New York Medical College, and became one of the city's most fashionable gynecologists, such a woman was "a drag on the energy, spirits and resolution of her partner." [105] So serious was this condition that some doctors, when examining women suspected of harboring it, took particular pains to manipulate the clitoris and breasts in an effort to elicit "positive amorous signs." [106] Oliver Wendell Holmes had taught: "A woman of flesh and blood and with infinite variety will, like a vampire, drain a man, *nolens volens*, of his life's blood." [107] Holmes was referring specifically to hysterical women, but other doctors extended the characterization to all members of the sex and used it to justify the extreme corrective measures which they began to impose.

One of them was clitoridectomy. Abandoned by many of the African tribes which had at one time or another practiced it, the removal of the clitoris was introduced as a formal surgical procedure by the British gynecologist Isaac Baker Brown in 1858. The London Obstetrical Society reviewed Dr. Brown's results and put a stop to

* Except for their usefulness as horrible examples, the poor were generally ignored by Acton and his followers and left to wallow in their brutish, sperm-squandering ways.

the operation in 1866, but it continued to be performed in the United States until the 1920s.* Another treatment, invented by Dr. Robert Battey of Rome, Georgia, in 1872, consisted of the "extirpation of the functionally active ovaries." Removal of one or both ovaries had occasionally been performed in cases of organic disease, but Battey named his procedure a "normal ovariotomy" to reassure surgeons that the mere apparent health of an ovary need not stay their scalpels. "Normal ovariotomy" became the operation of choice for such conditions as "troublesomeness, eating like a ploughman, masturbation, attempted suicide, erotic tendencies, persecution mania and simple 'cussedness.' " [109] Some doctors claimed with pride that they had removed more than 2,000 ovaries and at medical meetings handed samples around on plates as if they were so many trophies. One reported that "patients are improved, some of them cured; . . . the moral sense of the patient is elevated; she becomes tractable, orderly, industrious and cleanly." [110] By the end of the 1890s the operation had become so prevalent that the *Journal of the American Medical Association* felt obliged to warn that it had reached the proportions of an "epidemic," a "thriving industry," and, perhaps most unconsciously appropriate, a "rage." [111] Nevertheless, "normal ovariotomy"—or female castration, to give it a less technical name—continued to be practiced in the United States until 1921.

Viewed in psychological perspective, the motives of the doctor— and of the husband in handing his wife over for castration—are understandable. So intense were their fears, in fact, that they were able to impose them on their women. Far from resisting the operation, many patients pleaded with their gynecologists for castration, "fully convinced that all their grief emanates from their pelvis." [112] As Dr. Ely Van der Warker, a critic of wholesale castration, pointed out in 1906, "So constantly have they been held up before her as the one evil spot in her anatomy, that she has grown to look with suspicion on her own organs." [113]

Other societies have been satisfied with trying to cope with male

* In general, it was reserved for cases of acute, incurable "nymphomania"— an exercise in restraint that must be viewed with the knowledge that Dr. Horatio R. Storer of Boston Lying-in Hospital referred to a patient as a "virgin nymphomaniac." [108]

penile anxiety, but ours has the distinction of going one step farther and making a thriving industry out of it. The Playboy clubs and Gaslight clubs, and, for less affluent, less upwardly mobile males, the dirty magazines, the topless and bottomless waitresses and dancers, constitute the ultimate, logical marriage between the Thousand and One Nights and the free enterprise system. At last, the guest is being made to pay for his Barmecide feast.

Recall Kinsey's men—in all more than a third of all American males—who copulate with their clothes on. They, or others like them, can be found leafing through the offerings of pornographic book-shops, feeding quarters into peep-show machines that promise "Three girls and a man: hard rear-end action," and patronizing burlesque shows, where they crowd up to the runway for a better, unimpeded view of the female nudity which in other circumstances they profess to find indecent or obscene. Clearly it is not nudity which is threatening, but its context. Once the ground rules—"Don't touch the merchandise"—are established and accepted, the only permissible performance which remains is masturbation. And that, as has been noted, is an encounter at which men almost never fail. *Hustler* magazine, which pioneered the near-clinical display of split beavers,* claims that its photographs are so inviting that readers report licking them.

As one of the earliest, most conspicuous successes of the commercialization of male anxiety, *Playboy* has received its full-size share of attention. Commentators have cited the magazine's preoccupation with the trappings and symbols of virility—automobiles; fancy high-fidelity equipment; clothes; food; travel; beds that shake, turn, or vibrate. One needs only add the observation that the same words which appear in the magazine's ads for sports cars—"the smoothest pleasure machine on the road"; "You drive it—it doesn't drive you"—can also serve as captions for the Playmate of the Month, without the least distortion in meaning. Rollo May summed it up when he said that *Playboy*, for all its pioneering of sexual freedom, had merely "shifted the fig leaf from the genitals to the face." [114]

Advertisers have not overlooked the opportunity of leavening their messages with a dash of anxiety relief. For women, they created

* A beaver is, in the trade, the term for female pubic hair.

Mr. Clean, Mr. Glad, and the Ajax White Knight, with his ever-ready lance.* For men, they pour glasses of beer with stately, rising foam, which, they promise, "will last as long as the pleasure." For smokers, they hold out the reassurance "It's not how long you make it, it's how you make it long." More recently they have even begun suggesting that male anxiety over sexual intercourse may be a thing of the past. Max cigarettes, which prides itself on its "long, lean, all-white dynamite look," presents a smiling girl who says, "Max, I can take you anywhere." Or, in another ad in the series, "Hello, long, lean and delicious."

These two ads, with their clear allusion to fellatio, strike a particularly contemporary note. Although its origin as what Kinsey calls a "sexual outlet" is lost in history, fellatio has apparently never been as popular with men as it is now. Reporting the preferences of prostitutes' customers, Charles Winick writes in *The New People*: "A quarter-century ago, the typical customer wanted coitus. Perhaps one or two percent wanted fellatio, and a brothel with 20 prostitutes might have one who performed fellatio or oral stimulation as a prelude to coitus (half and half). Today, however, approximately four-fifths of the customers want fellatio." Closer to home, Winick notes: "The most thorough early study of marital sex [by G. V. Hamilton in 1929] concluded that only eight percent of the husbands engaged in any oral sexual activity." [115] Kinsey's findings, published nineteen years later, were that about four out of ten married men said they had ever been fellated by their wives. And bringing returns up to date, Morton Hunt discovered in a survey of 2,026 men and women conducted in 1972 that the number was up to 58 percent. Hunt also found that among men under twenty-six, 72 percent had been fellated by a female partner, compared to less than 33 percent in the Kinsey study. [116]

Hunt's explanation is:

> . . . the increase in the use of such techniques . . . [he includes cunnilingus and anal sex in his discussion] owes much to the general education of wives and (even more so) of husbands as to the usefulness of precoital activity in making coitus more successful for the female. It is also attributable in part to the desire, now common to both men and women at almost all

---

* "The longest, stiffest prick in America" is how one of its creators described it to this writer.

levels, to see themselves as sexually expert. But beyond this, liberation has undoubtedly given many people the internal freedom to relish such acts in themselves. . . .[117]

At least the first of these reasons seems more applicable to cunnilingus than fellatio, and in any case none of them would explain the preference of prostitutes' customers. Winick is more convincing when he writes: "Fellatio's new popularity suggests an increased passivity and fear of the vagina in many men." * And he observes:

> Their decreased forcefulness also emerges in the growing popularity of men's use of the fatalistically passive verb "to get laid" to describe sexual intercourse. A generation ago, the definitive dictionary of American slang did not even mention the phrase, and men were far more likely to use an active verb.[118]

One contemporary phenomenon which supports Winick's view is the proliferation of massage parlors, not only in such fleshpots as San Francisco, New York, and London but in cities large and small across the United States and Europe (Asia, presumably, has had them for centuries). Characteristically, they bear such names as Tahitia, Taj Mahal, The Casbah, The Garden of Eden, Moulin Rouge, The French Quarter, The Barbary Shore, evoking the ineffable delights of pliant, exotic maidens and the raunchy, two-fisted masculinity of a prospector dropping his lode. Their advertising tries hard to encourage such visions: "Be an Emperor for a Day"; "Select your personal slave girl—she will hand bathe you while your body rejoices in a golden whirlpool of fragrant milk bubbles . . ."; "Our provocative hand maidens (carefully trained in our Paris establishment) await only your command to begin *The Ritual of Ecstasy* . . . a wanton ritual involving soothing body anointments using special aphrodisiac oils. . . ."[119]

Depending on their quality, massage parlors provide such amenities as saunas, whirlpool baths, sunlamps, waterbeds, stereo, color TV, complimentary drinks, mirrored walls, sunken bathtubs, and female attendants who, as promised, will wash, dry, stroke, rub, and anoint—all for prices that may range from $10 to $100. It is also possible, if one is insistent and willing to tip like an emperor, to "get

---

* The mouth is, in fact, more "dentata" than the vagina, but because it is not associated, in childhood fears, with genital activity, it poses no threat to the penis.

laid" in most massage parlors, but the practice is neither encouraged nor often requested. The usual demand, which the personal slave girls generally satisfy without removing their skimpy costumes, is for a hand job or a blow job, after which the patron is encouraged to linger—but not too long—in "the spectacular opulence of our Maharaja Lounge," where he can reflect with quiet satisfaction on a piece of work well and truly performed. It is either through happy chance or shrewd insight that the Tahitia, one of the most elaborate and expensive parlors, call itself "a 'pleasure island' in New York's sea of anxiety."

Male preferences for fellatio appear to derive from complicated motivation. To some degree, the "forbidden" aspects of the act are attractive. All studies of prostitutes and their clients routinely cite this as a reason—"I can't get it at home." But current indications are that the clients now can and do. We have seen, in discussing the role of the penis as a weapon, that it can serve to establish dominance, express aggression, and inflict degradation. One of the common English terms for fellatio—"going down"—suggest that, to some men at least, the act satisfies these ends. A third reason, already noted, is men's passive attitude toward sex. But passivity is only a clinical symptom, which still requires explanation.

Most men, and all prostitutes, know that a penis which falters during conventional sexual intercourse can usually be restored to operational rigidity, and sometimes even be encouraged into an encore, by oral ministration. In a paper entitled *"Phallic Passivity in Men,"* the psychoanalyst R. Loewenstein says:

> It is well known that, in many men who suffer from disturbances of potency, inhibitions such as collapse or total absence of erection make themselves felt in certain circumstances only. In some cases this occurs whenever the sexual partner makes the slightest show of resistance, while in others coitus is impossible unless the woman not merely consents but takes the initiative.[120]

He goes on to suggest that this inhibition derives from castration fears associated with childhood episodes during which the expression of early sexuality was met with rebuff or threat:

> The adult man seems to wait for the woman's "permission" to have intercourse with her, for the effects of the prohibition

imposed in childhood have to be counterbalanced. For some young men suffering from inhibitions it is enough if "permission" is given on one single occasion by a woman who is a substitute for the female "castrator" of their childhood; their genitality is then set free, once and for all. . . . But, as a rule, the woman has to repeat her "permission" and even to extend it to important details of the sexual act itself, e.g. to the introduction of the penis by her help.[121]

For this purpose, the mouth, which had none of the frightening connotations of the vagina, is a far more effective orifice.

Another response to the fear of sexual intercourse, admittedly atypical, is the practice of autofellatio. Kinsey estimates that only 2 or 3 men out of 1,000 are able to achieve this objective, although he adds: "A considerable portion of the population does record attempts, at least in early adolescence . . . and there are 3 or 4 case histories of males who had depended upon self-fellation as a masturbatory technique for some appreciable period of time."[122] Kinsey did not speculate on why men should select so strenuous a technique, and for once the psychoanalytic literature is not very helpful. The first reported case of autofellatio, published in 1927, concerned a thirty-three-year-old depressed apprehensive man who was remorseful concerning his practice but maintained that he could not control the impulse, which he said overtook him on the average of once a month. He also said that his interest in autofellatio was stimulated by watching circus contortionists perform. Having presented his case, the author concludes, inarguably but uninformatively: "These morbid inclinations no doubt indicate an extreme degree of sexual maldevelopment."[123]

In 1938 two psychiatrists described the case of another man, also thirty-three years old, who began to think of autofellatio when he was nineteen years old and, after considerable endeavor, managed to consummate the act, which he then repeated on the average of every two weeks. He occasionally dressed as a woman and spoke of a fantasy of self-impregnation, the accomplishment of which he felt would make him the center of attraction. The authors report that the patient also engaged in other forms of deviant behavior such as "fellatio, sodomy, mutual masturbation, exhibitionism, fetishism, algolagnia, and voyeurism." Faced with such a rich menu, they shy away from specifics and simply conclude: "From an early time onward inclining toward the position of black sheep in his overreligious family, he appeared to have utilized his sexual perversions as his own method of rebelling against his family and their moral standards." [124]

Finally, writing in 1971 in the *International Journal of Psychoanalysis*, Frank Orland, whose case histories include a female patient, concludes that autofellatio is a "multilevel oral-genital auto-erotic phenomenon manifested by acts, fantasies and dreams, with their associated instinctual drive derivatives and related objects." [125] Here the matter rests for the present. As refuge from the threat of woman, autofellatio remains as an option which, if still not satisfactorily clarified, at least has the virtue of not being illegal—unless there is somewhere a statute prohibiting unnatural acts between one consenting adult.

Autofellatio, as was noted, is an atypical response. Far and away the commonest expression of male sexual anxiety is concern over penile size. Questions regarding what is normal and abnormal appear regularly not only in *Playboy* and *Penthouse* but also in *Medical Aspects of Human Sexuality*, a professional journal edited for and read by physicians. No writer on the subject has failed to reassure men. Albert Ellis has even suggested that a man with no penis at all can make a successful lover. Masters and Johnson authoritatively state in *Human Sexual Response*:

> Another widely accepted "phallic phallacy" is the concept that the larger the penis the more effective the male in coital connection. . . . The delusion that penile size is related to sexual adequacy has been founded in turn upon yet another phallic misconception. It has been presumed that full erection of the larger penis provides a significantly greater penile size increase than does erection of the smaller penis. This premise has been refuted by a small group of men selected from the study-subject population for clinical evaluation.[126]

The next chapter will deal with penile size—average and extraordinary—and performance. It will consider what can go wrong, why, and what can be done about it—a technological profile of the penis at work. But it must be noted that technology is only part of the problem. The biggest and most crucial erogenous zone, for women as well as men, lies between the ears. Although she undoubtedly endorses her coauthor's views quoted above, Virginia Johnson Masters also said in an interview: "If a female believes that a large penis is the most exciting and stimulating thing for her, then it is. Perhaps she's told this, perhaps she picks it up from popular lore, perhaps a past pleasurable experience has conditioned her to believe this. But the difference can be real in her mind. It may even be used by her to provide the crucial difference when her own response to a partner is less than she would like." [127]

Pointing out that "Myth and misinformation is shared by the female," another investigator hazards the opinion that "many females find a small penis to be less psychologically arousing during foreplay than an average or large penis . . . [which] symbolizes aggressivity, power, strength and masculinity. Also, where the penis is larger than normal, the woman may find the prospect of intercourse more exciting and thereby achieve higher levels of sexual arousal." [128]

Again, hard clinical data are scarce in this area, but one study did attempt to come to grips with the problem. Thirty-six male and twenty-four female college students were shown slides of, among other objects, a large penis and a small penis. They were then asked to rate their reactions on various adjective scales. The large penis was described as stronger, more active, and more virile than the small one. It also was rated as harder, sharper, and more handsome.[129]

In their discussion of these results, the authors state:

> It should be emphasized that . . . subjects were young college students, fresh from or still struggling with the rigors of adolescence and, for the most part, still naive and inexperienced. Perhaps as they get older, have new and different experiences, and leave adolescence, the stereotype of . . . the large penis does not hold.[130]

Perhaps. But perhaps, after all has been said and properly analyzed, it may just be that the size of his penis *is* something for a sensible man to worry about.

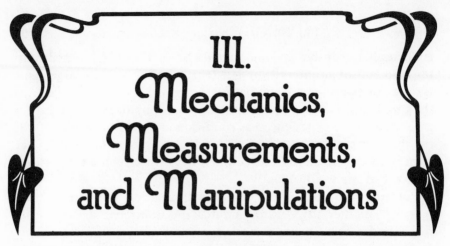

III.
Mechanics,
Measurements,
and Manipulations

As bodily organs go, the penis is relatively simple in structure and operation. Gray's *Anatomy*, for instance, disposes of it in five and a half columns, while devoting seven to the tongue and twelve and a half to the large intestine.[1] This chapter will consider how the penis functions and all too often malfunctions. It will review the causes of these failures to function and also the remedies, old and new, that have been devised to correct them. Under this heading, it will summarize the effects of various drugs on sexual performance, from such tried-and-true preparations as cantharides to glossy, potent new agents such as p-chlorophenylalanine. It will report on mechanical and other devices intended to enhance penile performance —a collective testament to man's ingenuity, cupidity, and indestructible credulity. And finally, it will then take a look at a body of current scientific work which holds out the promise of relieving the anguish of millions of men.

The bulk of the penis consists of three cylindrical masses of spongy tissue. Two of them, the corpora cavernosa, lie parallel to each other and just above the third, the corpus spongiosum, which also contains the urethra. Upon engorgement, the corpora cavernosa have the far greater capacity, thus giving the erect penis its characteristic shape of a triangular prism with rounded angles. Gray's *Anatomy* notes than the skin covering the penis is "remarkable for its thinness, its dark color, its looseness of connection with the deeper parts of the organ, and its absence of adipose tissue."[2] But at least as remarkable is the thick, fibrous membrane, the tunica albuginea, which surrounds the spongy masses and therefore causes them to lengthen as they fill up with blood, rather than simply to balloon out.

The mechanism of erection is sufficiently intriguing to have instigated a number of early attempts at explanation. Among the most fetching is that offered by Constantinus Africanus, who practiced medicine in Sicily around 1070, in his *De Coitu*:

> Three things are involved in intercourse: appetite (created by the fancy), spirit, and humor. The appetite comes from the liver, the spirit from the heart, and the humor from the brain. When appetite arises in the liver, the heart generates a spirit which descends through the arteries, fills the hollow of the penis and makes it hard and stiff. The delightful movements of intercourse give warmth to all the members, and hence to the humor which is in the brain; this liquid is drawn through the veins which lead from behind the ears to the testicles and from them it is squirted by the penis into the vulva.[3]

Modern understanding began with the work of the German Christian Eckhardt, who in 1863 reported that electrical stimulation of certain visceral branches of nerves from the sacral spinal chord—the *nervi erigentes*, as he called them—produced penile erection in dogs.[4] Subsequent research has attempted to trace the path of these nerve impulses more accurately, but meanwhile, an important contribution was made by two Americans, Drs. James H. Semans and Orthello R. Langworthy, to the understanding of the mechanical aspect of erection. It was believed, just as Constantinus Africanus had proposed, that the penis became "hard and stiff" because of an inflow of arterial blood. But it was also thought that the veins collaborated by somehow shutting down and preventing the accumulated blood from escaping. Semans and Langworthy, who were working with cats, cast doubt on this hypothesis with a simple demonstration. They placed a loop of thread around the animal's aorta and tightened it. No amount of stimulation of the sacral roots could then produce an erection. "Then," they note, "the thread was released and the roots were again stimulated; this time the usual erection occurred. When the arterial supply was interrupted during excitation, the erection subsided within two minutes."[5] All well and good so far, but then they dissected away the muscles which normally serve to keep the outgoing veins closed. The penis should have collapsed like a punctured bag. Instead, they report, stimulation of the roots still brought about full erection.

That a similar principle governs human erection was neatly demonstrated by Dr. Herbert F. Newman. He applied an infant's blood pressure cuff to the base of the penis of each of ten normal adults and inflated it to just below diastolic pressure, thus closing off the veins but not the arteries, for five minutes. The result was that the penis became puffy and cyanotic, but not erect.[6] So much for all the devices, store-bought or homemade, which attempt to preserve or prolong an erection by preventing the blood from escaping.

It has now been fairly well established that the small arterioles which pass through the spongy tissues of the penis have valvelike structures which open upon neural stimulation and allow blood to fill up the vacant spaces and distend them. This in turn causes the penis to enlarge, until an equilibrium is reached in which the rates of inflow and outflow are equal.[7]

Erection, then, depends upon a continuance of the blood supply, which in turn depends on a neural impulse, and this is where the story becomes complicated. Part of the difficulty is that there are two kinds of erection, functionally equivalent but different in inspiration. There is the "reflexogenic" erection, which arises from direct stimulation or manipulation of the genitals and sometimes of the rectum or bladder, and there is the "psychogenic" or "no hands" erection, which is caused by visual, auditory, olfactory, tactile, or purely imaginative stimuli. Reflex erections are believed to be triggered from nerve centers located well down on the sacral part of the spinal cord. Psychic erections, obviously, originate somewhere in the brain.[8] It has been observed that patients who have suffered complete destruction of the sacral spinal cord could still have erections in response to erotic psychic stimuli but not in response to genital manipulation.[9] Conversely, more than 90 percent of patients whose sacral cords had been cut above the sacral level were able to achieve erection in response to manipulation but not in response to psychic stimuli.[10]

It would seem that nature was unusually thoughtful in providing a backup system for a function which is essential to the preservation of the species, but unfortunately its bounty seems to work both ways. As Dr. Howard Weiss points out, psychological factors, such as fear, guilt, or hostility, are by far the most common causes of impotence.[11] "Apparently," he adds, "these psychological factors activate inhibitory neural pathways that are capable of suppressing the spinal erection centers, thereby preventing erection. The neuroanatomy and physiology of these inhibitory pathways are not known." This missing knowledge, Dr. Weiss notes, has more than theoretical interest: "Elucidation of the neurotransmitters responsible for this inhibition could, theoretically, lead to the development of drugs that antagonize central inhibition and thereby constitute a pharmacologic treatment for psychic impotence"—much as high blood pressure is now controlled by drugs which are believed to block certain neural impulses.

There are other essential patches of ignorance in our understanding of the process. Detumescence, the mechanism whereby an erection subsides, is not clearly understood. Neither is priapism, the very painful refusal of the erect penis to subside. The whole phenomenon of ejaculation, which is quite separate from erection, has yet to be explained. It can occur spontaneously, without any genital stimulation, and in fact does occur that way to the more than 80 percent of all males who, according to Kinsey, report having experienced a wet dream. Kinsey attributed them to "psychic stimulation during sleep," [12] but it has since been established that paraplegics have wet dreams, despite the complete functional disruption of their spinal cords. Ejaculation can occur without orgasm or even without sexual stimulation of any kind. It is, for instance, a fairly common occurrence among men who are executed by hanging.[13] Conversely, orgasm can be experienced without ejaculation. Under certain circumstances, ejaculation can occur but be retrograde—instead of being propelled outward, the seminal fluid is forced backward into the bladder.[14] Constantinus Africanus was hampered by the imperfect anatomic understanding of his day, but in some respects we have not improved much on his explanation.

In their first book, *Human Sexual Response*, Masters and Johnson observe: "The size of the male organ both in flaccid and erect state has been presumed by many cultures to reflect directly the sexual prowess of the individual male."[15] A reason for this presumption may be the general notion that "bigger is better." But it probably also betrays a fundamental sense of inferiority or at least insecurity. In response to a question, Dr. James F. Glenn notes, in the *Journal of the American Medical Association*: "It can be safely said that the adult male population suffers an almost universal anxiety in regard to penile size." [16] More specifically, one urologist has reported that more than three-quarters of his male patients are convinced that their penises are smaller than average.

And what is average? Considering how crucial the matter appears to be, it may be surprising that no one tried seriously to answer the question until 1949. Dr. Robert Latou Dickinson, one of the most distinguished gynecologists of the century, endeavored to do so if only to make his *Atlas of Human Sex Anatomy* complete. He reported: "After a vain hunt for such measurements, both here and abroad, in libraries and in departments of anatomy, I gave carte blanche to the most expert of our library searchers, the late Edward Preble, M.D. He reported that in the long list of volumes consulted and the standard indexes 'there is little or nothing to unearth.' " [17] Combining the nine studies which the search had produced, Dickinson came up with the following dimensions: The average length of the flaccid penis was 4 inches (10 centimeters), within a range of 2⅜ to 4½ inches (6 to 11.5 centimeters); the average circumference was 3⅜ inches (8.5 centimeters) within a range of 3 to 4⅛ inches (7.5 to 10.5 centimeters). The average length of the erect penis was 6 inches (15.5 centimeters), within a range of 4¾ to 8¼ inches (12 to 21 centimeters); its average circumference was 4⅜ inches (11 centimeters), within a range of 3⅜ inches to 4¾ inches (8.5 to 12 centimeters).

To these reports Dickinson added his own findings, that "very exact measurements" on 1,500 American white males yielded an average erect penile length of 6¼ inches (16 centimeters) and an average circumference of 4 inches (10 centimeters). He also reported that 90 percent of his sample fell within the range of 5 to 7½ inches (12.5 to 19 centimeters). These dimensions, he noted, correspond with the 3,500 measurements collected in the Kinsey study.[18]

Masters and Johnson measured penile length along with everything else, and with their usual meticulousness: "All 80 penises were measured on three different occasions both in flaccid and erect states by the same individual. Only one clinical investigator conducted this clinical measurement so that any idiosyncrasy of measurement would be common to all results.* One of the measurements of penile erection was taken during automanipulation, and two measurements were initiated immediately upon withdrawal of the plateau-phase penis from active coition.") [19] For some reason, these data were not published. Dr. Masters said in an interview that they were "safely

---

* The measurement was taken "from the anterior border of the symphysis at the base of the penis along the dorsal (upper) surface to the distal (far) tip of the glans."

under lock and key." [20] They did report, however, that measurement in forty men disclosed that those with the smaller phallic proportion —3 to 3½ inches—averaged an increase in length of 3 to 3¼ inches upon erection, while those men with larger flaccid penises—4 to 4½ inches—averaged an increase of only 2¾ to 3 inches. The largest increase in size (3½ inches) occurred in a man whose flaccid penis had measured less than 3 inches. The smallest increase (2¼ inches) was observed in a penis which had been 4¼ inches long. "At full plateau-phase erection," Masters and Johnson note, "the two organs were measured at identical lengths on three separate occasions," demonstrating, one supposes, that nature tries to compensate for its own deficiencies. Presumably as additional reassurance, Masters and Johnson note that the size of the penis has less constant relation to general physical size or development than that of any other bodily organ, a fact first noted in the literature by Heinrich Loeb in 1899 [21] and probably confirmed by a good number of women since then.*

Next to size, the penile property most prized by men is durability. In the fantasy world of pornography, the universal wish-fulfilling hero is tirelessly and unflaggingly erectile. Greek mythology took disparaging note of premature ejaculation in the story of how the ugly, lame Hephaestus, spurned by his wife, Aphrodite, attempts to embrace Athena but succeeds only in dropping his seed on her leg.[23] *The Perfumed Garden* describes several categories of men who are to be held in contempt and includes this one: "Scarcely has he commenced when he is already done for; he makes one or two movements, and then sinks upon the woman's breast to spend his sperm; and that is the most he can do." [24] Contemporary men's magazines, addressing themselves to the same problem, carry ads which promise: "Now You Can Prolong Sexual Relations As Long As You Wish. . . . A learned sexologist has discovered an easy to use, uniquely new sex miracle that INSTANTLY allows you to maintain the same erection . . . ," [25] or "Stay harder longer with our special *Prolong Pills*, and be still in there where the action is when ordinary men would have had to quit. . . ." [26]

A number of commentators have proposed that male concern for female sexual response is a relatively new cultural acquisition. In-

---

* New parents may possibly be interested in still another study completed by two physicians at the University of Washington School of Medicine. They took penile measurements of 37 full-term male newborn infants and found them to be 3.5 cm ± 0.7 cm in length and 1.1 cm ± 0.2 cm in diameter.[22]

deed, one of them has written: "It is presumed, in heterosexual coitus, that female orgasm depends on male performance. It is this issue of male responsibility which creates the category of the sexual incapacity called premature ejaculation." [27]

It would be nice to believe that the male's preoccupation with his sexual staying power is, in fact, so selfless in origin, but there are obviously other motives at play—such as, for instance, the wish to prolong his own pleasure and perhaps the desire to demonstrate and hammer home his dominance. Whatever the reasons, it would seem that men have grounds for concern. Kinsey's findings, which have not been invalidated by subsequent research, were that some 75 percent of American men ejaculate within two minutes of penetration and after a total of some forty to fifty thrusts. Reasoning as a biologist, he argues that such a pattern of rapid response is not only normal but actually "a superior mammalian trait." And still as a biologist, he adds: "The idea that the male who responds quickly in a sexual relation is neurotic or otherwise pathologically involved is, in most cases, not justifiable scientifically." [28]

Nevertheless, the phenomenon had attracted the attention of psychoanalysis as early as 1913, when Karl Abraham, one of Freud's earliest and most faithful disciples, leveled the full artillery of the fledgling science against it.[29] He begins by equating ejaculatio praecox with bed-wetting: "The same individuals who acquired normal control of bladder function only late or only incompletely also tend toward a premature, precipitate seminal emission." But there is also the specter of castration anxiety: "We are dealing with the phobia of being unable to withdraw the penis from the body of the woman and having to leave it behind." Then there are the oedipal overtones: "The patient would like to surpass his father, who is coarse and brutal, by means of refinement, and thereby supplant him with his mother." And the shock of the primal scene: "The normal sexual act then appears to be a brutal act. The *ejaculatio praecox* to a certain extent makes an appeal to the female tenderness of the mother; it wishes to express: 'See, I approach you more tenderly than father.'" On the other hand:

> The patient is permanently dependent upon his mother and struggles against his dependency, which arises from his unconscious. The struggle to defend himself is manifested as a struggle against all womanhood. But in this struggle the patient does

not command the resources of powerful, masculine activity. He must confine himself to disappointing a woman, and, in this way, he avenges himself on every woman for the erotic disappointments to which he was exposed, as a child, at the hand of his mother, and which in later years repeat themselves.

Commenting on this polymorphic formulation, Wilhelm Stekel notes in his *Impotence in the Male*: "Abraham unfortunately was unsuccessful in solving the problems of *ejaculation praecox*." [30] * His own explanation is far simpler and seems to have better stood the test of time:

> We may consider the sexual act the resultant of two groups of forces. The first group is of libidinous origin; it represents the demands of the sexual impulse. The other group comprises all inhibitions, safeguards, protective functions, of the inner man. When the struggle is strong, the inhibition is more easily overcome. With a very strong inhibition (the voice of conscience) the libido can only assert itself with difficulty. *Ejaculatio praecox* is a compromise between both tendencies.[31]

All this was theory. The first factual, statistical study of premature ejaculation was completed in 1943 by Bernard Schapiro, who over a period of twenty years personally observed 1,130 cases.[32] In 56 of them, less than 5 percent, he found some physical cause for the disorder, which could easily be corrected. As for the rest, he notes:

> The important part played by psychic processes is evident. . . . There are always fears and inhibitions, conscious or unconscious, spoiling the sexual act. The fear may be connected with the act itself, such as fear of infection, fear of pregnancy, fear of hurting the woman, fear of failure, or, sometimes this fear seems to be unrelated to sex.

Schapiro identified two distinct types of patients: the "hypotonic," who suffered from general nervous exhaustion, insomnia, fatigue, and digestive and circulatory disorders; and the "hypertonic," whose condition was brought about by excessive sexual tension, which he likened to a "high electric charge." For the first group he prescribed prolonged sexual rest, nerve tonics, and brisk exercise. The second,

---

* Parenthetically, he adds: "His comparisons . . . will not be conducive toward spreading an understanding of psychoanalysis into wider medical circles."

he suggested, would respond well to drugs, such as belladonna and papaverine, which "act upon the vegetative nervous system" to slow down the transmission of erotic impulses. In addition, he made an observation so self-evident that it apparently had escaped some of the deep students of psychic mechanisms: "Potency stands in a class all by itself because it is the only bodily function that requires the presence of a second individual."

It had all along been taken for granted that loss of control over ejaculation was caused by excessive stimulation and excitement. Home remedies included—and still include—diversionary maneuvers such as biting one's tongue, pinching one's arm, or tightening the anal sphincter during intercourse. Men making love forced themselves to review the day's business events or to count backward from 100. They discouraged their partners from fondling or even touching their genitals; some put on multiple condoms to deaden sensation; a few took the precaution of masturbating before starting intercourse. Physicians gave tacit support to this strategy by experimenting with various topical anesthetics applied to the most sensitive portions of the penis. Some success was reported for this procedure, but it entailed considerable premeditation.[33] The anesthetic had to be applied "copiously" some two or three hours before the penis was to be used. If it were not completely removed before intercourse, it would begin to act on the vaginal tissues and undo its own purpose. Moreover, the very act of advanced planning was counterproductive for some men because it focused attention on the precise source of their anxiety. But most important, it was fundamentally antithetical. If a man complains of an earache, you don't send him to a concert wearing earmuffs.

In 1956 Dr. James Semans, the urologist who had helped trace the mechanism of erection, proposed a new idea. Far from being oversensitive, he argued, the premature ejaculator suffers from a decrease or an absence of sensation as he becomes aroused. There is, as every man knows, a distinct moment when he feels himself coming. For control purposes, this sensation arrives too late. Ejaculation is a reflex response, and once it begins no act of will—and no anesthetic—can delay it. This being the case, Semans writes:

> The procedure recommended for prolonging the . . . reflex mechanism of the ejaculation is extravaginal stimulation of the penis during erection, until the sensation premonitory to ejacu-

lation is experienced by the patient . . . stimulation is then interrupted until the sensation has disappeared. Penile stimulation is repeated until the premonitory sensation returns and is then again discontinued. . . . By repeating this procedure, the response of ejaculation becomes no longer premature; that is, it can finally be delayed indefinitely.[34]

In practice, Semans instructed his patients' partners to stimulate the penis manually, at first in the dry state and later lubricated to simulate more closely the moist environment of a vagina. His original paper reported on eight cases, ranging in age from twenty-five to forty-two and in occupation from an IBM salesman to a dining-car waiter. All of them achieved control within a month.

Semans was not a psychiatrist—indeed, he warned that "psychiatric symptoms related to sexual activity, such as hatred and fear, are contraindications to use of the method"—but the impact of his technique seems to be directed as much to the mind as to neuromotor reflex mechanisms. By obliging the female to become actively involved in the problem as a helper rather than as a potential enemy or humiliator, the method automatically tends to reduce the male's possible hostility and relieve his anxiety or guilt—the main inhibitory forces which Stekel identified.

The widely publicized Masters and Johnson "squeeze" technique for the treatment of premature ejaculation is, as its authors readily concede, an elaboration of Semans's procedure. The mechanics of the squeeze itself, which Semans left up to his patients' discretion, is specifically described:

> The female partner's thumb is placed on the frenulum, located on the inferior (ventral) surface of the circumcised penis, and the first and second fingers are placed on the superior (dorsal) surface of the penis in a position immediately adjacent to one another on either side of the coronal ridge. Pressure is applied by squeezing the thumb and first two fingers together for an elapsed time of 3 to 4 seconds. If the man is uncircumcised, the coronal ridge can still be palpated and the first and second fingers correctly positioned. An approximation of frenulum positioning must be estimated for thumb placement.[35]

Masters and Johnson also added three new factors to the treatment. The first was the introduction of a mixed-gender cotherapy team which works intensively with patients and their partners over a two-week period. Semans saw his partners for a total of only three and a half hours. The second factor was the use of "sensate focus" exercises as a means of giving and receiving pleasure without raising preoccupation over performance. The third was to prescribe a specific position:

> Stimulative techniques are best conducted with the wife's back placed against the head-board of her bed (possibly supported by pillows), her legs spread, and with the husband resting on his back, his head directed toward the foot of the bed, and with his pelvis placed between her legs, his leg over hers, so that she may have free access to his genital organ.

Nowhere in their book do the authors of *Human Sexual Inadequacy* give the reasons for adding these three factors, but all of them seem to be based on simple psychological principles. The presence of a therapy team, for instance, encourages the development of transference on the part of the patient. Transference has been described as "not simply the attribution to new objects of characteristics of old ones but the attempt to re-establish and relive, with whatever object will permit it, an infantile situation much longed for because it was once either greatly enjoyed or greatly missed." [36] More specifically, as the psychoanalyst R. Michels observes:

> The new sex therapy would appear designed to maximize the patient's transference response to the therapist's authority. In this way the therapist can replace the patient's internalized authority figures, and substitute benign, permissive, encouraging and even demanding attitudes toward the patient's sexuality . . . for previous unconscious prohibitions and injunctions, stemming from the patient's childhood images of his parents. The patient thus gets better for the same reason that he got sick, his desire to please and his fear of disapproval by authorities.[37]

In specifying the physical position of patient and partner, it is possible that—intentionally or not—Masters and Johnson are mining a still deeper Freudian vein. Dr. Louis J. Ripich suggests:

> We know that some of the early manifestations of love for the child on the part of the parent are the cleansing ministra-

tions of the mother. And certainly, if one looks at the diagram of the recommended position in Masters' and Johnson's work, one sees a recapitulation of that position in which genitals are presented to the mother, and for the moment the man receives exclusive attention, a situation in which the self-love is temporarily reinforced and gratified. The pleasure in exhibition of the penis, so typical of childhood, is again reflected in the technique that is suggested by Masters and Johnson in which the woman fondles the penis. Certainly, the position that is recommended is one in which there is maximum exhibition of the penis. Therefore, by gratifying some of the early desires and impulses of the individual, and by allaying the early fears associated with those impulses, one is able to bring about the inhibition of premature orgasm.[38]

The third Masters and Johnson innovation—the introduction during therapy of sensate focus exercises—seems to owe its inspiration to a more recent psychological movement: behavior therapy, or the application of the theory that neurotic behavior is acquired through learning and that it therefore can be modified by appropriate techniques without resolving or even necessarily understanding its underlying dynamics. Masters and Johnson contend that premature ejaculation, or "rapid sexual patterning," as they term it, is the result of poor early learning. Particularly in the case of men now in their thirties and forties, they point to such educational factors as youthful experience with prostitutes, sex in drive-ins and on parental living-room couches, and the contraceptive practice of pulling out just in time, all of which tend to condition the male to rapid response. The sensate focus exercises, the gradual approach toward intercourse, the squeeze itself are all, in behavioral terms, means of counterconditioning and reinforcement within a hierarchy —a stepped program of increasing anxiety-arousing situations.*

* The requirement of having couples come to stay in St. Louis during their treatment, which was part of the original Masters-Johnson program, may have been merely a matter of convenience for the researchers, but it also served a behavior therapy purpose. The behaviorist I. Goldiamond notes: "One of the most rapid ways to change behavior is by altering the conditions under which it usually occurs." [39] It may be a coincidence, but Masters and Johnson report that those of their patients who already lived in the St. Louis area and therefore did not need to leave their homes while undergoing treatment required three weeks of therapy instead of the normal two.

There is more than academic interest in identifying the theoretical basis of the Masters-Johnson technique. As of 1970, the publication date of *Human Sexual Inadequacy*, the authors reported success on the part of 98 percent of the 186 men they had treated for premature ejaculation. Subsequent reports from other therapists who have used the technique confirm this near-perfect record. If they are accurate, then the means exist to provide training for the tens of millions of men who, according to Kinsey, could make excellent use of it. Unfortunately this training has up to now been time-consuming, expensive, and limited in availability. However, if the therapy is largely based on learned responses and the modification of behavior, why can it not be incorporated into a programmed learning course—a course, moreover, which one could take in the privacy of one's own home?

This question has now been answered—provisionally in the affirmative—by two psychologists at the University of West Florida in a paper entitled "Use of Written Material in Learning Self-Control of Premature Ejaculation." [40] The subjects consisted of ten heterosexual couples selected on the basis of meeting three criteria: that the male ejaculated either upon penile-vaginal contact or within three minutes of intromission; that the female agreed to cooperate with the program; and that there were no apparent intrapersonal problems with the couple that needed to be treated first. Five of the males were then given an eighty-page program consisting of instructions, diagrams, and five quizzes which had to be correctly answered before they proceeded. The couples were instructed to complete the program at their own speed. The remaining five couples became the control group and were put on a waiting list.

Before treatment, the first five experimental males had a mean ejaculatory control of 1.8 minutes. After treatment, which lasted an average of three weeks, their mean control was 39 minutes. The control males began at a mean of 1.4 minutes and reported no changes while on the waiting list. After treatment, however, their mean control rose to 20 minutes.

The authors are quick to point out that all their subjects were volunteers and therefore well motivated. Furthermore, the sample was small and in no way demographically representative. There was also no provision to evaluate the permanence of the change. On the other hand, they note that the program was a first attempt and that suggestions for improving it have already emerged.

Some cases of premature ejaculation stem from factors so deeply rooted that they require the intercession of a therapist, if only to permit transference to operate, but it appears that the great majority can be dealt with much more simply and quickly. Premature ejaculation is a source of great humiliation for many men. It is a frequent precursor to impotence. It is the cause of considerable marital discord and no small amount of female infidelity. Why then, since the necessary knowledge is available, can it not simply be made part of the high school curriculum? Surely, in terms of social utility, such a program would have almost as great value as driver education.

Premature ejaculators, by definition, cannot control themselves. At the other end of the spectrum there are some men who cannot achieve ejaculation at all. They will respond to sexual stimulation with erotic feelings and a firm erection. But however hard they try and however urgently they desire release, they cannot trigger it.

Retarded ejaculation is a relatively uncommon disorder—Masters and Johnson came across 17 cases among 510 couples they treated—and may even appear to be something of a blessing in disguise, if not to the sufferer, then at least to his partner. In practice, however, it is often damaging to both. Dr. Lionel Ovesey, who has written the most comprehensive account of it, says: "The patient may struggle to ejaculate with such desperation that he may physically exhaust himself, and sometimes even his partner, in the attempt." [41] Furthermore, the partner may well suffer mental anguish as well. Sex therapist Helen Singer Kaplan notes: "The wives are usually as deeply disturbed about this as they would be about any other sexual dysfunction, and tend, in a paranoid manner, to interpret their husband's problem as a personal rejection." [42]

The immediate cause of retarded ejaculation is the specific inhibition of the ejaculatory reflex. This, in turn, can be brought about by disease, organic damage to the nerve apparatus, or as a side reaction to some drugs. [43] The far more frequent underlying cause, however, is entirely psychological.

Again, the psychoanalytic pioneers have proposed a rich range of interpretations. Ferenczi reported the case of a patient with retarded ejaculation who was also afraid of falling off bridges, and made the classic aquatic connection: "We are thus enabled to understand the patient's apprehension . . . and his incapacity for complete sur-

render to a woman, who always meant for him, though unconsciously, deep water with the menace of danger, water in which he
must drown. . . .[44] Bergler, on the other hand, attributed retardation to the opposite fear: "In this form of disturbance, the defensive,
pseudo-aggressive anal pleasure of retaining is combined with the
also defensive pleasure of 'harming' the object, arising from the
notion that the woman may be hurt in some way by protracted intercourse." [45] Fenichel blended both theories, attributing retardation
to fears of death and castration as well as to "strivings, anal (retaining) or oral (denial of giving), sadistic or masochistic in character." [46]

In his paper, Ovesey concedes that "there is merit in all these
propositions" but points out that "without exception they lack
adequate documentation." He then suggests, on the basis of his own
clinical experience, that a striking feature of retarded ejaculation
is its occurrence in patients with marked paranoid tendencies: "The
central conflict in these patients, as in all paranoid males, was their
hostile rivalry with other men. Psychodynamically, in retardation,
this competitive struggle was symbolically displaced to the sexual
act with women, where ejaculation was equated with the violent
destruction of male competitors." But in order for this formula to
work, the patient must maintain his self-confidence, which is precisely what the paranoid lacks. Instead, his doubts mobilize the
threat of retaliation. To avoid it, the patient withholds his ejaculation but simultaneously denies his impotence by maintaining an
erection.

Occasionally retarded ejaculation can be traced to a single trau-
matizing experience. One of Masters' and Johnson's cases involved
a strictly Orthodox Jew: "One night, at the age of twenty-four
years, totally breaking with traditional behavior for the first and
only time of his life, he not only forced physical attention upon,
but tried to penetrate a young woman somewhat resistant to his
approach. She stopped him with a plea that she was menstruating." [47]
Four years later the man married a young woman of the same
religious background as his own. Both rigorously adhered to Orthodox demands of celibacy within menstrual and postmenstrual
periods. Nevertheless, so haunting was his fear of contamination that
he could not bring himself to ejaculate into her. Another of Masters
and Johnson's patients was a man who had caught his wife in the
physical act of adultery and who subsequently could not ejaculate
intravaginally because "he was faced with the vivid but castrating

mental picture of the lover's seminal fluid escaping his wife's vagina."

Neither of these patients responded to the Masters and Johnson treatment—two of seven failures they reported out of seventeen cases. Ovesey's rate of success was 50 percent—five out of ten cases.

The relatively poor results of therapy suggest that, whatever their dynamics, the causes of retarded ejaculation lie deep within the personality. Occasional success has been claimed for purely behavioral techniques,[48] but in general, the condition remains a puzzle. Perhaps the best hope, statistically anyway, lies with the induction of ejaculation by electrovibration. The procedure consists of subjecting the tip of the penis to stimulation by means of a specially adapted electric massage vibrator. One of the groups to use this method states that "ejaculation and orgasm may follow after three to six minutes. A few artificially provoked ejaculations make the patient conscious of what he is expected to do, and enable him to have normal intercourse." [49] Using a fairly representative sample, they report that the method proved successful for fifty-five out of seventy-two patients.

Regrettably, no such simple, reliable mechanical aid is available to victims of the fundamental male sexual disorder. Although firm figures are not available, impotence appears to be as prevalent as the common cold. Stekel believed that "there is hardly a marriage where the husband has not at some time experienced a period of temporary impotence,"[50] and Ernest Jones, the British Freudian, writes that "only the minority of men pass through life without showing signs of it." [51] Freud himself went even further: "I shall . . . put forward the proposition that psychical impotence is far more widespread than is generally supposed, and that some degree of this condition does in fact characterize the erotic life of civilized peoples." [52]

Freud's description of psychical impotence is broad. He says, for instance, that "it would comprise, to begin with, all those men who never fail in the act but who perform it without special pleasure." [53] For practical purposes, the definition given by Donald Hastings in *Impotence and Frigidity* seems more acceptable: "that condition wherein the male cannot obtain or maintain penile erection satisfactory to him for purposes of heterosexual coitus." [54] At least, it has the virtue of focusing on the agony of the afflicted. You *want* to get it up and put it in, but you can't.

Considering the many delicate mechanisms involved, it is not surprising that there should be a long list of organic causes of impotence. Severe damage to the central nervous system through disease or accident can result in impotence,[55] as can conditions which cause interference with the blood supply to the penis.[56] Endocrine disorders can result in lack of potency, as can diabetes, the removal of the prostate, pelvic fracture, and various physical anomalies of the genitalia, including agenesis, the unusual circumstance—1 in some 10 to 30 million cases—of a male child being born without a penis.[57,58]

Many of these physical conditions are incurable or require complicated and uncertain treatment. Fortunately, however, most of them are rare. Kinsey concludes that "impotence in a male under fifty-five years of age is almost always the product of the psychological conflict." [59] Howard and Scott, the authors of a basic textbook on endocrinology, report that "by far the greatest number of patients seeking medical advice for impotence are found to have no demonstrable organic disease, but to have clear-cut psychiatric problems," [60] and D. Stafford-Clark, a leading British expert on sexual disorders, holds that "at least ninety percent of all cases of impotence are psychogenic in origin." [61] Psychogenic, and therefore at least theoretically remediable.

Freud thought as much, for he wrote in 1912—and, in retrospect, rather offhandedly—that "we are usually able to make a confident promise of recovery to the psychically impotent." [62] In the classical psychoanalytic view, psychic impotence arises out of the smoldering ashes of a poorly resolved oedipal conflict. The patient's intense sexual attachment to his mother in childhood leads to guilt and fear of castration. Reactivation of these fears in adult sexual life by a woman who is identified with the mother causes sexual inhibition and impotence. This inhibition protects the individual from indulging in a symbolically incestuous relationship. The identification, however, is not as likely to occur with a mistress, a prostitute, or, in fact, any woman of lower social standing. Freud is never more stuffy or Victorian than when he states:

> . . . full sexual satisfaction only comes when he can give himself up wholeheartedly to enjoyment, which with his well-brought-up wife, for instance, he does not venture to do. Hence comes his need for a less exalted sexual object, a woman eth-

ically inferior, to whom he need ascribe no aesthetic misgivings, and who does not know the rest of his life and cannot criticize him.[63]

Other interpretations abound. Abraham [64] and Jones [65] believed that childhood fears of the father overshadow sexual potency. Stekel claimed that a bipolar component of hatred is essential to every love and that the first expression of that hatred may be a temporary impotence.[66] Freud himself proposed the additional explanation that impotence is due to the feeling of disgust which men experience when they discover that women do not have a penis.[67] Jones pointed to fear caused by punishment, or the threat of punishment, for childhood sexual activities.[68] Fear of social or divine retribution has been proposed, as have fear associated with prior sexual experiences, fear of disease, fear of pregnancy, and fear of inflicting injury on the partner. Some authors have maintined that impotence results from a fear of expressing hostility and sadism.* Finally, many agree that impotence is the result of a self-fulfilling prophecy—that it is caused by the fear of impotence itself, based on a conviction of sexual inadequacy.[70]

Masters and Johnson emphatically endorse this final formulation. They write: "It should be restated that fear of inadequacy is the greatest known deterrent to effective sexual functioning." [71] For once, Soviet thinkers appear to agree with their Western colleagues. The magazine *Zdorovye*, which has a monthly circulation of 10 million copies, testily told the readers of its December 1970 issue that "the majority of men who complain about lowered potency are not suffering from any organic condition. It is functional and can be overcome. The men are always preoccupied with self-observation and self-analysis and are plunged into such gloom that their condition can only worsen."

* One commentator has even blamed the design of wallpaper. A. Salter reports in *Conditioned Reflex Therapy* on the case of a thirty-five-year-old man who complained that he had suffered from impotence at home for six months, although he was entirely competent when he and his wife were in hotel rooms. During the course of therapy the patient described a traumatic incident prior to his marriage when he had been caught in bed with a woman. It transpired that the wallpaper in the bedroom of his new apartment, which he and his wife had occupied for half a year, was identical with that of the bedroom in which he had been discovered. A change in decor was the extent of the therapy needed to restore his potency.[69]

But sadly, not even an ukase from the Central Committee can prevent a man from brooding over a permanently limp penis. The problem is aptly stated by the psychiatrist Joseph Wolpe: "The key to the problem of impaired sexual performance is the subtraction of anxiety from the sexual encounter." [72] How to do it is not so clear.

Psychoanalysis still claims to offer a solution, even though Freud was obliged to modify his earlier optimistic view and, by 1919, warn his colleagues that "we are accustomed confidently to promise recovery to psychically impotent patients who come to us for treatment, but we ought to be more guarded in making this prognosis so long as the dynamics of the disturbance are unknown to us." [73] There are numerous published case histories of successful analytic treatment of impotence, but because psychoanalysts seldom write up their failures—or, as some of them would have it, their patients' failures—there is no way to evaluate their rate of success.* Furthermore, analysis requires considerable amounts of time, money, and psychic energy—more than most prospective patients can invest in the process.

Success has also been claimed for more rapid and superficial treatments. The English physician J. F. Tuthill believed that most cases of impotence could be ascribed to severe inhibition and culturally imbued taboos. He recommended to his patients that they "retrace the steps of courtship, which in some cases they may have never trod at all." [76] Specifically he advocated that the couple spend more time in bed together and urged the male to concern himself with experiencing and enhancing the sensual pleasure of the act, rather than dwell on his performance. He also urged abandoning restraint, increasing sexual experimentation, and incorporating sexual fantasies into actual sexual practices. Tuthill, who rarely saw his patients more than a few times, nevertheless claimed on the basis of a postal return that 136 out of 257 of them—53 percent—declared themselves satisfied with their improvement. Another Englishman, Stafford-Clark, emphasized the importance of "positive motivation" in treatment and reported that "at least fifty percent of impotence presenting in the psychiatric clinic can be

---

* Any claims should be viewed in the perspective provided by the studies of Denker [74] and Eysenck [75], which show that the rate of success in treating neurotic disorders by therapeutic means is approximately the same as that resulting from spontaneous remission.

satisfactorily treated with a dozen interviews." [77]

More carefully controlled clinical studies have not supported this optimism. Alan J. Cooper followed the progress of forty-nine patients who faithfully completed a ten-month course of treatment and reported the following results: [78] Seven recovered their potency, twelve said they felt they had improved, twenty-one were unchanged, and nine claimed they were worse off than when they started.* John Johnson investigated forty patients who had, between 1950 and 1959, received various treatments including testosterone and psychotherapy. His findings were equally discouraging: Twenty-five said the disorder had persisted or had got worse.[79]

A different approach was advocated by still another English physician. Confronted with a patient who complained of impotence, he prescribed the following regimen:

> I told him . . . that he was to go to bed to this woman, but first promise to himself that he would not have any connections with her for six nights, let his inclinations and powers be what they would; which he engaged to do, and also to let me know the result. About a fortnight after, he told me that this resolution had produced such a total alteration in the state of his mind that the power soon took place, for instead of going to bed with fear of inability, he went with fears that he should be possessed with too much desire, too much power . . . and when he had once broken the spell, the mind and powers went on together, his mind never returning to its former state.[80]

The name of the doctor was Joseph Hunter, and one reason why his successful technique was not reported in the medical literature is that it took place in 1781.

By 1961 the idea behind Hunter's treatment—that human behavior can be modified by appropriate conditioning—had blossomed into a new psychological discipline. Reviewing its progress in a paper entitled "Sexual Disorders and Behavior Therapy," S. Rachman begins by postulating that impotence is the result of neurotic behavior, which he defines as "any persistent habit of unadaptive behavior acquired by learning in a physiologically normal organism." [81] Because it was acquired by learning and not innate to the

---

* Treatment consisted of "an optimum combination of: a) deep muscular relaxation; b) provision, as far as possible, of optimal sexual stimulation for the male; c) sexual education; and d) psychotherapy."

organism, it follows that such behavior can be changed. All that is needed is the proper combination of reward and punishment.

Manipulating the form and intensity of this reward and punishment—in their own vocabulary, reinforcement and extinction—is the central concern of behavior therapy. An extreme example of the punishment mode, used to treat a rape-prone gang of young thugs, was demonstrated in the film *A Clockwork Orange*. In attempting to cope with impotence, therapists prefer to hold out the carrot of reward. One of their techniques is positive conditioning, which "identifies some condition which is capable of eliciting sexual responsivity in the subject, and then arranges that the appropriate transfer of sexual arousal occurs through an associative process." [82] Another is systematic desensitization, which "inhibits the anxiety responses provoked by phobic or noxious stimuli. The lasting inhibition of these responses is gradually evoked by the controlled and systematic reduction of anxiety followed by relaxation. The therapist begins by presenting only modestly disturbing visual images. Each presentation of a noxious image is followed by deep relaxation. When the emotional effects of the milder images has been considerably reduced or eliminated, the therapist then presents slightly more disturbing images until even the most anxiety-provoking situations can be pictured without disturbing the patient." [83]

Early reports of success through behavioral therapy were encouraging: In one instance, five out of seven patients were apparently cured of their impotence after an average of 14.4 sessions each; [84] in another, eight out of ten men reported satisfaction. [85] But more recent, and perhaps more rigorous, studies have shown a falloff in batting averages. More significant, they tend to show that the control groups, which go through the motions of interviewing and history taking but receive no treatment, react in approximately the same fashion as those under active therapy—a circumstance which can perhaps be attributed to the Hawthorne effect. [86]*

Possibly influenced by male chauvinism, early writers on im-

* So called after a pioneering experiment in industrial psychology conducted half a century ago by Elton Mayo at the Hawthorne Works of the Western Electric Company in Chicago. The investigators were trying to find out whether output could be increased by altering working conditions, and if so, how. They discovered that *any* change—the very evidence that someone appeared to be interested in them—caused the women on the assembly line to produce more.

potence accorded women no contributing part in the problem. Tuthill, for instance, stated that "to assume that [impotence] is caused by a failure of emotional relationships and that treatment should be directed to adjusting these relationships is, I am sure, unwise." [87] This view, which in retrospect appears strange because sex, most of the time, takes place with a partner, has now been rejected. Writing about the attacks of occasional impotence which afflict virtually all men at some time, Martin Goldberg suggests that "most sexual disorders exist not inside one person, but between two people." [88] In a comprehensive review of women's role in male impotence, Henry J. Friedman raises an interesting point:

> Because of the high visibility of the male genital, most likely the impotent male patient, his wife, and the psychiatrist focus the attention upon him. It is more than an accidental finding that when a woman fails to achieve orgasm, one of the first questions by both the educated layman and the psychiatrist is "What kind of a lover is your husband?" No such question seems to be raised for the male suffering from impotence.[89]

Finally, Masters and Johnson complete the circle when they insist that "there is no such entity as an uninvolved partner in a marriage contending with any form of sexual inadequacy. Sexual dysfunction is a marital-unit problem, not a husband's or wife's problem." [90]

The Masters and Johnson technique for dealing with impotence employs an eclectic mix of behavior modification, insight-oriented psychotherapy, educative counseling, and just plain heart-to-heart talk. More than any prior discussion of the subject, it has received wide publicity which includes three full-dress translations into lay language.[91] Part of this attention is probably due to their utilization of female "surrogate-partners," but part must also be ascribed to their reported 72 percent rate of success—176 out of the 245 men in their pilot study.

Some critics have complained that Masters and Johnson may have loaded the dice in their own favor by their method of selecting couples for therapy. To be eligible, candidates had to be willing to devote two uninterrupted weeks to their treatment; they had to present themselves as a pair, willing to cooperate in helping each other; and most of them had to travel to St. Louis. These conditions, one of the critics noted, effectively screened out all but the most highly motivated.[92]

To this, defenders of Masters and Johnson point out that another of the conditions they imposed was that the prospective candidate had to have undergone a previous unsuccessful therapeutic venture of at least six months' duration.

The most persuasive argument in favor of the technique is that it has repeatedly passed the basic scientific test of replication both in the United States and abroad. Its crowning acceptance, in fact, may be that at least one group of investigators has used it as a reward for volunteers in their own study. Reporting the results of some less than successful attempts at treating impotence through behavior modification, three German doctors note that "when this project was completed the therapy strategy was changed. Those patients who had shown no improvement in this study were then treated using a modification of the Masters and Johnson technique combined with sex education. Twelve patients have been treated by this method. Of these twelve patients, eight are cured or improved. . . ." [93]

As sex research has poked deeper into the intimate corners of the bedroom, scientists have recognized that what they sorely needed was a reliable, objective method of measuring sexual arousal. In the wake of the publication of Kinsey's first volume, with its then-astounding statistics on such touchy matters as masturbation and homosexual contacts, the question most often asked was: How do you know they're telling you the truth? Kinsey had tried to anticipate this with a lengthy description of his sampling and interview techniques,[94] but when he was pressed further, his stock answer was: "We just look them straight in the eye." Subsequent work has validated so many of his findings that perhaps Kinsey did have a faculty for eliciting truth which any schoolteacher would envy, but even so the gift has not necessarily been inherited by other investigators.

In their search for a valid, measurable indicator of sexual arousal, scientists have fairly exhausted the range of bodily processes. They have tried such accessible variables as blood pressure, pulse, respiration rate, and body temperature and more sophisticated factors, such as pupil dilation, secretion of adrenaline and other hormones, inhibition of gastrointestinal activity, and galvanic skin response—the accurate measurement of sweaty palms.[95] None has proved satisfactory because while all of them did register change upon sexual arousal, similar change could be induced by other means of arousal —fear and anger, to name two—and by nonsexual stimuli, such as pain, disgust, and even surprise.

So far as men are concerned, there has been, all along, another indicator. It is not infallible because, as has been shown, sexual arousal does not necessarily produce an erection, nor are all erections the result of sexual arousal. But these exceptions are easy to recognize and account for. The difficulty was one of measuring the degree of response.

The distinction of solving the problem belongs to a Czech psychiatrist named Karl Freund, who invented the penile plethysmograph. He demonstrated this device by showing pictures of nude men and women to a test group of thirty-nine homosexual and thirty-one heterosexual males. Simply by measuring their penile response, he correctly identified every one of them. Then, using the same technique but varying the pictures, he was able to pinpoint the homosexuals' individual predilections for adults, adolescents, and children.[96]

Freund's plethysmograph worked on a volumetric principle. The flaccid penis was inserted through a flat rubber ring into a glass cylinder, which was then inflated with air and sealed off. Any subsequent increase in penile volume would affect the air pressure inside the cylinder, which in turn could be measured and recorded. The device was accurate enough to distinguish changes so slight that even the subject was not always aware of them. This qualified it ideally for its first field assignment—to spot men who tried to fake homosexuality in order to evade military service in Czechoslovakia —but still left it too bulky and obtrusive for many experiments. This objection was overcome, in 1966, by a simple strain gauge consisting of a thin silicone rubber tube filled with mercury. Once fitted around the shaft of the penis, it could electrically detect and record changes in circumference on the order of one-half millimeter —a highly sensitive measurement considering that the average increase in full erection is about twenty-five millimeters.[97]

The female counterpart—a vaginal photoplethysmograph—was not far behind. Based on Masters and Johnson's demonstration that sexual arousal in woman is accompanied by an increase in vaginal blood volume, it consists of a Plexiglas cylinder, 4.5 mm long and 1.2 mm in diameter, containing a small lamp and a photoelectric cell. The instrument is inserted into the vagina as if it were a tampon. As blood collects in the surrounding tissues, the amount of light reaching the photo cell is affected, and this in turn can be readily measured and recorded.[98]

To judge by the number of papers published in recent years, clinicians have been as happy with these new toys as any six-year-old birthday boy. They have used them for diagnosis, for monitoring change, and for determining methods of treating sexual deviation.[99] As a side effect, they have also succeeded in shaking one of man's most stoutly held beliefs. Busy as he was, Leonardo da Vinci took time to observe in one of his notebooks that the penis "has intelligence of itself, and although the will of the man desires to stimulate it, it remains obstinate and takes its own course, and moving sometimes of itself without license or thought by the man, whether he be sleeping or waking, it does what it desires; and often the man is asleep and it is awake, and many times the man is awake, and it is asleep. . . ."[100] Or, as one feminist champion, her wrath surer than her grasp of anatomy, puts it: "The penis is the only muscle man has that he cannot flex."[101]

It now appears that under certain circumstances, he can not only flex it but unflex it as well. The latter part of this proposition was demonstrated in an experiment during which four male subjects were shown "motion pictures chosen for their erotic content"—the technical euphemism for stag movies—three times in succession. Before the first presentation, subjects were instructed to do nothing to inhibit their sexual response. Before the second, they were instructed to try to avoid an erection by any means they wished except not watching the film. (To make sure that they did, they were requested to respond to brief, random flashes of light which appeared at the top and bottom of the projected image.) Then, to eliminate the possibility that the film's erotic effect had worn off with repetition, it was shown a third time, and the subjects were again instructed to avoid attempts at inhibition of response.[102]

The initial finding of the experiment was that the films had been well chosen.* During the first showing, "every subject produced a

* This is not always the case. In a long review of psychosexual testing procedures, Marvin Zuckerman comments on the routine use of *Playboy* nudes as the erotic stimulus and reports that "in more than one study, the subjects found them monotonous and tedious." And he adds: "Hugh Hefner, take note!"[103]

full erection within three minutes of the onset of the film. In three of the four subjects, almost full erection was maintained for the duration of the film." During the second showing, when they had been told to try to prevent an erection, the subjects were 86 percent successful. Results for the third showing were a duplicate of the first.

During the postexperiment discussion, all four of the subjects reported that their basic strategy, when instructed to control their erections, had been to concentrate on neutral or disagreeable thoughts—multiplication tables; bits of verse; unfinished work or school assignments. To determine whether this, in fact, had made any difference, the experiment was repeated with another group, but with an additional feature. During the inhibition showing, the men were required to give a running, verbal, blow-by-blow account of the film's action.[104] The change did not affect the results, suggesting that some mechanism other than conscious thought accounted for the inhibition.

In a subsequent experiment, still another feature was added.[105] The subjects were again instructed to suppress their erections, in this case in the face of "erotic passages extracted from popular pornography and tape-recorded by a female narrator." But this time part of the group was provided with contingent feedback: A red light was automatically triggered to go on whenever the subject experienced as much as a .5 mm increase in penile diameter. The notion behind the study was that feedback had proved instrumental in helping control other involuntary body functions such as heartbeat. It proved very successful in this instance as well. Subjects receiving the feedback were three to four times more successful in inhibiting their erections than the control group.

While the voluntary suppression of erection has theoretical interest and even some practical applications, the preponderance of market demand lies in the other direction. The next step, therefore, was to apply what had been learned to the voluntary induction of erection. For this test, there was no erotic stimulation of any kind, save what the twenty-four test subjects could conjure up for themselves. They were comfortably seated in private sound- and temperature-controlled rooms containing an orange light bulb and a white light bulb.* All of them were told that when the white light

* There was no need to observe the subjects because they could not cheat. Manual or other physical stimulation shows up on the plethysmograph's tracings in a characteristic, identifiable pattern.

went on, they would be rewarded with a bonus of twenty-five cents. One group of twelve was given the additional information that the intensity of the orange light would go up in proportion to the increase in penile volume they could achieve and that the white light would signify that they had reached the goal set for that trial. The control group was not given this explanation. Over a wide range of tests, with goals set increasingly high, the test group outperformed the control group by a ratio of approximately two to one. Obviously, feedback and reward made a big difference in performance.[106]

All these tests had used as subjects men with normal sexual function—to ask a man who cannot produce an erection to suppress it will not add to human knowledge. But once it had been demonstrated that erections can be induced by these techniques, the next logical step was to try them on men suffering from psychogenic impotence. The first study of this kind was carried out in Australia in 1976. Six patients suffering from erectile impotence, in one case for ten years and in no instance for less than six months, were subjected to both erotic stimulation and self-generated fantasies. Tests were conducted for a period of eight days. From the outset, it was found that feedback produced improvement in all but one of the subjects. More significant in terms of learning was the fact that all but one of them also showed progressive day-to-day improvement.[107]

Much still remains to be learned about how mental processes can improve sexual performance, and progress continues to be slow and uncertain. For the impatient, other methods have been proposed, written about, touted by word of mouth, and sold over the counter for thousands of years. One of the earliest, discovered on a Babylonian cuneiform tablet dating to the eighth century B.C., promised that "if a man's potency comes to an end . . . you behead a male partridge, put its blood into water, swallow its heart, and set that liquid out overnight. When the sun comes up you give it to him to drink and then he will get potency."[108]

The search for an effective aphrodisiac—one which would simultaneously promote libido, increase sexual activity, and heighten its pleasure—has been one of man's abiding quests. The Greek physician Dioscorides wrote glowingly about a plant called satyrion, which had "a double bulbous root, as big as apples and red, but within white as eggs. . . . One ought to drink it in black wine if he will be with a woman, for they say that this doth stir up courage in the conjunction." [109] Reputedly the family physician to both Cleopatra and Antony, he may have stumbled onto something because other classical writers such as Plutarch, Petronius, and Pliny all confirmed his claim.*

Unfortunately modern botanists have been unable to identify satyrion, beyond placing it in the *Orchis* genus. The loss is more academic than practical, however, because the plant's description suggests that it owed its properties largely to the workings of sympathetic magic—the belief that substances which have physical similarities will have similar effects.

One of the other plants to have its virtues thus recognized was the mandrake, or mandragora, whose knobbed, furcated root often bears a startling likeness to the human form.† The Bible mentions mandrakes twice, once in the Song of Solomon and again in the account of how Leah came to bear Jacob his fifth son.[111] Its properties as "the Root that serveth to win love" were recorded in medical texts, and its magic power has at various times been celebrated both by Machiavelli, in his *Mandragola*, and in a popular comic strip.

Similar powers were ascribed, for similar reasons, to the root of the *panax ginseng*. Although most eagerly sought after in the Orient, where it has been a staple of Chinese erotic pharmacopoeia for more than 1,000 years, the plant seems to thrive better in the climate of the New World. The Iroquois, whose name for it meant "man's thighs separated," used it sparingly, and only for such ailments as muscle cramps and menstrual disorders. By the middle of the nineteenth century, Yankee merchants were exporting more than 200 tons a year to the Far East, either unaware of or uninterested in the ineffable delights they were trading away.

The Western world's best-known aphrodisiac is prepared by heating to pulverization an insect which, despite its fame, is neither a fly nor native to Spain. *Cantharis vesicatoria* is a sparklingly shiny green beetle found throughout southern Europe, Africa, and even western Siberia. Its mode of action was described by the Italian physician Hieronimo Cardanus in 1554: "In moderate quantity,

* Pliny, who habitually embroidered stories, wrote that the mere holding of the root in the hand was enough to arouse sexual desire.

† A likeness noted by Shakespeare in *Romeo and Juliet*: "And shrieks like mandrakes torn out of the earth,/That living mortals, hearing them, run mad." [110]

it causes lust and the greatest erection of the penis; in larger quantity it excoriates the bladder and causes bloody urine." [112] Yet as late as 1896 Murrell's *Manual of Therapeutics* still claimed that "large doses of cantharides are useful in impotence, especially in the impotence of elderly men." [113]

Of the two, Cardanus was the more observant practitioner because the active chemical agent of Spanish fly, cantharidin, is now known to be a powerful irritant. When ingested, it causes acute inflammation of the urinary tract, particularly of the sensitive membranes of the urethra, accompanied by dilation and possible rupture of local blood vessels.*

The *Manual of Therapeutics*, and many subsequent textbooks of materia medica, also list as aphrodisiacs two other substances which have at least theoretical credentials for the title: nux vomica, the active ingredient of which is strychnine, and yohimbine, the alkaloid extract of the bark of a West African tree. It has been theorized that their erotic action, if any, may be due to their ability to increase the sensitivity of the parasympathetic nervous system, which is involved in the mechanism of penile erection. No direct cause and effect have ever been demonstrated, however, and both substances are known to have a number of other effects on the body, including extremely disagreeable death by poisoning. Nevertheless, an American drug company—Bentex Pharmaceutic Company of Houston, Texas—not long ago concocted an "anti-impotence" agent consisting of equal parts of nux vomica extract and yohimbine, with a little testosterone thrown in for good measure. Four glowing accounts of the effectiveness of the drug, whose trade name was Afrodex, were published between 1963 and 1967. Unfortunately the authors were obliged to concede that "the evaluation was subjective and based on the patients' and physicians' judgment as to the degree of effect produced." [114] Nothing further has been heard about Afrodex.

Not surprisingly, the sexual parts of animals were a staple in the early preparation of aphrodisiacs. Pliny recommended "the testicles of a horse, dried so they may be powdered into a drink." An Elizabethan medical text listed "a confection made of the stones of a fox,"

---

* Apparently any irritant powerful enough will do as well. "Sloan's Liniment" has all but vanished from drugstore shelves in the United States but still sells briskly in parts of West Africa. Purchasers are not seeking relief from sore muscles, however. They drink small quantities of it and claim it does wonders for their sex lives.

and the *London Dispensatory* of 1672 suggested that "cock stones nourish mightily, . . . increase seed, and help such as are weak in the sports of Venus." [115]

The popularity of such recipes had waned with the increasing sophistication of medical science, but it was given fresh impetus on June 1, 1889, by a distinguished French physiologist named Charles Brown-Séquard. During a lecture before the Société de Biologie in Paris, the seventy-two-year-old scientist described some experiments he had just performed on himself: "I removed the testicles of a very vigorous 2-3-year-old dog. After cutting the entire organ into little pieces, I put them into a mortar, adding a little water . . . then mashed the pieces to obtain as much juice as possible. . . ." [116] The audience, whose average age was only slightly less than the speaker's, listened politely as Brown-Séquard went on to describe how he injected himself with the filtrate he had produced. But they all sat up in their chairs when he went on to state, as an additional clinical observation, that after ten years of involuntary abstinence he had, that very morning, been able to *rendre visite* to the much younger Madame Brown-Séquard.

Daily newspapers as a rule did not bother covering the doings of the Société de Biologie, but in this instance *Le Matin* not only reported the gist of the lecture but even organized a Rejuvenation Institute Fund. A geriatric horde descended on Brown-Séquard's laboratories at the Collège de France. Hundreds of others too infirm to travel sent money with their pleas for an injection of the precious elixir. Foreign publications, however, remained skeptical. The *Deutsche Medizinische Wochenschrift* muttered about "senile aberrations," and the *Wiener Medizinische Wochenschrift* observed that "the lecture must be seen as further proof of the necessity of retiring professors who have attained their three score and ten years." [117]

In the end the skeptics proved to have been right. Several researchers followed Brown-Séquard's procedures to the letter, but none was able to duplicate his results. A scientist of unimpeachable integrity, he had become the happy victim of autosuggestion and the placebo effect.

Despite this setback, the pseudoscience of glandular engineering continued to flourish under the leadership of what Patrick McGrady, in his *The Youth Doctors*, called "the Erector Set." They included such competent scientists as Dr. Eugen Steinach, whose results found their way into the highly reputable *Medical Journal and Record*, and Dr. Serge Voronoff, who abandoned a brilliant career in experimental surgery to graft strips of monkey testicles into more than 2,000 male patients.* They also included charlatans such as Dr. Clayton E. Wheeler, whose mail-order "glandular extract suppositories" turned out on government examination to be desiccated hamburgers, and John Romulus "Billy" Brinkley, who in 1912 received his doctor's diploma from the Eclectic Medical University of Kansas City, Missouri, and over the next twenty-seven years managed to amass $12 million by selling the testicles of 6,000 billy goats to eternal optimists in the Bible Belt.

His marketing triumph, carried on from the safety of a radio station just across the Mexican border, prompted the American Medical Association to warn that "these frauds make their appeal to a class of individuals lacking in ordinary intelligence. Some of them appeal only to the feeble-minded or at least completely unintelligent individuals, while others, including impotence 'cures,' have a wider, but only slightly higher class of clientele." [118]

But maybe Dr. Brinkley's clients knew what they were doing, after all. In 1940 a group of scientists headed by Dr. H. T. Carmichael performed what is still the definitive investigation of the effect of testosterone on impotence. Their primary finding was that, out of eighteen men who complained of impotence and who had no obvious disease of the central nervous system, testosterone injections proved effective in seven cases and useless in the other eleven. Their secondary finding was that exactly the same results were obtained when sesame oil, their control placebo, was substituted for the testosterone without the subject's knowledge. "It was concluded," the authors write in their summary, "that the successful results were probably explained by psychological factors." [119]

Psychological factors of a different kind govern the ancient relationship of alcohol and sex. Shakespeare neatly summed up the clinical evidence in the famous knocking scene of Macbeth: "What three things does drink especially provoke?" Macduff asks the drunken porter. He replies, "Lechery, sir, it provokes, and unprovokes; it provokes the desire, but it takes away the performance." [120]

---

* Many of them world-famous and all of them rich, because Dr. Voronoff's rock-bottom fee for his operation was $5,000.

The first part of the statement can be confirmed by a visit to any college fraternity party, singles bar, or business convention. Although no proof exists, it is generally assumed that the aphrodisiacal action of alcohol consists of nothing more than a relaxation of moral inhibitions and a reduction in the level of anxiety. Until recently the second part of the statement rested on empirical evidence. With the refinement of penile strain gauge techniques, however, two separate studies have now not only demonstrated that ingestion of alcohol does in fact inhibit erection but also measured the degree of that inhibition in terms of amplitude, rate and duration.[121] * A third study, this one conducted with vaginal photoplethysmographs on sixteen college women, produced similar results.[122] Female sexual arousal, at least as measured by physical evidence, decreases under the influence of alcohol. So much for Ogden Nash.

Impelling as these findings may be in favor of abstinence, they must be tempered with the observation that the laboratory conditions under which the tests were performed, with their sterile little private cubicles, pornographic films, and careful measured-out drinks, have little relation to the real world. In fairness, some of the investigators make this point, and two of them even go further to write:

> ". . . an individual whose threshold for penile erection and/ or ejaculation has been raised by the ingestion of alcohol may consider this depressant effect to be an enhancement of sexual abilities because it increases the time available for sexual stimulation of his partner, which could well increase the probability of her being brought to orgasm. To him, the depressant effect of alcohol leads to enhancement of his abilities.[123]

The concept betrays certain male chauvinist overtones. What seems certain, however, is that despite the weight of evidence to the contrary, men with sexual aspirations will undoubtedly continue to fuel them with a few stiff drinks and coax their prospective partners to do the same.

The association of sexual pleasure with the taking of drugs extends

* Because of the number of variables involved, it is difficult to summarize these findings, but they suggest that, for acceptable performance, two hefty drinks should be the limit.

back at least to Dionysian rites and the carryings-on described by Petronius in the *Satyricon*. Indeed, much of the current preoccupation with perception-altering drugs on the part of the vast majority who have never used them is probably due to their imagined view of the rich and varied sex lives of those who do. Harry J. Anslinger, the former commissioner of the United States Bureau of Narcotics, did nothing to dampen speculation of this kind when he stated in 1969:

> "There isn't any question about marijuana being a sexual stimulant. It has been used throughout the ages for that. . . . A classical example is contained in the article 'Hashish Poisoning in England' from the London Police Journal of 1934. In this remarkable case, a young man and his girl friend planted marijuana seeds in their backyard and when the stalks matured they crushed the flowering tops and smoked one cigarette . . . and then engaged in such erotic activities that the neighbors called the police and they were taken to jail." [124] *

By contrast, the Indian Hemp Drugs Commission of 1894 reported that hemp drugs have "no aphrodisiac power whatever; and, as a matter of fact, they are used by ascetics in this country with the ostensible object of destroying sexual appetite." [125] Théophile Gautier, then an ardent young romantic, tried smoking hashish during one of his voyages and noted that "the hashish user would not lift a finger for the most beautiful maiden in Venice." [126] More recently investigators at Dr. William H. Masters's Reproductive Research Foundation in St. Louis found that chronic marijuana use —defined for purposes of the study as four days a week for a minimum of six months—was associated with decreased plasma testosterone levels in young men, a finding that was reversible when the marijuana was discontinued. [127]

Because of its relative availability, marijuana has commanded the widest interest among students of the effects of drugs on sexual activity, but other agents have received their share of attention as

---

* In the same interview, Mr. Anslinger, who ex officio was then the leading authority on drugs in the nation, also stated the view that "As to LSD . . . the principal side effect of taking it is pregnancy. . . . We should call LSD 'Let's Start Degeneracy.' "

well: hallucinogens, opiates, barbiturates, amphetamines, cocaine, amyl nitrate.* Some of their reports, under titles such as "Sex in the 'Drug Culture'" and "Drug-Sex Practice in the Haight-Ashbury, or 'The Sensuous Hippie'" provide interesting and occasionally gaudy reading, but none of them satisfactorily answers the basic question of whether drugs improve sexual performance or make sex more enjoyable.[128]

One problem is that the assertions of participants are inevitably subjective and therefore difficult to confirm. Another is that there is little or no opportunity to set up control groups or to study cumulative effects over time. Still another, and probably the most serious, was noted by Dr. Stephen Levine of the University of Kentucky Medical Center:

> Any investigator of the interaction between drugs and behavior faces the danger of confusing causes and effects. Because individuals using a specific drug engage in certain behaviors does not necessarily mean that the drug caused the behavior. Possibly individuals who engage in certain behaviors are more likely to use certain drugs.[129]

Even if the aphrodisiac action of any of these drugs could be indisputably demonstrated, there would remain the problem that they are hard to obtain, expensive, usually addictive, and frequently illegal. Recent work, however, has pointed to still another drug which has none of these disadvantages, yet seems to have the desired effect. Like many other important advances of modern medicine— X rays, sulfa drugs, antibiotics—its discovery was due not to design but to happy accident.

In 1961 scientists attempting to find a nonsurgical treatment for paralysis agitans—Parkinson's disease—began experimenting with a drug called L-dihydroxyphenylalanine, or L-dopa. Their work was

---

* Amyl nitrate, commonly known as poppers, is pharmacologically an unlikely candidate for use as an aphrodisiac. Its sole action is to cause relaxation of smooth muscle, which accounts for its former use as a rapid vasodilator for patients suffering from angina. Its unpleasant side effects—severe headaches, dizziness, and a sudden drop in blood pressure—have caused it to be replaced by newer drugs in medical practice. As a sex aid, it is inhaled just prior to orgasm, usually by the breaking of a small vial. Although used heterosexually, the drug is especially popular with male homosexuals perhaps because one of the smooth muscles it relaxes is the interior anal sphincter.

successful, to the extent that L-dopa in combination with other drugs has now become the preferred treatment for the disease. Like other powerful pharmaceuticals, the drug has side effects: nausea; vomiting; mood elevation; a change in patients' sense of taste and smell. In addition, one report notes: "A clear-cut visually evident increase in libido occurred in at least four male patients. . . . It is difficult to evaluate the presence or absence of this effect in our female patients, but we believe it is present in them as well." [130] Subsequent studies have confirmed this supposition. One reports that a female patient receiving L-dopa became so insistent in her sexual advances toward male members of the hospital staff that it became necessary to request her husband to visit her regularly. Another cites the case of an eighty-year-old man who, after L-dopa therapy, began experiencing nocturnal emissions and erotic dreams.[131]

Patients suffering from Parkinson's disease are not ideal candidates on whom to test a possible aphrodisiac. Nor was L-dopa intended to be one. The drug's effectiveness apparently was due to its ability to stimulate the production of dopamine, a neurohormone whose depletion is one of the symptoms of Parkinsonism. Dopamine in turn is related to another neurohormone, serotonin, which apparently numbers among its effects the inhibition of sexuality. In the body, the two substances act somewhat like the two teams in a tug-of-war, pulling toward opposite poles of behavior. If L-dopa can affect sexual behavior by favoring dopamine in this tug-of-war, scientists reasoned, why not make the contest even more one-sided by introducing an agent which blocks the production of serotonin altogether?

Animal tests with such an agent, p-chlorophenylalanine (PCPA), seem to bear out this logic. Castrated rats treated with PCPA will successfully fight off intact but untreated specimens for access to females; male rabbits will attempt to mount each other, as well as cats or small dogs of either sex.[132] So far only a few small-scale studies of PCPA in human males have been reported, and none in women. The findings have not been spectacular possibly because the drug's toxicity has mandated dosages one-third or less than those given to animals. But even at these levels the specific effect of PCPA on sexual behavior has been confirmed.[133] "This as yet incomplete knowledge," one medical writer notes, "suggests the likelihood that drugs can be developed which will produce sexual stimulation reliably."[134]

In the absence of such drugs, men have tried to improve on nature by means of mechanical contrivances. Many of the early efforts in this direction, like the "appliance for assisting anatomical organs" for which Horace D. Taggert was awarded United States Patent 594,815 in 1897, consisted of devices intended to apply pressure to the base of the penis and thus restrict the outflow of blood from the engorged organ. Others tried to provide simple mechanical support for a flagging penis by means of splints, tubes, sleeves, or even spiral springs. Still a third category, more gallant in inspiration, sought to improve the organ's stimulative faculties, in the manner of the *ampallang* or *guesquel.**

Although more than 100 such devices were deemed original enough to merit a patent, none of them have earned wealth or fame for their inventors. The clamplike devices were doomed to failure because, as is now known, the mere trapping of blood in an engorged penis will not alone sustain an erection. Splints and sleeves, however ingenious, are of limited means to a man who cannot produce an erection in the first place.

More recent inventions such as those described in United States Patents 3,744,486 ("Apparatus for obtaining an artificial erection") and 3,631,853 ("Genital Erector") overcome these difficulties. Both operate on the same principle as a plumber's plunger, creating "a vacuum . . . to which the penis is subjected to induce a flow of blood thereinto." The "genital erector," for instance, includes "a tube that fits over the organ and abuts the scrotum, and a hand-operated pump connected to the tube by a flexible hose which

---

* The *ampallang*, which is favored by men in Borneo, the Celebes, and Philippines, is a matchlike piece of copper, gold, or ivory some two inches long with flattened or rounded ends. It is inserted through a horizontal perforation made in the end of the penis and, by stimulating the vaginal canal during coitus, reputedly enhances the female's enjoyment of the sex act. The *guesquel*, which is used by Patagonian Indians, is composed of the stiff hairs of a mule's mane, attached to a thread and formed into the shape of a comb. Prior to intercourse, the device is wrapped around the end of the penis like a wreath, but with the hairs sticking outward. Its effect, according to one traveler, is so overwhelming that women on whom it is used "foam at the mouth and have such a paroxysmal orgasm that they lie around stupefied and exhausted after intercourse."[135]

allows the pump to be operated discreetly by the patient or an assistant." As an added convenience, "the tube that fits over the organ is transparent so that the enlargement of the organ can be observed and controlled."

Clearly, this still does not constitute everybody's cup of tea. A neater solution—indeed, one which comes close to actually improving on nature—is offered by the "penile erection system" described in United States Patent 3,954,102, issued on May 4, 1976. It consists of "a pair of expandable cylinders which are implanted in the penis, replacing the two corpora cavernosa. Supplying fluid to the expandable cylinders is a fluid transfer mechanism that is also implanted in the patient's body so as to permit inflation of the cylinders when an elasatomeric bulb is squeezed through the person's skin." The system also includes a series of valves which permit its possessor to select the desired degree of erection, to maintain it for whatever length of time he wishes, and eventually to bring it back to quiescence.

Patent 3,954,102 appears to solve the problem with remarkable discretion and efficiency. The text notes that all the components, once installed by means of relatively minor surgery, are permanently concealed from view. At the same time, they are "simple, compact, long-lasting . . . and will function without medical supervision once implanted in the body." Some complications may still occur, as the patent itself suggests when it specifies that the fluid in the system should contain a radiopaque dye because it "affords a ready means of determining where the leak occurred and also the magnitude of such leak, thereby localizing and thus minimizing the extent of surgical repair." But even with this small cloud hanging over it, the "penile erection system" seems to work well. A paper presented at the 1976 Symposium on Urodynamics of the Mayo Clinic and Mayo Foundation reported the complete satisfaction of thirty-four out of thirty-six patients who had been fitted with an implanted penile prosthesis.[136]

The ultimate device of its kind would appear to be a completely new penis, replacing one lost through accident, amputation, or congenital oversight. The earliest mention of such restoration occurs in the work of Ambroise Paré, the brilliant and innovative sixteenth-century surgeon. He writes: "Those that have their yardes cut off close to their bellies, are greatly troubled in making of urine, so that they are constrained to sit downe like women, for their ease.

I have devised this pipe or conduit, having a hole through it as big as one's finger, which may be made of wood. . . ." [137]

Paré does not give any postoperative reports on his conduit, nor does he comment on its effectiveness in performing other functions associated with the organ. The first modern successful penile reconstruction was reported by a Soviet surgeon in 1936,[138] and the technique was refined and made part of the surgical repertory by the Englishman Sir Harold Gillies in 1948.[139] In this procedure, abdominal skin is used to construct a tube within a tube, the internal one eventually to serve as the new urethra. To provide rigidity for the new organ, a cartilage graft taken from a rib is later inserted into a pocket which had previously been prepared for it.

Gillies's operation was originally intended to repair the effects of prior radical surgery for malignancy, wartime wounds, self-inflicted mutilations, and other traumatic loss or to compensate for congenital abnormalities. More recently, however, a new class of potential patients has materialized. "In the female transsexual who is attempting to become a male," a group of surgeons working in the Stanford Gender Identity Program notes, "the objective is to construct a penis and all the external male genitalia, including the scrotum with implantation of testicular prosthesis." [140] They then go on to describe the technique they developed to satisfy this objective. It is relatively simpler than that of Gillies because no attempt is made to construct a new urinary tract. The penis is structured *in situ* out of a flap of abdominal skin. The female organs are removed, except for the clitoris, which is left to serve its sexual function, and the labia majora, which are fused to create a scrotal sac. Erection is achieved by means of a special removable T-shaped device which is inserted prior to intercourse. Reporting the results of twelve operations, the authors state that ten of the patients were able to perform intercourse and nine said that they had attained "climax."

It had been known for more than a decade that ordinary and apparently uneventful sleep is punctuated by recurring periods of rapid vertical and horizontal eye movement—invisible because it occurs behind closed lids, but readily measured and recorded by an electro-ocularograph.[141] Subsequent study has also shown that other changes occur during these periods: increased and irregular pulse and respiration rates; a different pattern of brain waves; changes in galvanic sking response. Two investigators had shown that most dreams occur during the periods of rapid eye movement.[142] In 1965, Dr. Charles Fisher of Mount Sinai Hospital in New York demonstrated that these changes are also accompanied by erections. Nor were these erections quick up-and-down phenomena. Describing one of the test subjects,* Dr. Fisher notes: "Erection periods were full and sustained, the strain gauge indicating increases in circumference of approximately $2\frac{1}{2}$ cm. . . . These full erection periods were sustained for periods of 15, 17, 27 and 21 minutes, respectively, approximately the full duration of each rapid eye movement period." [143]

Fisher offers no explanation for his findings. He proposes that the erections are somehow connected with the dreams which also accompany rapid eye movement periods and notes:

> Dreaming sleep constitutes a special organismic state, a third state, in some way intermediate between the other two, namely, waking and nondreaming sleep. . . . It is a state of very markedly physiological activation, respiratory, cardiovascular, and other physiological changes approaching those of the awake organism in a state of alertness. But in the end he concedes:

"It is difficult to conceptualize what the functional or adaptive value of such extensive periods of nocturnal erection can be." [144]

Additional findings shed no new light. If anything, they compound the mystery. An obvious question was whether sexual activity just prior to sleep had any effect on the number or duration of nocturnal erections. The answer, arrived at by comparing the performances of ten men on a night following ten days of sexual abstinence and another night immediately after an evening of sex was that "sexual abstinence did not . . . increase the amount of nocturnal tumescence" [145]—or, to put it the other way, sexual activity did not inhibit nocturnal erections. Another question was whether the whole erectile cycle was somehow related to the familiar phenomenon of morning erections, which laymen and even a number of doctors had for years attributed to a distended bladder. Again, a simple test sufficed: Ten subjects were asked to void their bladders and bowels before going to sleep. Five of them

* The study included seventeen subjects, who were observed during twenty-seven nights.

were wakened two hours before their usual time, asked to urinate, and sent back to sleep. The other five were allowed to sleep undisturbed. No difference in erectile pattern could be observed in the two groups.[146]

Still another question, more difficult to answer, was whether the nature of the dreams had any effect on the erections. By waking up the subjects some five to fifteen minutes after their dreams had begun—which is to say, after periods of rapid eye movement had begun—the investigators were able to collect the dream content while they were still fresh in the subjects' minds. Then, by using standard objective checklists, they attempted to evaluate the subjects' attitude toward the dreams. After everything was measured and weighed, the conclusion was that anxiety on the part of the subject had a slight effect on erections, but that the nature of the dream itself did not.[147] *

Dr. Ismet Karacan, one of the pioneers in the field, conducted the most ambitious study yet undertaken in 1975.[148] It consisted of 125 subjects, divided into ten age-groups from three to five years old to seventy to seventy-nine years old. Each of them was monitored in the sleep laboratory for at least three consecutive nights, and the majority for seven or eight. Again, all previous results were confirmed. But the most unexpected finding of all was that even men in their seventies could consistently produce four or more erections per night, each lasting some twenty minutes or more. Indeed, the total time the subjects remained tumescent, as a proportion of their sleep period, did not decline greatly from the age of twenty onward. As a general rule, it averaged approximately one and a half hours per night, or 20 percent of the total sleeping period.

A final finding of the study, no longer startling because it had been observed earlier, was that men who suffered from impotence when awake were as capable as anyone else of producing repeated erections when asleep. This faculty has led to the only practical application yet devised for nocturnal penile tumescence—its use as a diagnostic tool to distinguish between psychogenic and organic

---

* The study also inadvertently confirmed the fact that recent sexual activity has no effect on nocturnal erections. One of the test subjects had a nocturnal emission during one of his rapid eye movement periods, then proceeded to produce an erection on schedule during the next period, approximately an hour later.

impotence. This differentiation, which heretofore had to rely ultimately on the subjective appraisal of patient and physician, can be of importance in selecting methods of therapy. Patients selected for the inflatable prosthetic devices described above, for instance, were determined to be organically impotent before being subjected to what otherwise would have been technically unnecessary surgery.

But although its significance is still unexplained, the mere observation that a nonresponsive, nonfunctioning penis seems to have independent power of its own is too tantalizing to file away as a medical curiosity. Few men, and none who have suffered the anguish of impotence, will disagree with Dr. Karacan when he proposes that "nocturnal penile tumescence is a phenomenon worthy of further investigation." [149]

We have now covered in broad strokes the extent of present-day understanding of how the penis works and the ways and means available to improve upon its performance. We have also seen that aggression and anxiety—the first caused in no small degree by the second—have a considerable role in determining the quality and nature of that performance. We will go on to look at how the interplay of these two drives has been reflected in art and literature. But first, no account of man's relations with his penis would be complete without at least a passing reference to his custom, as peculiar as it is persistent, of subjecting it to surgical alteration.

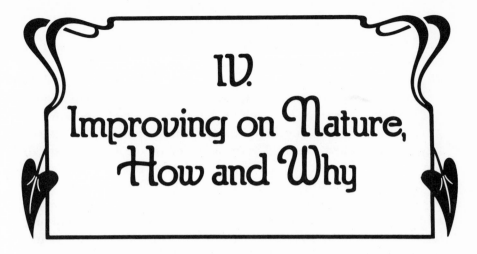

IV.
Improving on Nature, How and Why

On one of the walls of the tomb of Ankh-ma-Hor at Saqqarah, near Cairo, there is a bas-relief which shows a man kneeling in front of a young child whose hands are firmly held by an assistant standing behind him. The man holds the child's penis, foreskin extended, in his left hand and an instrument that appears to be made of stone or shaped flint in his right hand. The hieroglyphics which accompany the scene read as follows: "Hold him so that he doesn't faint." [1]

Circumcision is by far the most common surgical procedure ever devised, performed on some one-sixth of the world's population, including 80 to 90 percent of all newborn male babies in the United States. The discovery of the bas-relief in Saqqarah, which dates from the Sixth Dynasty or about 3000 B.C., also proved it to be one of the oldest. It has been found to be practiced in cultures ranging from the most primitive to the most civilized—indeed, it may be one of the few experiences which central Australian aborigines and Nobel laureates have in common.

Anthropologists speak of diffusion as the mechanism whereby the customs, practices, or beliefs of a given group may be assimilated by their neighbors. The global distribution of circumcision rules out this explanation for its prevalence. Jews, of course, practice circumcision, as do Arabs, who did so for centuries before the appearance of the Prophet. It is practiced throughout Africa, Asia, and Oceania. Some of the inhabitants of the New World encountered by Christopher Columbus were circumcised. Clearly, the practice had independent origins, and clearly, too, since it is not an action one would undertake as a whim, its performance must reflect some deeply felt human need. What this need might be is the subject of this chapter, which also considers an even more elaborate form of penile mutilation—subincision.

The Egyptians left no clue to why they practiced circumcision, but Herbert Spencer, the nineteenth-century social philosopher, provided a rationally inspired explanation: Originally the ancient Egyptians castrated captured warriors prior to consigning them to slavery. However, given their imperfect knowledge of surgery and postoperative care, this procedure resulted in a high incidence of death or disability. Circumcision was therefore devised as an alternative method which would still mark a man as a slave while preserving his ability both to work and to generate offspring, who in turn would be suitably identified as slaves.

However practical-sounding, the explanation was dealt a severe blow by the discovery of statues, and later of actual mummies, of high priests and even pharaohs who had undergone circumcision. Scholars also noted that one of the myths preserved in *The Book of the Dead* describes how the sun-god Ra mutilated himself and how the blood that fell from his penis gave rise to the gods Hu and Sia. Others pointed out that when the Greek philosopher Pythagoras visited Egypt in the fifth century B.C., he was obliged to submit to circumcision before being allowed the study in the temples. Summing up this and other evidence in an article in the *Encyclopaedia of Religion and Ethics*, George Foucart concludes that circumcision was "in the final analysis, the mark or sign of affiliation" and that it "arose in Egypt from the idea of the ceremonial purity of the people in the service of their god." As an explanation, this is still unsatisfactory because it misses the central point. Why this particular mark or sign, inflicted on this particular part of the body?[2]

The Bible is not much more helpful. The first allusion to circumcision occurs in Chapter 17 of Genesis. God appears before the ninety-nine-year-old Abram and says: ". . . I will make my covenant between me and thee. . . ." He first describes the bounty that he proposes to bestow: ". . . thou shalt be a father of many nations. . . . And I will make thee exceeding fruitful, and I will make nations of thee, and kings shall come out of thee. . . . And I will give unto thee, and to thy seed after thee, the land wherein thou art a stranger, all the land of Canaan, for an everlasting possession. . . ." Then God states the terms of the covenant: "Every man child among you shall be circumcised."

The ritual, which, as in ancient Egypt, apparently was originally performed with a sharpened flint,* was abandoned during the forty years of wandering in the wilderness. It was reinstated by Joshua at the hill of the foreskins [4] and has continued to be observed by Jews throughout the world. St. Paul, though he had been circumcised and himself had performed the rite at least once,[5] came to believe that the physical evidence of allegiance was unnecessary: ". . . circumcision is that of the heart, in the spirit, and not in the letter." [6] This, of course, is the view that was accepted by Christians.

Again, neither in describing the origin of circumcision nor in discussing its necessity does the Bible give an indication of the reasons for the practice. Philo of Alexandria, a contemporary of St. Paul's, attempted to rectify this omission by proposing not one but five reasons:

> It secures exemption from the severe and almost incurable malady of the prepuce called anthrax or carbuncle. . . . It promotes the cleanliness of the whole body. . . . It assimilates and makes those who are circumcised alike. . . . The most vital reason is its adaptation to give fertility of offspring, for we are told that it causes the semen to travel aright without being scattered or dropped into the folds of the foreskin and therefore the circumcised nations appears to be the most prolific and populous.

These four reasons, according to Philo, are all implicit in the writings of Moses. The fifth reason was the product of Philo's own Hellenistic training: Circumcision is the symbol of the excision of pleasures which bewitch the mind and thus reminds man that he "should know himself and banish from the soul the grievous malady of conceit." [7]

A study of the literature reveals that, except for one school of thought which will be considered shortly, some twenty centuries of speculation have not added materially to Philo's list. The explanation of circumcision as a hygienic measure, which was in fact proposed by Herodotus almost 500 years before Philo, appears at first to be supported by geographic evidence. Most of the primitive cultures which observed the practice lived in warm or hot climates,

---

* "Then Zipporah took a sharp stone, and cut off the foreskin of her son, and cast it at his feet. . . ." [3]

where the likelihood of discomfort or infection resulting from non-circumcision was greater. Militating against this hypothesis, however, is the fact that these same cultures in other respects demonstrated—and, where they have survived, still demonstrate—broad disregard for hygienic concepts.

Except among Jews, who perform the operation on the eighth day of the male child's life, circumcision is usually connected with puberty rites. This context led some early anthropologists to believe that it was somehow intended to prepare a youth for sexual life. Ernest Crawley, for instance, proposed that it was meant to protect against the peril inherent in sexual relations. According to Crawley, primitives feared the female genital organs and believed them capable of generating a dangerous emanation. "Its retention," he writes, "is prevented by cutting away separable parts which would easily harbor it." [8] A somewhat similar theory, proposed by several writers, is that circumcision was a form of sacrifice, a willing surrender of a small part of the penis in exchange for the safety of the rest. Sir Richard Burton, translator of the *Arabian Nights* and connoisseur of erotica, believed that Philo had got it all wrong. Far from inhibiting sexual pleasure, circumcision was intended to increase it: "Removal of the prepuce blunts the sensitiveness of the *glans penis* and protracts the act of Venus." [9]

Still, none of these or other explanations of circumcision as a form of initiation, a test of endurance, a tribal mark help us understand why it should be practiced among so many different kinds of cultures which have little or nothing else in common.

The very universality of circumcision, as well as its inescapable sexual connotations, made it impossible for the Freudians to ignore it. Freud himself first alludes to the relationship of circumcision to castration in a footnote to the celebrated case of Little Hans:

> The castration complex is the deepest unconscious root of anti-Semitism; for even in the nursery little boys hear that a Jew has something cut off his penis . . . and this gives them a right to despise Jews. And there is no stronger unconscious root for the sense of superiority over women. . . . From the standpoint of [the infantile complexes] what is common to Jews and women is their relation to the castration complex.[10]

Later Freud elaborates upon the relationship:

> Circumcision is the symbolical substitute of castration, a punishment which the primeval father dealt his sons long ago out of the fullness of his power; and whosoever accepted the symbol showed by so doing that he was ready to submit to the father's will, although it was at the cost of a painful sacrifice.[11]

But castration anxiety, which circumcision was supposed to reinforce, was difficult to account for solely in terms of patients' personal experience. Freud therefore postulates the existence of a primal horde whose effect is perpetuated by memory traces:

> When I further took into account Darwin's conjecture that men originally lived in hordes, each under the domination of a single powerful, violent and jealous male, there rose before me out of all these components the following hypothesis, or I would rather say, vision. The father of the primal horde, since he was an unlimited despot, had seized all the women for himself. . . .[12]

Later still, in what turned out to be his last writings on psychoanalysis, Freud combines these concepts:

> The possibility cannot be excluded that a phylogenetic memory trace may contribute to the extraordinarily terrifying effect of the threat—a memory trace from the prehistory of the human family, when the jealous father would actually rob his son of his genitals if the latter interfered with him in rivalry for a woman. The primeval custom of circumcision, another symbolic substitute for castration, is intelligible if it is an expression of subjection to their father's will.[13]

Presumably, at some point between the passing of the primal horde and the beginning of recorded history, outright castration yielded to circumcision, but the purpose served by the two rituals remained the same: to support the repression of incest.

   This, at any rate, has become the classical Freudian interpretation of circumcision. Three writers—Geza Roheim, Theodor Reik, and C. D. Daly[14]—studied a variety of primitive societies and came up with what was substantially support for Freud's formulation. A fourth, Herman Nunberg, used clinical evidence gathered from his own patients to propose an alternate explanation. Among the most significant manifestations of the castration complex, Nunberg pointed out, are doubts about one's own sex as well as the wish to be, and the fear of being, of the other sex. He noted that dissatisfaction with one's own sex is widespread among primitive as well as highly civilized cultures, suggesting that circumcision could well be an expression of this dissatisfaction. But the pull of orthodoxy was still so strong at the time of Nunberg's writing—1949—that he concluded his paper by restating the official doctrine of symbolic castration and molding his own findings to conform to it.[15]

Several of the Freudian hypotheses—penis envy, castration anxiety, the oedipal complex, infantile psychosexual development—have in recent years been subjected to empirical test, with varying results.[16] One of these tests sought to prove or disprove the circumcision-as-symbolic-castration explanation by examining the behavior of a group of 111 societies.[17] The investigator began by making the assumption that if circumcision is a symbolic substitute for castration, and therefore a means of reinforcing the incest taboo, the nature of the relations between son and mother should have something to do with its presence or absence:

> If the relationship between mother and son is indeed very close, the latter is likely to develop a very strong attachment to the mother, and this may increase the likelihood of circumcision. On the other hand, if this relationship is more distant, the incidence of circumcision is likely to be less frequent. In brief, the presence or absence of circumcision can be studied in terms of the intensity of the son's oedipal attachment.

To measure the degree of this attachment, another assumption was made: that it is likely to be greater in those societies where mother and son sleep in the same bed during the nursing period—in some instances for two or three years—and greater still if the father during this period sleeps in separate quarters altogether. The 111 societies were then divided according to the sleeping arrangements they practice. It was found that circumcision is twenty-two times more common in groups in which mother and son cohabit and the father is absent than in those in which all three sleep in separate beds under the same roof—results which the investigator characterized as "not incompatible" with the Freudian theory of circumcision.

Against this evidence, however, some considerations must be noted. "Natives" have been known on more than a few occasions to try to ingratiate themselves with visitors by telling them what they think they want to hear. Sometimes, too, the arbitrary classifications imposed by the investigator for statistical purposes do not properly represent what takes place and may in fact reflect the opposite. Thus, one of the societies included in the study within the group "child sleeps with mother" was Samoa. Possibly the child does spend its sleeping hours with its mother, but as Margaret Mead has written about the Samoans: "From the first months of life, when the child is handed carelessly from one woman's hands to another, the lesson is learned of not caring for one person greatly. . . ." [18] Hardly the sort of upbringing that is likely to induce heightened oedipal feelings or require the corrective measure of circumcision.

Another flaw in the study—and many others like it—is that its conclusion violates the statistical axiom that "correlation does not demonstrate causation." What is missing, as one critic puts it, is "evidence that the rites relieve the tensions or resolve the conflicts." [19]

It is possible, after all these reservations, that circumcision is still a symbolic form of castration, but one final bit of conflicting evidence must still be noted. In the United States, where very few one- or two-year-old boys sleep with their mothers, and very few fathers sleep in quarters separate from their families, circumcision is practically universal.

A final, fundamental objection to the circumcision-castration analogy is that while many of the cultures which practice the custom incorporate them into puberty ceremonies, others do not. The covenant between God and Abram specified that circumcision should be performed on the eighth day after the child's birth—a rule so explicit that it is scrupulously observed by Orthodox Jews if that eighth day falls on the Sabbath or even on the Day of Atonement. Moslems observe no designated time but normally perform the operation between the child's second and tenth birthdays. In Turkey it is generally done before the boy starts school, and some societies in Africa and Australia wait until he is sixteen or seventeen years old.

One writer, Dr. Frank Zimmerman, has proposed an explanation for the Jewish rite of circumcision which not only explains the insistence on the eighth day but also proposes a psychological explanation that has nothing to do with castration or incest taboos:

To the ancient Hebrew, as to all other groups, the events of dying and death . . . were an ever-present and stark reality. Death meant grief, terror, loss of life, decay; after death had only dark surmise and apprehension. . . . There was one alternative, one consolation, even one great hope. If a man could produce a son in his image who would be a projection of himself, so to speak, who in the image of himself would walk the earth after he is gone . . . then to some extent the finality of death could be mitigated, assuaged.[20]

To produce sons, as the Bible and subsequent writings bear out, was the supreme concern of the Hebrews and a matter of great anxiety to them. Zimmerman continues:

Within this context we come now to the importance of circumcision. . . . When an uncircumcised male has sexual intercourse, the sexual gland, in erecting, presses through the foreskin, so that before the ejaculation of semen and immediately thereafter, the penis would look as if it was circumcised, i.e. the head of the penis is disclosed and the foreskin is retracted. . . . The intent of circumcision therefore becomes clear. A circumcised penis is a copy of a penis in erection. In other words, the ancient Hebrew unconsciously thought as follows: "May the penis of this infant now circumcised be always sexually potent and fertile, and ready to fertilize as if in perpetual erection." Circumcision in essence stems therefore from deep-seated anxiety, the anxiety that one may be left without children.[21]

As for the timing of the ceremony, Zimmerman points out that according to the original Talmudic law, it was the responsibility of the father himself to perform the circumcision. The *mohel*—the professional circumciser—is a later invention.* Because the operation was—and is—painful, it is possible that fear of retaliation might have been a factor. A youth circumcised at puberty would certainly remember the operation and the man who had performed it. An infant would not. Therefore, it was desirable to perform the operation as soon after birth as possible. But the Bible also states: "If a woman have conceived seed, and born a man child: then she shall be unclean seven days"[22]—she and presumably whatever had touched

* Even today in the Orthodox ritual the *mohel* is required to turn to the father and specifically ask whether he is appointed his agent for the task.

her. Hence the choice of the eighth day. Indeed, Talmudic law specifies that it be done "early in the morning of the eighth day."

So much for Jewish circumcision. As regards the ritual among other cultures, a provocative explanation was advanced by Bruno Bettelheim in a book entitled *Symbolic Wounds*. Himself a practicing psychoanalyst, Bettelheim takes firm exception to the Master:

> No evidence has yet been presented to show that man ever lived in an organization such as the primal horde, or that such a horde was ruled by a father who was so recognized. Even if there once was such a father, we do not know his thoughts on any matter. To present these speculations as facts, simply because they originated with Freud, is not science but mythology.[23]

Rather, Bettelheim suggests, Nunberg was on the right track when he saw circumcision as an expression of man's dissatisfaction with his own sex. On the basis of his observations of a group of young patients who spontaneously devised and enacted their own "initiation rites," he notes: "As my study progressed, I became more and more impressed with a . . . psychoanalytic premise for an understanding of the deeper meanings and functions of initiation rites: the premise that *one sex feels envy in regard to the sexual organs and functions of the other*." [24] And: "But in regard to what counts most, nature *permits* each person only one sex. Hence a desire for the bodily characteristics and functions of the other leads to a psychological impasse: to become like the other sex (which is desired) implies giving up one's own sex (which is feared)." [25] One of the purposes of "rites" is to satisfy the desire to possess both male and female functions and bodily characteristics. Circumcision in particular accomplishes this in three ways: It makes men feel more male by exposing and freeing the glans; it provides them with a sign of sexual maturity and with potent blood from the genital; and it satisfies their desire to become like the other sex by giving them symbolically the capabilities of women.

In 1966, while preparing an article on the purely medical aspects of circumcision, a physician at the Kingston General Hospital in Kingston, Ontario, did something which, in the years of speculation on the subject, apparently had not occurred to anyone before. He thought to ask 100 sets of parents whose newborn children had just been circumcised why they had requested or consented to the operation.

Nineteen cited reasons of hygiene or cleanliness. Fifteen said that friends or relatives had been obliged to undergo the operation later in life, and ten pointed to uncircumcised people whom they knew to be experiencing "trouble." Seven requested it so that the child would "match" his siblings. Four assumed that the operation was performed automatically. Two believed it would prevent masturbation, and another two thought that it would eliminate the possibility of rupture. Still another two said that stories in women's magazines had recommended the operation. Other reasons cited included the belief that it was a requirement for admission to the armed forces, that it prevented excessive crying, and that "it just looks better." One interesting additional finding was that, in the vast majority of cases, it was the mother who had made the decision in favor of circumcision. "In general," the author found, "the fathers were indifferent." [26]

Whatever the reasons, circumcisions are now performed in United States hospitals on such a routine basis as to prompt one physician to warn: "Any recently delivered mother who is eccentric enough to wish her child to retain his prepuce would be well advised to maintain permanent guard over it until such time as they both leave the hospital." [27]

Hospital records do not reveal when the practice of circumcision began to gain momentum, but one of its earliest proponents was a Dr. P. C. Remondino, who in 1891 published a volume entitled *History of Circumcision from the Earliest Times to the Present.* The historical aspects, however, were merely a pretext for the author's real purpose, which was to expand upon the "moral and physical reasons for its performance." In a series of chapters entitled "The Prepuce, Syphilis and Phthisis," "The Prepuce as Outlaw," "The Prepuce, Phimosis and Cancer," "The Prepuce and Gangrene of the Penis," and "General Systemic Diseases Induced by the Prepuce," he attributes all these and much of the world's other ills to that single bit of skin:

> The prepuce seems to exercise a malign influence in the most distant and apparently unconnected manner . . . like some of the evil genii or sprites in the Arabian tales, it can reach from afar the object of its malignity, striking him down unawares in

the most unaccountable manner . . . later on beginning to affect him with all kinds of physical distortions and ailments, nocturnal pollutions, and other conditions calculated to weaken him physically, mentally and morally; to land him, perchance, in the jail, or even in a lunatic asylum.[28]

Against all this, however, there is a simple remedy which Remondino recommends with all the fervor of an insurance salesman: "Circumcision is like a substantial and well-secured life-annuity; every year of life you draw the benefit, and it has no drawbacks or after-claps. Parents cannot make a better paying investment for their little boys. . . ." [29]

Not as flamboyant but, one suspects, infinitely more influential, was the endorsement which circumcision received from Dr. Benjamin Spock in his *Common Sense Book of Baby and Child Care*, which has been the blueprint for a generation of babies.* Said Spock: "I think circumcision is a fine idea, especially if most of the boys in the neighborhood are circumcised—then a boy feels 'regular.' " [30]

One of the first medical voices raised against circumcision was that of an English pediatrician named Douglas Gairdner.[31] He reviewed the classic medical arguments in favor of circumcision—the prevention of penile cancer for the male and of cervical cancer for his sexual partner—and showed that they had little basis in fact. (Using better statistics, a later investigator evaluates the prophylactic value or circumcision as follows: "A surgeon performing one circumcision every ten minutes eight hours a day, five days a week, could be reasonably certain of preventing one penile carcinoma by working steadily for between 6 and 29 years." [32]

As for the other supposed benefits of circumcision, Gairdner has this to say:

> Moreover, if there were sensible disadvantages in being un-circumcised, one would expect that the fathers of candidates for circumcision would sometimes register their feelings in the matter. Yet in interviewing the parents of several hundred infants referred to circumcision I have met but one father who wished his son circumcised because of his own disagreeable ex-

* Commenting on the cast of the London production of *Oh! Calcutta!*, the sharp-eyed reviewer for the *Guardian* noted that "they are all American and therefore Spock-marked, or they are all Jewish."

perience of the uncircumcised state. The rest of the fathers were equally indifferent about the matter, whether they themselves had been circumcised or not.

And he adds: "Indeed, so little of the father's personal experience seems important that one quarter of the mothers did not even know whether their husbands were or were not circumcised." [33]

The purely hygienic arguments in favor of circumcision have also come up for medical evaluation. One physician writes:

> Circumcision may facilitate cleaning of the distal penis, but is operation a legitimate means of improving hygiene? To advocate newborn circumcision because small boys go camping for three weeks without ever bathing raises other possibilities of operation in lieu of soap, water and instruction in cleanliness. . . . Simple vulvectomies of newborn female infants might facilitate cleanliness and diminish the risk of vulvitis in young girls as well as carcinoma of the vulva in older women. Fingernails loom as yet another repository of filth and potential disease vector.[34]

And another notes: "The argument is also put forth that the circumcised organ is more hygienic for the prepuce collects nasty secretions. So does the ear, but the removal of this rather ugly appendage is frowned upon." [35]

In 1971 and again in 1975, the Committee on Fetus and Newborn of the American Academy of Pediatrics found that "there are no valid medical indications for circumcision in the neonatal period." [36] In 1978 an article in the *American Journal of Obstetrics and Gynecology* came to the same conclusion.[37] * In reviewing the pros and cons, the article again notes that fathers tend to be indifferent about the circumcision of their sons. The frequency with which this observation has been made has prompted one writer to hazard, possibly tongue in cheek, a final explanation for the practice: "Perhaps not least of the reasons why American mothers seem to endorse the operation with such enthusiasm is the fact that it is one way an

---

* Circumcisions are generally performed in hospitals by the mother's obstetrician rather than the infant's pediatrician. Noting this practice, the article points out: "Commenting on limitations of practice for candidates, the American Board of Obstetrics and Gynecology, Inc., warns that physicians who assume responsibility for the health of male patients for operative or other care will not be regarded as specialists in obstetrics-gynecology. . . ."

intensely matriarchal society can permanently influence the physical characteristics of its males." [38]

Advocates of routine circumcision have tended to describe it as a harmless, if not wholly benign, procedure. Complications such as hemorrhage and infection do occur, they concede, but they are statistically insignificant among the more than 1 million circumcisions performed annually in the United States.* Little has been said about the possible psychological effects of the operation on the patient. Neonatal circumcision is generally performed without anesthetic. The procedure is quick but hardly painless. As described by one physician: "Marked flushing frequently occurs during circumcision and the propensity of newborn infants to vomit under the stress of circumcision is well appreciated by nursery personnel. The alteration in pitch and intensity of cry when the first crushing clamp is applied to the foreskin is unmistakable." [39]

It has been known for some time, largely through eye movement studies, that circumcision does have a direct effect on infant behavior.[40] The exact nature and duration of this effect still need clarification, but three investigators have rather ingeniously demonstrated that it may well be more extensive and permanent than had been assumed.[41] Any number of American studies, they note, have reported gender differences in the response of newborn babies to various stimuli. While these results may indeed show that very young boys and girls are not equally well equipped to cope with their environment, they do not take account of the fact that the large majority of the male subjects—some 80 to 90 percent—had already in their brief lives undergone one rather forceful experience not shared by the female subjects. They then surveyed the results of similar tests performed in England, where circumcision is not routinely practiced, and discovered that no comparable gender differences had been found. This alone, they hasten to point out, is not proof that the act of circumcision caused the difference, but it does suggest that "circumcision requires more study in its own right." As for the duration of the effects, they again make no claim, but point to the numerous studies showing that the human brain is particularly susceptible to influences during the period of its maximum growth, from the latter part of pregnancy through the

---

* Gairdner reported that about sixteen deaths a year as a result of circumcision occurred in England and Wales, but this relatively high incidence has not been substantiated by subsequent studies, at least not in the United States.

first eighteen months of life. "We would be unwise," they note, "to assume without empirical demonstration that the circumcision effects are short-lived."

Circumcision, in one form or another, is practiced around the world, but a few groups, notably among the Australian aborigines, also ritually perform another more drastic form of penile surgery—subincision. Herbert Basedow, the first anthropologist to report on it in detail, describes it as follows: "The actual operation consists in slitting the whole or part of the penile urethra along the under side of the canal. The initial cut is in most cases from 2 cms. to 2.5 cms. long, but on subsequent occasions it is extended, bit by bit, right up to the edge of the scrotum." As for the actual method:

> The surgeon's assistant, who sits astride the novice's body on an operating table composed of the bodies of initiated men, holds the penis firmly between the fingers of both hands near its point and base. He steadies his grip by resting either his elbows against his thighs or his arms upon the novice's hips. This position secure, he draws the *corpus penis* longitudinally, with its dorsal surface downwards. . . . The operator, who stands between the initiate's legs, uses this natural line as his guide and makes his incision. . . .[42]

The traditional instrument used is a sharpened stone or flint, although the more progressive now prefer a piece of broken glass. Postoperative treatment is simple. Still according to Basedow: "Blood flows in considerable quantity and often spurts. The sufferer is immediately released and told to sit over a wooden receptacle. . . . If the bleeding persists, a handful of hot ashes is thrown over the wound."

Whites in Australia who come in contact with aborigines sometimes refer to them as whistle-cocks, but because the operation is performed on the dorsal, or under, side of the penis, its trace is not visible under ordinary circumstances. Upon erection, however, the organ balloons out to twice or more what would have been its normal width. And, of course, men who have undergone subincision and therefore have lost their urethra must urinate in the squatting position, as women do—a necessity which has loomed large in the attempts to explain the purpose and significance of the operation.

Basedow lists some of these explanations: "Some writers have advanced the theory that the operation of subincision is the outcome of lustful motives. . . . The idea, no doubt, originated through the statement one may elicit from the women to the effect that a mutilated organ gives them more enjoyment than one not so treated." But, he notes, "proof in support of this is wanting." To the contrary, there is little in the way Australian aborigine men treat their women to suggest that they have any extraordinary concern for their pleasure or well-being.* Furthermore, as a later writer notes, "the suggestion seems to be an extension of the common (but erroneous) male myth in Western communities that the larger the penis the greater the female pleasure derived." [44]

Another explanation, proposed by the anthropologist Hermann Klaatsch, was that the operation is performed for homosexual purposes—a conclusion he drew after observing a peculiar form of masturbation in which one youth made use of the incised urethra of another in the place of a female. There would seem, if homosexual pastime was the intent, to be enough naturally available orifices to preclude the need for rather violent surgical intervention. Furthermore, as Basedow observes, "One can scarcely imagine how a youth could lend himself, even passively, to an indulgence such as this without becoming himself excited; and so soon as this happens, the swelling of the *corpora cavernosa* does away with the slit or groove, and the theory collapses." [45]

Still a third explanation was that subincision is intended as a means of checking or controlling the natural increase of population—because the absence of the urethra would decrease the chances of the semen's finding its way into the inner reaches of the vagina. Dutifully Basedow set about testing this hypothesis—but not before voicing a reservation about early methods of anthropology:

> I do not mean to dispute the accuracy of early investigation, but it is a well-known fact that men of low character used to make a habit of giving quantities of rum, gin, and other spirituous liquors to the natives who would then, in a semi-intoxicated condition, be persuaded or forced to perform in a way which may have satisfied the lustful humour of the white

* One observer reported this exchange with a male Australian aborigine: "When you want to . . . . . your wife, do you ask first?" "Yes." "Does she refuse?" "No." "Does she ever refuse?" "No." "What would happen if she did?" "I'd beat her." [43]

villain, but was opposed entirely to the sense of decency and modesty of a primitive people.[46]

Without the aid of rum or gin, and presumably from the shelter of a neighboring eucalyptus tree, Basedow noted the following ethnographic data:

> When a couple is about to indulge, the female, by request or by habit, always takes her position by lying with her back upon the ground. The man squats between her legs facing her, and lifts her thighs on to his hips. Leaning forwards, he steadies his body with his knees on the ground and accommodates the parts with his hands. This accomplished, the woman grips him tightly around his flanks or buttocks with her legs, while he pulls her toward his body with his hand around her neck or shoulders.[47]

The description does not quite have the poetic lilt of contemporary sex manuals, but it is adequate to make Basedow's point: that subincision is not an effective form of population control because the semen, even if not impelled by ejaculation, can hardly fail to drip or fall by gravity into the upwardly pointed vagina.*

Having knocked down these various explanations and elicited nothing useful from the aborigines themselves—their answer was: "We do it because we have always done it"—Basedow was left with only one theory which he conceded was not overwhelmingly persuasive, that "A naked hunter, hotly pursuing his game through the bush cannot altogether avoid the risk of occasionally finding a foreign body (splinter, bur, grass seed, insect, grit, etc.) lodged in his urethra." [48] Given the state of medical care available, such accidents would lead to complications. Subincision, therefore, was a prophylactic measure.

M. F. Ashley Montagu, the very prolific author-anthropologist who had done his doctoral dissertation on Australian aborigines, approached the problem differently. The effusion of blood, he says, was the central act of subincision. Another observer has already noted this, he concedes, "but it seems never to have occurred to him that the peculiar means adopted to produce this effusion, namely

---

* In fact, even this demonstration was not absolutely required to demolish the theory. Basedow and other students of Australian aborigines were well aware that they practice two other forms of population control—abortion and infanticide—which do not require men to undergo any physical discomfort whatever.

the . . . incision of the male copulatory organ might in some way be connected with the analogous natural effusion of blood in the female from a similar source." From this, Montagu reasons, "Sub-incision in the male was originally instituted to cause the male to resemble the female with respect to the occasional effusion of blood which is naturally characteristic of the female, and possibly also with respect to producing some feminization in the appearance of the male organ." [49]

But why would men want to go to considerable trouble just to be able to simulate menstruation? Is not menstruation so unclean as to be everywhere considered as the pretext for the most stringent taboos? Precisely so, continued Montagu:

> Menstrual blood is a noxious humour of mysteriously strong potency, this much is clear. Is it not possible, therefore, that judging this to be the natural or normal or the most efficient way of getting rid of the bad 'humours' within one's body, some early aborigines, upon the principle of like producing like, essayed to produce an artificial menstruation within their own bodies, and seeing that the blood came in the female from the vulva, what more natural than make it likewise come from the organ in one's body which most closely corresponds to that organ in the female? [50]

Montagu's central insight was original, brilliant, and apparently supported by previously unexplainable behavior: Not only did aborigines submit to subincision, but they would subsequently on ritual occasions pick away at the scar in order to cause blood to flow. But the motive proposed by Montagu—a restatement of Frazer's old formula for sympathetic magic—was weak. Or so, at least, it seemed to practitioners of the Freudian school of psychoanalysis. Geza Roheim, in particular, constructed an entire psychic family edifice on the practice of subincision, complete with "phallic mothers," "vaginal fathers," [51] and children who assert: "We are not afraid of the bleeding vagina, we have it ourselves. It does not threaten the penis, it is the penis." [52] And for Bruno Bettelheim, of course, sub-incision was prime evidence of male envy for the female's role and equipment.[53]

All these explanations—Basedow's, Montagu's, Roheim's, Bettel-heim's—fail to take into account one essential characteristic of sub-incision. With very minor exceptions, which can be accounted for, it is practiced nowhere on earth except in Australia. Is it possible that something in the climate or water of that subcontinent induces in men an irresistible compulsion to slice away at each other's penis?

This possibility has yet to be investigated, but meanwhile, J. E. Cawte, a psychiatrist at the University of New South Wales, has made an interesting contribution.[54] In common with many primitive cultures, Australian aborigines possess numerous myths involving the animals around them—in their case, kangaroos and other marsupials. Cawte took the trouble to investigate some aspects of the anatomy of marsupials, and found:

> Whilst the female reproductive system has aroused great interest and is represented by scores of papers in the literature, little attention has been paid to the male. The classic account of gross anatomy is that given by Richard Owen in his article "Marsupalia" in *Todd's Cyclopaedia of Anatomy and Physiology*. . . . This author draws attention to the original observation by Cowper in 1704, that the male opossum possesses a doubled or forked glans penis. Owen's own treatise confirms that many marsupials possess a grooved penis. . . . In the koala, the glans penis terminates in two semicircular lobes and the urethra is continued by a bifurcated groove. . . . In the wombat, there is a similar expansion of the urethra into two divergent terminal grooves. . . .

As for the kangaroo, Cawte himself caught two males and satisfied himself that they conformed to the same characteristics.

Animals, as a source of food and as evidence of an alternate form of life, play important parts in primitive cultures—and the more so in rude environments, such as the Australian interior, which offer few diversions. Cawte writes:

> It seems incredible to Western observers that animals should occupy a position of influence in the child's psychic development remotely resembling that of the parents. But from the aboriginal point of view the formative influence of animals should not be underestimated. In addition to the animal's totemic significance, much of the everyday play and education of children is devoted to them. . . .

That subincision should merely be an attempt on the part of men to identify themselves more closely with their totemic animals may seem a farfetched and, to the sophisticated, simplistic explanation. But as explanations go, it has one strong factor in its favor: Except for zoos, there are very, very few kangaroos, koalas, or wombats outside Australia.

V.
The Artist's View

In the vestibule of one of the houses excavated from the ruins of Pompeii there is a remarkably well-preserved painting of a man wearing a short cloak and a rakish red Phrygian cap. His right hand holds a balance, one of whose pans is weighted with a bag of gold. With his left hand, he is delicately raising the hem of his cloak to permit his penis to protrude and rest on the balance's other pan. The whole composition is deft, stylish, and, except for the grossly exaggerated proportions of the organ which is made to be longer and thicker across than the man's forearm, joltingly lifelike.

Despite the fact that the painting is now shielded from public view by a battered green shutter, which a caretaker will cheerfully open for a surreptitious coin or two, there is nothing obscene about it. Its sole purpose was to ward off evil and invoke good fortune—which, judging by the size and opulence of their house, Aulus Vettius Conviva and Aulus Vettius Restitutus enjoyed in more than modest measure. Other phallic representations of this kind abounded in Pompeii, as they undoubtedly did in other Roman cities, in the form of statuettes, pendants, lamps, mosaics, and even the carved sign above one baker's shop which, along with the stylized form of an erect penis and testicles, bore the legend *Hic Habitat Felicitas*.

All these, as discussed earlier, are expressions of the nonsexual or pseudosexual attributes of the penis. However, by A.D. 79, when Pompeii was fixed in time, another motive for its depiction had also emerged. An example of this new context can be found elsewhere in the same House of the Vettii. Many of the building's rooms are richly decorated with frescoes portraying mythological episodes or scenes from Homeric legend, but there is also one small chamber the walls of which are covered with scenes of men and women copulating. None of the guidebooks, and very few of the scholarly works

160

about Pompeii, even mention the existence of this room, but it served a very special purpose in the household. Although very rich, the Vettii brothers were also somewhat past their vigorous prime. Apparently, they used the little room to quicken their flagging spirits before moving on to the evening's disportments.

An even better example can be found three blocks away in the house which has been identified as the *lupanar* of Victor and Africanus. Even if the peculiar arrangement of the building's hallways and small cubicles, each with its own stone bed, had not given archaeologists a strong hint, they had no trouble deducing the nature of the establishment's business from its interior decorations. Not only did the murals provide patrons with a vivid *carte du jour*, but they demonstrate that in this particular form of enterprise, man has devised few fresh ideas over the past 1,900-odd years.*

Writing about the graphic representation of explicitly erotic subjects, the art historian Otto Brendel has observed: "There is cause for surprise that the history of this theme began, as apparently was the case, so late in the universal history of the world's art. Other themes, such as the hunt, or battle, or the tending of herds, precede it by far."[1]

This chapter will deal with the erotic representation of the penis in graphic and plastic art. It will show how, like most of the cultural baggage we still carry, it originated in classical Greece and was modulated and put to commercial use by the Romans. It will consider how the moral strategists of the early Christian Church, with their odd notions about the nature and causes of sin, attempted to cope with the awkward presence of the human body, especially of its sexual parts. It will note how, after a millennium's absence, the body was allowed to emerge again with the Renaissance. It will trace the development of the erotic image at the hands of a variety of artists from Hogarth to Picasso, and, finally, it will attempt to explain why in this most sexually liberated of ages, when virtually anything can be shown, done, and described, one final taboo should still seem to prevail.

Scenes depicting sexual intercourse do occur in neolithic and Bronze Age art. However, they are usually intended to celebrate the

---

* The surly tone of some of the graffiti left by patrons also suggests that then, as now, there was often wide disparity between what was promised and what was delivered.

enactment of the *heiros gamos*, the sacred marriage which annually united the Earth Mother and Sky God to generate the summer's bounty. Frequently the artist took pains to indicate the divine nature of the participants by endowing them with their attributes or even by rendering them fully or partially in animal form. At best, these matings evoke the coming together with yet-unreckoned consequences of elemental forces. In sheer sexual impact, they display all the libidinous impulses of the men and women in James Thurber's drawings.

In contrast is a Greek red-figured cup, dated to the sixth century B.C. and now preserved in a Berlin museum. Its frieze shows ten men and seven women, all unclothed, in a variety of postures. One woman is leading a man by his erect penis; one pair is copulating standing up; one man reclines between the legs of a standing woman. He is staring at her vulva, which he has exposed by raising one of her legs, and is evidently on the point of performing cunnilingus. All the participants are young, attractive, unmistakably human, and clearly enjoying what they are doing.

Similar cups, and also vases, bowls, and dishes, repose in the collections of most of the world's major museums—if not on public display, then in curators' locked cases. The Louvre owns a cup which depicts another group encounter. A woman, nude and belly down, has stretched herself across a four-legged stool to practice fellatio on a man bending over her from the left, while another man prepares to enter her from the rear. To the right of this group, another woman has gone down on her knees to perform the same service to a man who is holding his penis with one hand and her chin with the other.

A drinking bowl, also in Berlin, shows four fashionably dressed men delicately dallying with four younger boys. One couple is embracing. Another is kissing, while one member is fondling the other's testicles with his fingertips. From the athletic equipment shown hanging in the background, it is evident that the scene is taking place in a *palaestra*, and the whole composition seems to confirm what everybody knows about the sexual habits of the ancient Greeks. But the reverse side of the same bowl shows another group of four men—possibly the same ones, judging from their clothing— but this time in the company of four elegant young ladies.

Still another orgiastic scene shows a group of Satyrs gifted with prodigious erections, which they are, all but one of them, in the process of inserting into the various orifices of a tangled mound of maidens. The last lonesome fellow, excluded by the others or pursuing his own design, has his back turned to the company and, penis ready in hand, is sneaking up behind the figure of a crouching Sphinx.

Such erotic scenes are so frequent on Greek pottery, and the artists have taken such care in developing their themes that art historians have been able to trace a line of stylistic development and even to hazard interpretations regarding motivation. The earliest examples center on the doings of Satyrs and Sileni who, as their hooves and tails indicate, are not yet completely detached from their animal antecedents. They were associated with the person of the wine god, Dionysus, who presided over all manner of revels, but the device of using them to comment on sexual practices provided the artist with opportunity for satire, ridicule, and caricature much in the same spirit which moves us to characterize a lusty lover as a young buck and, later in his life, as an old goat.

The nature of the objects chosen for decoration is significant. Painted vases, bowls, and other vessels were among the comparatively few objects of Greek art that were turned out primarily for private use. Many of them have been ascribed to painters and workshops of high reputation. Clearly, they were articles made for affluent connoisseurs, and possibly intended as gifts, if not for wives, then for the *hetaerae* toward whom classical Greek social and intellectual life gravitated.

The fact that the setting of many of the scenes is social—banquets, parties—and the further fact that many of the objects themselves were expressly used for drinking are also significant. An art historian has noted: "Apparently, in the Bacchic religion traces of an early cult of vegetative growth were combined with a deliberate emphasis on enthusiastic psychic conditioning." [2] A psychic conditioning not much different, one would guess, from the kind that takes place nightly in contemporary singles bars.

Within the limitations of their medium and subject matter, the artists achieved an astonishing range of expression. A small, elegant black and red jug shows a pretty and very young couple, naked and about to make love. He is sitting on a low chair; she is facing him, her arms around his neck preparatory to sitting down on his erect penis; she has leaned forward so that their foreheads touch and their gazes meet in a look of melting bliss. Another scene, this one drawn on the bottom of a two-handled cup, shows a pretty young woman, half lying and half kneeling on a bed, face downward. Her right hand is stretched out and reaching behind her toward the flaccid penis of her partner, who is kneeling between her legs. His beard, and the embarrassed expression on his wrinkled face, complete the telling of the story. Still another scene, one of many of its kind, shows a solitary but smiling young woman holding an enormous dildo in one hand and an even larger one in the other.

There is in all this art a total lack of the prurience or of the sniggling which characterizes much of pornography, and certainly none of its sadomasochistic resonances. Sexual activity, in all its variety of postures and participants, was a theme at least as important to classical Greeks as the hunt, the battle, or the tending of flocks. Penises and vulvas were the bodily parts principally involved in this activity, and the artists represented them with no more self-consciousness than they accorded to the flexed right arm of a discus thrower or the straining limbs of a Laocoon.

Being themselves fascinated by the broad possibilities of sex, the Greeks not surprisingly ascribed the same interest to their gods. Bulfinch's *The Age of Fables* records more love affairs, seductions, abductions, and *ménages à trois* than a year's worth of gossip columns: Apollo and Daphne, Artemis and Actaeon, Pluto and Persephone, Orpheus and Eurydice, Psyche and Eros, Apollo and Hyacinth, Echo and Narcissus. In particular, the incessant philanderings of Zeus with assorted nymphs and mortals, and his heroic efforts to circumvent his wife's suspicious eye, stirred the imagination of Greek mythmakers. Time and again, he is represented in the guise of a serpent, a bull, or even a shower of gold, as he woos and wins his Ios, Europas, Danaës, and Pasiphaës. But it is in the form of a swan, and in pursuit of Leda, the wife of King Tyndareus of Sparta, that he appears most frequently.

By the third century B.C. profound changes had taken place in Greek society and been reflected in even the minor forms of artistic expression. Gone were the highly detailed, amusing scenes of the earlier pottery, to be replaced by crude depictions of copulating couples. The vehicle for the art had changed, too. Typically, it was now the terra-cotta oil lamp, a simple everyday utensil which was mass-produced in molds and exported to every corner of the Hellenistic world. Erotic art had gone wholesale.

Looking at examples of both, one sees immediately the great difference. The act portrayed and the positions of the participants are essentially the same—human anatomy accounts for that—but there is in the one a lyrical and celebratory quality, as well as a sense of personal comment, which is totally lacking in the other.

This same celebratory quality is largely absent from Roman depictions of sexual scenes. Otto Brendel notes:

> The traditional Roman sense of gravity was apt to frown on any manner of frivolousness, for either of two rather opposite reasons: because it was held to be an expression of aristocratic luxury, always suspect in ancient Rome, or because it was regarded as an entertainment tolerable, to an extent, among the lower classes but unbecoming to a person of rank and responsibility.[3]

Romans did make an important and lasting contribution to the tradition of erotic art—a contribution entirely in keeping with their reputation as master organizers and entrepreneurs. Its principal evidence consists of the vast quantities of Arretine pottery which archaeologists are still turning up in every corner of the Roman world. So called because it was first manufactured in the town of Arezzo, this red-glazed clay pottery is distinguished by its decorations of delicately molded reliefs. Various activities are portrayed in these decorations, but one recurring motif consists of erotic scenes. Each presents a single nude couple, invariably a man and a woman. Their facial features, although finely drawn, are stylized and unchanging. Except for a bit of drapery or the suggestion of a bed or couch, the characters appear to be in limbo, with no suggestion of context. The lines of the composition are fluid and frequently elegant, but as uncluttered and expository in intent as those of a mechanical drawing.

Individual pieces of Arretine pottery were, of course, untitled. But anyone studying them, or cataloguing them for a museum, is almost irresistibly tempted to label them "woman on her knees, male partner kneeling behind her," or "male partner on his back, female kneels in opposite direction, with double oral-genital contact." It is impossible to say for certain what the purpose of this pottery was. Much of it, however, consisted of bowls which served as drinking vessels. One can therefore imagine a collection of them, set out side by side on shelves like an illustrated manual or catalogue.

However passionate his interest in logic and the classification of things, no Athenian would have approached the pleasures of love with such mechanical determination. It is, however, entirely in keeping with the compulsive mentality of a civilization which built not only magnificent roads but built them arrow-straight, with no concession to terrain.

Assessing the consequences of Christianity's attempts, during its first millennium, to regulate the sexual behavior of its flocks, G. Rattray Taylor concludes in his *Sex in History*: "It is hardly too much to say that medieval Europe came to resemble a vast insane asylum." [4]

Ironically, there had been nothing in the early documents to presage this later preoccupation with sex. Neither the Old Testament nor the Gospels ascribed any special importance to chastity, and certainly none to sexual abstinence. Rather, their attitudes reflected the values one would expect to find in a patriarchal society. Chastity was important only to the extent that its absence reduced the property rights of husbands and fathers. Sexual license was seen essentially as a threat to the social order. Indeed, the words "fornication," "lust," and "whoredom" were used indiscriminately to describe any and all sins against God.*

The first intimation that there was more to sex than just a diverting pastime came with Paul's teachings regarding the dualism of body and spirit. "So then with the mind I myself serve the law of God; but with the flesh the law of sin,"[5] and ". . . the flesh lusteth against the Spirit and the Spirit against the flesh: and these are contrary the one to the other."[6] Obviously, such identification of the flesh with sin carried certain implications. Still, Paul recognized human frailty. The well-known passage which begins "It is good for a man not to touch a woman" goes on to observe: "But every man hath his proper gift of God, one after this manner, and another after that" and ends up conceding: "But if they cannot contain, let them marry: for it is better to marry than to burn."[7]†

---

* That sexual license was associated, at least in the minds of the Disciples, with other blandishments of competing religions is evident in Acts 15:20: "But that we write unto them, that they abstain from pollutions of idols, and from fornication, and from things strangled, and from blood."

† Moreover, a number of biblical scholars believe that Paul's precepts on marriage were local and temporary, relating only to the special circumstances of the Corinthians to whom they were addressed and who, for centuries, had borne the reputation of being unusually dissolute in their ways.[8]

Unfortunately the notion of dualism was not unique to Christianity. Faced with active rivals for Roman converts and not yet powerful enough to impose its brand of belief on others, the Church intensified the pitch of its message. As Geoffrey May notes:

> It could expand only by demonstrating in competition its claim to a higher sanctity and virtue. To effect this end, the Church came to phrase its doctrine more and more in the terms of dualism. In the process it came increasingly to accept the idea that mortification of the body constituted a triumph of the soul over the evil principle.[9]

Appropriately, the saints of this religion were chosen from among those men and women who showed the greatest perseverance, to say nothing of ingenuity, in inflicting harm upon themselves: Macarius, who went naked in a mosquito-ridden swamp and let himself be stung until unrecognizable; Ammonius, who tortured his body until he was entirely covered with burns; Simeon Stylites, who not only spent thirty years atop a pillar but used the time to ulcerate his flesh into maggot-infested putrefaction with an iron belt; Evagrius Ponticus, who spent winter nights in a fountain until his flesh froze.[10] If sex was the ultimate evil, the absence of sex was the ultimate good. Thus, Saint Ursula, with her 11,000 fellow virgins, chose death at the hands of the Huns rather than lose her chastity, and Saint Gorgonia, with "all her bodie and members thereof . . . broken and bruised most grievouslie," refused the help of a physician because she did not want to be seen or touched by a man.[11]

But the most characteristic aspect of the Church's attitude toward sex—and the aspect which pervaded much of the art it sponsored—was its reduction of the procreative act to the interplay of forbidden orifices and musty secretions. The early fathers devoted endless volumes to examinations of the question, but Saint Augustine summed it up in a single sentence: *Inter faeces et urinam nascimur.*

In Augustine's view, the Fall was the pivotal event in man's, and woman's, sorry history on earth. Their original sin, born of lust, was inexorably transmitted from generation to generation by sexual intercourse, which itself became the greatest of sins. The story served as the subject for countless representations. But despite the context of the scene, artists were not permitted to portray Adam and Eve as anything more than flat, stylized, and sexless creatures. All their imagination was therefore lavished on the third party to the guilty transaction, the serpent. In one instance, in the cathedral at Rheims, he is shown responding to Eve's caress in what can only be described as the act of tumescence. More often there are sadistic overtones to his presence. A twelfth-century relief in Moissac depicts a naked Eve with two snakes coiled about her, each reaching up to fasten its mouth around a breast. Another Eve, on the porch of the Abbey of Charlieu, is shown lying on her back as the serpent is in the process of devouring her vulva. Still another shows a naked woman looking down at her vulva from which the head and body of the serpent is emerging. The Freudian symbolism of all this herpetology is obvious, but if more evidence is needed, one has only to look at one of the marble panels which Jacopo della Quercia created for the main portal of the Church of San Petronio in Bologna. Here, Eve is again shown caressing the serpent with one hand while beckoning him with the other. To the right, Adam is looking at the scene with envious resignation as, with the fingers of his left hand, he measures his penis.

Christian art, like that of other authoritarian systems to come, was didactic. Its noblest monuments were not only tributes to God but, during an age of near-total illiteracy, elaborately illustrated object lessons in stone, stained glass, and carved wood. For the most part, they retell scriptural stories, illustrate parables, or recall events in the lives and martyrdom of the saints. Sometimes, however, their meaning is ambiguous. A twelfth-century relief at the Church of Sainte-Croix in Bordeaux shows a devil fondling a woman's breast; another, at the Chartreuse du Val de Bénédiction in Villeneuve-lès-Avignon, shows a woman copulating with a goat. A frieze on the façade of the cathedral in Fidenza contains a couple engaged in sexual preliminaries; one of his hands clutches her shoulder while the other, inserted in a slit at the side of her skirt, gropes for the cleft of her legs. Sin, judging by their smiling expressions, is not uppermost in their minds. Indeed, in all these depictions, it is hard to distinguish between moral indignation and sexual fantasy.

Frequently sexual expression took anal or scatological form. One of the bosses in the cloister of Norwich Cathedral consists of a bearded little man in the process of defecating. The cathedral at Freiburg im Breisgau and the Church of Saint-Lo in Rouen are decorated with gargoyles in human form which drain water through their anuses, penises, and vaginas. Even on the south portal of Notre

Dame in Paris, beneath the exquisite rose window, sharp-eyed visitors will be able to distinguish two female figures sticking their naked backsides out at the world.

Some examples of medieval ecclesiastic erotica defy explanation —save perhaps for wily artfulness on the part of the anonymous craftsmen who created them. Thus, the doorway of the Church of Saint-Martin in L'Isle-Adam is decorated with a carving which explicitly shows a man performing cunnilingus with his head between the thighs of a standing naked woman. One of the misericords in the Church of Saint-Materne, in the Belgian town of Walcourt, shows a woman leading a man by a rope which has been tied around his penis. Another depicts a man holding his erection in his hand and chasing after a woman who is about to extinguish it with the contents of a pitcher of water. In the great cathedral of Toledo, scenes carved into several of the capitals attest to the fact that sexual intercourse in the *seicento-nove* position was not only known but enthusiastically practiced in the thirteenth century.*

Also unexplained after nearly nine centuries is an erotic scene which appears, of all places, on the Bayeux Tapestry. It consists of a couple, the male of which is sporting a massive erection, facing each other and crouching like wrestlers. It has been suggested that the scene alludes to the violence which war brings in its wake or that it recalls the plight of the combatants, obliged to leave their grieving women. Save for the martial theme of the tapestry itself, which relates the story of William of Normandy's successful foray across the Channel, there is nothing to give credence to either interpretation.[12]

All these touches and details were the anonymous, idiosyncratic expressions of an attitude toward sex in general and the sexual act in particular. At the hands of a man of genius, this attitude inspired one of the most extraordinary works of art ever achieved: Bosch's "Garden of Earthly Delights." Hieronymus van Aeken was born around 1450 into a family of painters and craftsmen which had for several generations been established in the prosperous Flemish town of Hertogenbosch. As an artist he was prolific and highly regarded during his own lifetime, possibly because of the fantastic wealth of

---

* Although undiscovered, or at least undocumented, examples of this kind undoubtedly still remain, a heroic attempt to catalogue hundreds of them was made by G.-J. Witkowski and published in two books: *L'Art Profane à l'Église* (Paris: 1908) and *Les Licenses de l'Art Chrétien* (Paris: 1920).

detail and the distinctive medieval inspiration of his work. The "Garden of Earthly Delights" is a large triptych—seven feet high and nearly thirteen feet wide when opened—which was commissioned by a wealthy patron in Brussels. Its fame quickly reached Philip II of Spain, however, and he acquired it for his personal collection.*

The theme of the work is, again, the fall of man. The left-hand panel represents Eden, where God is presenting a newly created Eve to Adam. This is not the traditional bearded God the Father, however, but God the Son, and although His posture and gesture are those of blessing, there is a troubled look of warning on His face. One can guess why, too. Eve's eyes are modestly downcast, and her long blond hair is chastely combed, but there is strong erotic appeal to her high, neat applelike breasts, and even more so to the forward thrust of her pelvis and rounded little belly. The expression of the naked Adam, at once astonished and eager, leaves little doubt about what is on his mind. There are other details which suggest that all is not well in this paradise. Instead of lying peaceably together, a lion is shown devouring a deer. A cat is striding along carrying a mouse in its jaws. Bizarre animals with mismatched heads and limbs are crawling out of a dark pool in the foreground. The Fountain of Life is adorned with a crescent, a sign of unbelief and heresy.

The central panel depicts the terrestrial garden: a large parklike landscape teeming with nude men and women, who nibble at giant fruit, consort with animals and birds, frolic in pools and streams, and, above all, indulge in every variety of amorous sport, overtly and with unalloyed bliss. In the words of one critic, "Bosch's garden appears to be a sort of universal love-in." [13]

Another writer, expert in older Dutch literature, has pointed out that many of the forms in the scene are erotic symbols inspired by the popular songs, sayings, and slang expressions of Bosch's time.[14] For example, many of the fruits being eaten or proffered to each other by the lovers are metaphors for the sexual organs—the phrase "to pluck fruit" was itself a euphemism for the sexual act. Organisms such as oysters, mussels, and giant clams are suggestive, in their moist and secretive nature, of the bridal chamber. The egg, which occurs repeatedly, symbolizes the crucible of sexual union.

The fact that Bosch chose a great park for his setting is in itself significant because parks and gardens had for centuries served as the

---

* It is now in the Prado, in Madrid.

setting for lovers and lovemaking. The time of day is significant, too. In the first panel, the light has the crisp, dewy coolness of early morning. Here, it is lazy, sun-warmed afternoon, when bare bodies that touch are pliant and tend almost to stick together.

The center of the composition is occupied by a circular pool in which a dozen nude women are disporting themselves and making beckoning gestures toward a procession of men riding bareback around them. The antics of the riders, one performing a somersault on the back of his mount, suggest that they are excited by the presence of the women, one of whom is shown already climbing out of the water. Chivalry notwithstanding, the notion that it was woman who led man into sin and lechery, following the example of Eve, was common belief among medieval moralists. The act of riding an animal, and especially of riding it naked and bareback, is employed by Bosch, as it still is, as a metaphor for the sexual act.

As in other Bosch paintings, there are hundreds of individual scenes and vignettes which, once they are picked out of the mass, arrest the eye. A youth is bending over a reclining maiden while another youth is inserting a flower in his rectum. A couple which has crawled into a giant shellfish is being swallowed whole; the position of their protruding feet indicates that this imminent fate has not interrupted their activity. Other couples, and groups of three and four, are engaged in various states of preliminary play. One man, not yet mated, is standing on his head in a stream of water and protecting his exposed genitals from the long beaks of two colorful birds.

Elsewhere in his work one of the most imaginative of portraitists, Bosch has given the more than 100 human figures in the garden no individual characteristics. They all have the same face and body; not even their ages vary. This surrender to sexual desire has reduced them to a common denominator. It has also, according to the right-hand panel, condemned them to common punishment in a particularly fiendish hell. There are no devils or imps with pitchforks here. Rather, innocuous everyday objects, swollen to monstrous proportions, serve as instruments of torture. In a nightmarish trio, one nude figure is attached to the neck of a lute, while another is helplessly entangled in the strings of a harp, and a third has been stuffed down the neck of a great horn. On the lake, now frozen, a man fastened to an oversized skate is about to fall through a hole in the ice, where another man is drowning. Phallic symbols, such as knives and keys, have come to life in order to grind and mangle writhing sinners. A bird-headed monster seated on a toilet chair is gobbling up damned souls and defecating them into a transparent chamber pot. Bosch's hell is the final full-dress evocation of the anal-scatological vista enunciated by Saint Augustine.[15]

"The Renaissance era brought mankind one revelation in the true sense of the word: the revelation of the human body. For the first time in a thousand years, men saw themselves as nature had created them. They made this discovery not in the mirror but through old broken marble statues dug out of the earth." [16] So writes Richard Lewinsohn in *A History of Sexual Customs*, and he goes on to describe how one of the most celebrated male statues of antiquity was found buried in the gardens of a villa in the Roman hills. "Cardinal Giuliano della Rovere, the later Pope Julian II, on whose estate the statue had been found, was liberal and artistically minded enough to take the young god into his house, and afterward to give him a place of honour in the Pavillion de Belvedere in the Vatican, after which the statue has since been called."

It's a neat story even if not quite true. The "Apollo Belvedere" does occupy a place of honor in the Vatican, and in most art history textbooks, even though one of Julius II's less liberal successors saw fit to provide it with a strategically placed fig leaf. But Renaissance artists had not needed classical models to remind them of what a human body looked like. Donatello cast his bronze "David" around 1430, a half century before the discovery of the "Apollo." Now in the Bargello in Florence, the statue shows the future Hebrew king as an adolescent of twelve or thirteen. Clothed only in richly ornamented leather boots and a large hat crowned with laurel, he stands with his left hand on his hip and a great sword in his right. His right foot rests upon a wreath, while his left foot toys idly with the severed head of Goliath, one long wing of whose helmet caresses the inside of the boy's right thigh. The pose, and the boy itself, are so startling in their combination of sinewy angularity and feminine softness that Vasari, the archgossip and talebearer of his time, hinted that the figure had been cast from a living model.

The rediscovery of classical antiquity was one of the manifestations of a new spirit of inquiry regarding the world and man's place in it. Central to it, and to the Renaissance itself, was the exhilarating realization that, in the phrase of Jacob Burckhardt, "all the things of this world became possible." [17] In the arts, perhaps the most

startling effect of this new spirit was that painters and sculptors began to use their eyes again. In Venice, Giorgione looked at a beautiful woman and painted what he saw: a reclining nude, perfectly
proportioned and bathed in the golden light of a warm Italian
afternoon, one hand supporting her head and the other modestly—
or invitingly—curled over her mons veneris.

Still, Giorgione's "Dresden Venus" observed certain conventions.
She is shown against a highly idealized landscape and is therefore to
be enjoyed as "woman-as-nature," and not yet "woman-as-woman."
She also has her eyes closed, effectively dissociating her from com-
plicity in whatever erotic thoughts are evoked in the viewer. Both
these niceties were swept away by Titian. The pose of his "Urbino
Venus" is so similar that it is hard to imagine he was unaware of the
earlier painting. But here the woman's eyes are not only open but
looking directly out at the viewer with whatever feeling—invitation,
affection, desire, gentle challenge—one wishes to read into them. And
rather than recline in a *paysage*, she is in bed—precisely, as Lord
Clark observes, where you would expect her to be.*

Medieval teaching had single-mindedly equated sexual expression
with mortal sin. To Renaissance artists, it became the context for
exploring the full range of human relationships. Thus, Francesco del
Cossa executed a cycle of twelve frescoes for the Palazzo Schifanoia
in Ferrara, representing activities appropriate to the months of the
year. April, which is dedicated to the goddess Venus, shows a group
of young men and women in a garden. Apparently they have been
playing music together because some of them are still holding lutes
and recorders, but now their minds are turning to other pastimes.
One couple is embracing, and a young man has his hands draped
over the shoulders of two young ladies. In the foreground three
others are smiling approvingly as still another young man, bolder
than the rest, reaches with one hand for the breast of his companion

---

* Titian's "Urbino Venus" was in turn the obvious inspiration for the most
famous nude of the nineteenth century, Edouard Manet's "Olympia." Save for
the fact that Manet gave her a pair of slippers while Titian left her barefoot,
the model is shown in almost the identical pose, down to the bracelet on her
right arm. The arrangements of pillows, bedclothes, and draperies are the same,
as is the presence of a servant in the background and of a small pet at the model's
feet—a lapdog in Titian's painting and a black cat in Manet's. Yet by 1865
Titian's work had achieved the eminence of a masterpiece while Manet's, which
was exhibited at the Salon in Paris, provoked such indignation that it had to be
protected from irate visitors by means of a rail and two guards.

while the fingers of his other hand have found their way underneath her skirt. Standing naked and unashamed on a rock overlooking the scene, the three Graces leave little doubt about what is about to start taking place. Only one figure does not share in the easy and completely natural spirit of the moment. Kneeling in the foreground, she is intent on the beads which she is telling.

Occasionally, as in Botticelli's "Primavera," the erotic theme is expressed symbolically.[18] More often it is explicit, but dressed in biblical guise. The stories of Lot and his daughters, Susannah and the Elders, Joseph and Potiphar's wife, Judith and Holofernes—all served time and time again as a springboard for the representation of men and women caught in the grip of sexual drives. The Virgin, which had been a sexless, somewhat forbidding abstraction, became a living, feeling woman. Parmigianino painted her with breasts lightly covered by a filmy garment as she caresses a well-developed and nearly adolescent boy. To Fra Lippo Lippi, she was a blossoming young Italian girl, the real-life prototypes of which he could not, despite his vows, resist.* In his Roman "Pietà," Michelangelo made use of the centuries-old mystical abstraction of the Virgin as the bride of Christ. There is, however, nothing abstract and very little filial about either the composition's two figures or their juxtaposition. The fact that the mother is impossibly youthful for the son was pointed out by a contemporary and elicited the explanation it deserved: "Are you not aware that chaste women maintain themselves much more fresh than the unchaste? How much more so a virgin in whom there has never arisen the least lascivious desire that might have affected her body?" But so masterful is the work that it is still difficult to accept at face value what Michelangelo has set before our eyes: "a smooth marble group which, under cover of a devotional theme, displays an exceptionally beautiful naked youth in the lap of a girl."[19]

The figure of the other Mary, all the more exciting for her past, exercised a special fascination. As some men still do when in the presence of a woman they know to have been a prostitute, artists projected their own erotic feelings and fantasies onto her. Furini portrayed her as a full-length frontal nude in a state of high excite-

* Such was his skill as a painter that the Pope granted him special dispensation from celibacy, a privilege which he enjoyed to the extent of fathering a reputed eleven children.

ment. Titian showed her clutching long silken tresses which fall to her waist but still manage to expose both of her breasts.* In a painting by Sirani, she is holding a whip to her naked body, a nonscriptural note which was purely the invention of the artist. Most often, it is the crucifix which is used to recall her own cry: "Oh, most blessed Cross! Would that I had been in Thy stead, and that my Lord had been crucified in mine arms." [20] It was not until Rodin's "La Madeleine," in which a naked, despairing woman is shown pressing herself passionately against Christ's crucified body, that an artist dared give literal expression to the wish, but Renaissance painters such as Annibale Carracci made it clear that the crucifix could serve as an object of erotic fantasy. In one "Crucifixion" by Isenbrandt, Mary Magdalene is made to kneel in such a way that her thighs straddle the cross, while her hands caress it.

Still, for all the freedom they were permitted—or permitted themselves—there was a line which Renaissance artists were not supposed to cross. Leonardo da Vinci had made several drawings of men and women copulating, but they were anatomical sections more concerned with the mechanics of bodily organs than with any expression of passion. Raphael had come close, and the assorted Ledas and Ios and Olympias left little to the imagination, but no one had dared show a man and a woman in the simple, straightforward act of fucking.

It was finally done in 1524, and the eminence of the perpetrators, as well as the high artistic order of their achievement, caused the episode to become one of the great artistic scandals of the century.

It was again Vasari who piously reported the episode:

> After these things Giulio Romano had engraved by Marcantonio in how many diverse modes, attitudes and postures dishonest men lie with women; and, what was worse, for each mode Messer Pietro Aretino made a most dishonest sonnet; so that I do not know which was the more ugly, the spectacle of the designs of Giuliano to the eyes or the words of Aretino to

---

* It may have been this painting which inspired the anonymous limerick:

When Titian was mixing rose madder
His model posed nude up a ladder.
Her position to Titian
Suggested coition,
So he nipped up the ladder and had her.

the ears; which work was much blamed by Pope Clement . . . and because many of these designs were found in places where one would least think, they were not only prohibited, but Marcantonio was taken and put in prison. . . .[21]

Pietro Aretino once sat for a magnificent Titian portrait: an impressive broad-shouldered giant of a man clad in doublet and cloak, with a broad forehead, flowing beard, and uncompromisingly penetrating eyes. But he was also "an obvious blackguard, a blackmailer, a pornographer, a sycophant, malicious and ass-licking in equal proportions, a megalomaniac, a lunatic with nothing but a good prose style to commend him.[22] He used that style to turn out a torrent of pamphlets on every political, social, and artistic subject, as well as numerous biographies of saints, penitential psalms, and some of the most perceptive, amusing, and unredeemably obscene pornography ever composed. For his services, he was knighted by Pope Julius III and nearly made a cardinal. He enjoyed the esteem of Henry VIII, Francis I of France, and Charles V, the Holy Roman Emperor, who employed him as a personal diplomatic agent. In his youth, he was almost killed in a street brawl by a man whose mistress he had described too accurately. He spent much of his life in Venice, then the most liberal-minded city in Europe, and used the literary device of imaginary conversations between some whores to produce his best remembered work, the *Ragionamenti*. He died at sixty-five, as a result of a fit of laughter provoked by an obscene joke about one of his sisters.

Marcantonio Raimondi was, in an age of superb craftsmen, the most accomplished of engravers. Travel was difficult during the Renaissance, and public access to works of art limited. It was thus through the engravings of Marcantonio and his students that artists in Germany, England, Scotland, Poland, Sweden, and even Russia became aware not only of the ferment which had gripped Italy but also of the great rediscovered treasures of antiquity.

The third member of the trio, Giulio Pippi, was born in Rome— hence his name Giulio Romano—and at an early age became one of Raphael's apprentices. In quick succession he became his master's star pupil, surrogate son, and unacknowledged collaborator. The closeness between the two is suggested by the fact that Raphael, on his death, charged Romano with the completion of all his unfinished works and that the younger man named his only son Raffaello. In his own day, Romano's fame reached the ears of Shakespeare, who mentions him by name in *The Winter's Tale*. As for his work, Renaissance scholars recognize it in the Vatican and Farnesina murals "where the Olympian lucidity and grave balance of Raphael is gathered into a flash of theater, into a nuder nude, into a humanity that seems to leap out into your arms like a child jumping off the top step." [23]

It is not clear which of the three men conceived the idea for the project. According to one version, Romano had sketched a series of copulating couples on the unfinished walls of one of the Vatican *stanze*, either as a practical joke or for the amusement of Clement VII, who as a Medici could have been expected to appreciate them. Aretino heard about the episode and proposed the collaboration. Whatever their source, the "Modi" consisted of sixteen—or twenty, according to some authors—scenes each of which represented a man and a woman on the point of, during, or immediately after making love. They are indoors, quite naked, and usually on a bed or couch. Like others of Giulio Romano's figures, they seem imbued with high spirits and great energy—the very qualities which may have prompted Frederick Hartt, Romano's most authoritative biographer, to dismiss the series as placing "special emphasis on abnormal and spectacular attitudes, on acute physical strain and on frustration." [24]

One is tempted to reply, as in the joke about the scandalized village priest, "But what does he know about fancy fucking?" A few of the positions are, in fact, somewhat on the strenuous side for everyday use—notably number 10, in which the standing man has placed himself between the woman's thighs and has raised her up from a prone position by hoisting her onto his forearms. Several are immediately and powerfully erotic. In number 5 the woman, whose back is to the viewer, stands with legs well apart, one hand stretched between them to grasp the man's penis and plant it into her vagina, the other grasping his hair to keep her balance, while the man, supported on his hands, is poised to begin thrusting with all the strength of his body as soon as he is inside her. Number 15 is probably the most effective of all. It depicts the conventional missionary position, but the slight foreshortening of the perspective leads the eye to focus on the man's rigid penis which the woman holds in her hand and is rubbing delicately against the lips of her vulva. Above all— and this is the surest measure of Romano's success—there is nothing of the discouraging instructional or taxonomic aura which characterizes most illustrated manuals of sex. These people are not putting on demonstrations; they are enjoying each other.

Aretino's contribution was a series of sonnets, one per position. Number 4 reads, in part:

> Place your leg, dearest, on my shoulder here,
> And take my truncheon in your tender grasp,
> And while I gently move it, let your clasp
> Tighten and draw me to your bosom dear.
>
> My hand shall keep the turgid dart in place,
> Lest it might slip and somehow get away,
> And I should see a frown on your dear face.

With the greatest of charity, this can only be considered as well below his usual standard. Or, for that matter, that of Oscar Wilde, who is credited with providing the translation.

The most intriguing aspect about the "Modi" is that despite the storm they caused and their subsequent fame, no complete set is known to exist. The British Museum has, in its famous locked cases, one complete print and the pasted-up fragments of nine others. The Bibliothèque Nationale possesses a set of nineteenth-century copies which profess to be faithful but are, in this writer's opinion at least, poor adaptations done with a leaden hand. Even more disappointing is the series done by a Bohemian soldier of fortune and itinerant artist named Friedrich von Waldeck, who claimed to have come across a set of Marcantonio's engravings in a convent in Mexico City in the 1820s. Waldeck's version suffers from a leery salaciousness—partly as a reflection of his own time and probably partly of the fact that he was in his sixties or seventies when he made them. The version generally considered closest to the original—and used in this account—derives from a series of woodcuts produced in Venice during the sixteenth century.[25]

The fate of the three collaborators is better documented. Marcantonio Raimondi did, as Vasari reported, go to jail but was quickly released only to be caught and killed in the disastrous Sack of Rome in 1527. Aretino fled to the more congenial atmosphere of Venice, where he pursued his various careers for another thirty-four years. Giulio Romano hastily took advantage of a long-standing invitation from Federigo, Duke of Gonzaga, to do some work for him in Mantua. The most spectacular result of that work is the Palazzo del Te, whose centerpiece is the "Sala di Psyche." Here, to the complete satisfaction of his patron and the delight of countless visitors, the unrepentant Romano produced a memorable "Zeus and Olympia." She is shown reclining, one arm thrown back and a look of pleased anticipation on her face, as Zeus, poised between her legs and equipped with an erection fit for a god, is about to slide into her.

By the end of the sixteenth century the appearance of private buyers and collectors had helped free artists from reliance on ecclesiastic or monarchic support. To please their new patrons—and, to a growing degree, themselves—they could begin to explore a wide range of themes. In England, William Hogarth combined the naturalistic themes of Dutch genre painting with the theatricality of Watteau and added to them his own social commentary to create what he himself called "modern moral subjects." The best known of these exercises is "The Rake's Progress," which, in eight tableaux, records the progress of a miserly merchant's son who uses his father's money to establish himself in society, collects mistresses and art, engages in debauchery, falls into debt, marries for money, gambles himself into debtors' prison, and ends up in Bedlam. Earlier he had similarly traced the fortunes of a young country girl who arrives in London expecting to be met by a "loving cousin" but is collected instead by a pock-faced bawd, who promptly sets her up in business. The succeeding scenes of the series—"A Harlot's Progress"—serve both as an object lesson and as evidence of Hogarth's erotic imagination.

Earlier still, he had done a pair of paintings entitled simply "Before" and "After." The first shows a young couple, elegantly dressed and set against a woodsy background. He is delicately holding her hand and voicing a proposal which, judging by her expression, is quite out of the question. Clearly, however, perseverance has won the day because the second painting shows the same couple, now sprawled in dishevelment. The girl's elegant red satin dress is hiked up to reveal white petticoats and pink thighs. The young man's breeches are unbuttoned just enough to provide a peek at his sexual organs.

Despite the financial success of "A Harlot's Progress" and the decidedly nonpuritanical life-style of eighteenth-century English aristocracy, Hogarth was punished for his choice of subject by the withdrawal of an important royal commission. The "Before" and "After," which now hang in the Fitzwilliam Museum in Cambridge, were privately commissioned by "a certain vicious nobleman." Greater license was permitted to caricaturists and used to advantage by James Gillray. His "The Final Resource of French Atheists," inspired by the political maneuvers of Charles James Fox, shows George III receiving a foreign ambassador who is holding a gigantic scroll in a phallic position, with two seals hanging from it like testicles. Another of his drawings was inspired by the impending marriage of George's favorite son, the Duke of York, to a young lady whose only visible asset was the daintiness of her feet. It shows, from the calves down, a horizontal pair of feminine legs shod in tiny slippers and, between them, an outstretched pair of men's legs.

Hogarth's heir as social commentator was Thomas Rowlandson, who dutifully trained in oils at the Royal Academy but gave them up to concentrate on the watercolors and etchings which made him famous. His output was prodigious—he "etched as much copper as would sheathe the whole British Navy," [26] according to his obituarist —and almost exclusively devoted to representations of the ordinary pleasures of life: eating, drinking, gambling, and whoring. Apparently he practiced what he drew because the last decade of a very long life found him broken in health and pocketbook, turning out mounds of redeemable but utterly explicit erotic subjects. His best customer, it appears, was the Prince Regent because the best of these drawings, for some reason not included in the BBC's otherwise exhaustive series of programs on the Royal Collections, are preserved among George IV's acquisitions at Windsor Castle.

In this work, Rowlandson calls upon a far-ranging imagination. One drawing, entitled "The Swings," is a parody of Fragonard's celebrated canvas, with the exception that the young lady, whose skirts are flying well above her waist, is about to descend onto the waiting erect penis of a chortling, trouserless gentleman coming up to meet her on another swing. Another, entitled "The Gallop," shows a man and a naked lady mounted simultaneously on a running horse and on each other. The caption accompanying it reads:

> While mounted on a mettled steed
> Famed for his strength as well as speed
> Corninna and her favorite buck
> Are pleas'd to have a flying f--k.

There are theatrical scenes (street juggler entertaining a crowd by balancing a pyramid of glassware on his erect penis, while his companion raises her skirt to her waist in order to catch the proffered coins) and historical scenes ("The Empress of Russia Receiving Her Brave Guards" depicts a bearded, pipe-smoking soldier demonstrating his virility upon the person of a chubby, reclining woman; an endless line of his companions, their trousers at their ankles, await their turn). There are illustrations for well-known stories, such as "Les Lunettes" by La Fontaine which deals with a nun who manages to become pregnant in a convent. Rowlandson has portrayed the nuns, one of whom is a man, parading in front of the abbess with their robes lifted; the culprit has become so excited at the prospect of his inspection that his penis knocks the abbess's glasses off her nose.

To dismiss this work, as one critic has, as "mere accumulations of pictured filth, incredible elaborations of things chalked by guttersnipes on street walls or worse" [27] is to condemn the subject matter without looking at it. "Les Lunettes," for instance, is enriched with the touch of a skilled humorist: the shock and bewilderment of the abbess, the concern of the more pious nuns, the nervous giggle of some of the others, and the irrepressible reaction of one of them, who falls back in helpless laughter.

Despite the ostensible fun and frolic, however, there is a powerful, bitter taste to most of the drawings, the frustration of an old man reflecting on the pastimes of his youth. Impotence is a recurring motif, as in a drawing entitled "Helpless Desire, or Fumble-Cunt," and another entitled "The Miser," in which a young girl tries to stroke life into an old man's flaccid penis while he devotes similarly affectionate attention to some sacks of gold. "The Star Gazer" shows an aged astronomer at a long, cylindrical telescope too engrossed to notice that in the next room a much younger man is using its flesh-and-blood prototype on his wife. Voyeurism, as in "The Inexperienced Yokel," which uses the device of a country bumpkin in a brothel as pretext for showing a massed display of gaping pudenda, runs like a refrain through much of Rowlandson's work. Indeed, "The Inspection," in which a nude, reclining woman has put her left leg over the shoulder of her elderly admirer so that he can more easily study her vulva through his eyeglass can serve as a graphic definition of fixation—down to the bowl in the foreground which is filled with a cluster of cutoff phalli. Had he lived in the twentieth century, Rowlandson would have been one of those men who crowd the front seats of the raunchier burlesque theaters and jump up for a still closer look when the performer, near the end of her act, deigns to "show pink." As it is, he caught to perfection their impotent, castration-ridden fascination.

Like his royal patron, for whom John Nash built the improbable Brighton Pavilion, Rowlandson was attracted by what he had heard about the exotic East and its hothouses of sensual indulgence. Essentially a realist, however, he could not do better than show aging, rolypoly pashas being tended to by platoons of nude harem girls.

It is interesting that a totally different painter, Jean Auguste Dominique Ingres, could hardly do better with the same imaginary milieu. His "Bain Turc," the apotheosis of a long lifetime of odalisques, piles into one composition a mass of bare female bodies. Buttocks, legs, arms, breasts, and bellies intertwine, but the net effect is very much that of a surreptitious look into the ladies' wing of the establishment described by the picture's title—a sensation unfortunately reinforced by the work's circular shape.

There is an erotic element missing from both Rowlandson's satire and Ingres's neoclassicism, however obsessive its bent. To identify it—to be overwhelmed by it—one need only look at the masterpiece of Ingres's archrival, Eugène Delacroix. Its subject was inspired by Byron's drama about Sardanapalus, the legendary Assyrian king who chose to immolate himself rather than fall into the hands of his enemies. But Delacroix has added details of his own. We are shown the despot, reclining on what will be his funeral pyre and commanding his servants to destroy his favorite dogs, horses, and women. Our eye is led, as the painter intended it to be, to the pair of figures at right: the man brandishing a knife and the superb young concubine he is about to slay. Her arms are outflung, her back arched and thighs tensed. It is not fear, however, which drives her, but the onset of orgasm. An art historian has noted that, for the preliminary sketches of this figure, Delacroix used "licentious paintings" from India.[28]

The roots of this sadoerotic fantasy are manifest in Delacroix's *Journals*. One of his models offers herself to him, but he evades her by feigning a headache. Why? Because days earlier he had tried to make love to another one and found that "nature did not permit it." Another entry reads: "Disgrace! I could not."[29] Nor are these the infirmities of an old man. Delacroix was in his early twenties when these entries were made; "The Death of Sardanapalus," a tortured exercise in wish fulfillment, was completed when he was twenty-nine.

The same fear of women, expressed in terms of perverse violence, also animated Delacroix's fellow Romantic, Géricault. His major work, "The Raft of the Medusa," is on its surface a horrifying view of the survivors of a shipwreck. On closer examination, however, the true reason for the horror becomes apparent. The gigantic canvas is a detailed, lingering study of the physical effects of violence on every part of the human body. The nude couples which Géricault painted repeatedly and sculpted on two occasions are the nearest thing we have to representations of forcible rape. Moreover, despite the mythological titles of the works—"Nymph Attacked by Satyr" or "Jupiter and Antiope"—this is not the allegorical rape of gods coupling with coy maidens, but the punishing, pain-inflicting rape chronicled on police blotters. The earliest and abiding subject of Géricault's work as an artist was the horse. His first successful work, "Officiers de Chasseurs à Cheval," depicted a cavalry charge; he was at work on an equestrian statue when he died—at the age of thirty-three and, fittingly, as a result of a fall while riding. It is commonplace to observe that a horse, especially a rearing, prancing stallion, is a metaphor for sexual potency. On a less abstract level, it is also the instrument for headlong flight.

Charles Baudelaire wrote in his personal journal in 1851: "The unique and supreme pleasure in love lies in the certainty of doing evil. Both man and woman know from birth that evil lies at the root of all pleasure." It is extremely unlikely that men or women know any such thing, at birth or at any other time. However, Baudelaire's brand of decadence found expression in the work of two extraordinary artists of the late nineteenth century. The first, Félicien Rops, was a Belgian etcher and illustrator who gravitated to Paris in 1862. The son of a textile manufacturer, he married well enough to secure himself a comfortable livelihood, but his disposition led him to frequent the ateliers. and absinthe cafés. Although he dashed off great quantities of landscapes and character studies of peasants, it was as a book illustrator that he found his calling. A frontispiece for Baudelaire's banned collection of poems, Les Épaves, earned him the friendship of their author and entrée into the Parisian literary demimonde. For the Goncourt brothers, he made a drawing of the prostitute heroine of their novel Manette Salomon. They repaid him by noting in their Journal: "Rops is truly eloquent in depicting the appearance of cruelty taken on by the contemporary woman, her look of steel, her ill-will towards men which is neither hidden nor dissimulated, but shown in her whole appearance." [30]

In 1883 there appeared one of the most outrageous, superheated works of the Decadent period: Jules Barbey d'Aurevilly's collection of short stories *Les Diaboliques*. Perhaps the best way to characterize them is with a brief synopsis of one of the stories. During the course of a dinner a guest relates the account of the mistress of a vicious, drunken cavalry officer who conceives and bears a child which dies young. Remorseful and grief-stricken, the officer has the child's heart preserved in a glass casket. Years later, in the course of a quarrel, the mistress tells him that the child was not his. In a fury, he smashes the casket, hurls the child's heart at his faithless mistress's face, then strips her and seals her vagina with hot wax. At this point in the story one of the other dinner guests, who happens to be a brother officer of the deceived man, leaps up and transfixes the narrator with a sword. The illustration which Rops provided for this story, which was entitled "At a Dinner of Atheists," depicts a naked woman lying across a table, her head hanging over the edge. One of her hands clutches at her mutilated vulva. But the expression on her face is intentionally ambiguous. She could be in agony, but she could also be registering masturbatory ecstasy.

Decadence attempted to raise to the level of philosophy a mixture of sex, sin, and the kind of immature sadism which prompts nasty little boys to tear wings off flies. With the addition of the obligatory anticlericalism, these elements inspired Rops to his version of Mary Magdalene. It is contained in two drawings, the first of which shows a nude woman, lying on her back with one leg raised to make way for a masturbatory hand, while her head is turned to stare at a crucifix to which is attached an erect penis. In the second drawing, the woman is relaxed and the penis hangs limply. This, and similar works, inspired a contemporary Belgian critic, possibly overcome by nationalistic pride, to state:

> We are not dealing here with little erotic scenes made for the delectation of old rakes. It is a profound, terrifying, entirely spiritual vision of the damnation of guilty flesh. . . . Never has a Christian artist depicted with more vigor the ravages produced by evil. Rops is a true father of the infernal Church.[31]

Rops's own estimate of his work was less apocalyptic. As he wrote to a fellow artist, "All this is basically only an excuse to paint from life a pretty girl who . . . for the first time and after much persuasion, agreed to sit for her old Fély as Princess Borghese sat for Canova. I only changed the hairstyle. . . ."[32]

Elsewhere, Rops set down his credo as an artist:

> The love of brutal rut, pre-occupation with money, mean interest, have glued onto the faces of most of our contemporaries a sinister mask in which the perverse instincts mentioned by Edgar Allan Poe can be read in capital letters: all this seems to me sufficiently amusing and characteristic that well-meaning artists should attempt to render the look of their times.[33]

In fact, the faces of Rops's male subjects are fairly forgettable caricatures that say "lecher," "hypocrite," or "sensualist," and his women, whatever their age, all seem stamped out from the same pug-nosed, hard-eyed mold of the Parisian street *poule*. What did fascinate him, and claim his loving attention, were sexual organs.

At the height of his career, Rops fell victim to the occupational hazard of illustrators. He conceived some marvelous ideas for which no book had been written. Rather than simply file them away, he drew them and published them as *Les Sataniques*. The missing text presumably recounts the adventures of a woman who, while still in full possession of her sexual powers, is carried off to hell. The first plate shows a raised altar on which have been erected two gigantic phalluses. Between them is a grinning, armless statue of Satan, its lower body covered by a naked woman who has shinnied up to impale herself. Another shows her sprawled on a pedestal while Satan, in the form of a giant snakelike penis, penetrates her. The final plate, which is as far as Rops's imagination could carry his theme, shows Satan nailed to the cross, with an erection reaching halfway up his chest. The woman stands between his legs, with her arms outstretched to emulate his pose, as her pubic hair mimics his goatee. A pair of hands is strangling the woman with her own hair as, in the background, a forest of phallic tapers light the scene.

"I cherish my obscurity," Rops writes. "I don't exhibit in order to expose myself to receiving an honorable mention. I grant no one the right to honor me . . . I don't know if I will produce something which pleases me; as for pleasing others, I give no more a damn for that than for my last year's gloves."[34] In his lifetime he did please others, including the authors whose books he illustrated. Perhaps he did not quite, as a recent biographer put it, catch "the febrile sadness of the damned soul" [35]—whatever that may be. But he did influence others such as Toulouse-Lautrec and Munch, as well as the early German film directors, and his willingness to explore the darker side of the erotic impulse anticipated the torrent of post-Freudian art.

In 1893, when Rops's output was finally beginning to tail off, there appeared in London a new, illustrated edition of Sir Thomas Malory's *Morte Darthur*. The printing process had obliged the artist to limit himself to black-and-white drawings, with no intermediate tones. Far from inhibiting him, however, it had prompted the design of a strange world in which the laws of gravity, perspective, and anatomy ceased to pertain. Although they owed much to such influences as the Pre-Raphaelites, Japanese painting, Whistler —and precious little to the presumed Celtic virtues of its protagonist—the 350 drawings announced the unmistakable arrival of an original genius.

Its possessor was a frail twenty-year-old Englishman named Aubrey Beardsley. The son of a shadowy, and shady, figure who appropriated his young wife's fortune to pay off a paternity suit and subsequently became an infrequent visitor to his own household, Beardsley was reared by a doting mother and a sister one year his senior, who became his mentor in everything, including, according to one biographer, sexual experience. Diagnosed as tubercular when seven years old, he was too frail as a child to participate in the rough games which, at the height of Victorianism, constituted a major portion of proper masculine schooling. In compensation, an unusually perceptive master at the Brighton Grammar School encouraged him to draw caricatures, vignettes of school life, and, on one occasion, illustrations for a text of Virgil which he was supposed to translate. Upon graduation, he found a job as a clerk in a London insurance office, attended evening classes at the Westminster School of Art for a year, and clung to the fringes of the city's literary and artistic avant-garde.

The illustrations for the *Morte Darthur* had been strongly erotic, but not in a manner to provoke censorship. Rather, it was a question of recognition signals—a dreamy, half-lidded gaze here, a hand gesture or body posture there. For his next commission—to illustrate Oscar Wilde's dramatization of *Salome*—Beardsley stepped over the line. He won the job by submitting to the publisher, John Lane, a drawing of the play's dramatic climax. Entitled "J'ai baisé ta bouche, Iokanaan," it shows a triumphant Salome floating in space and gloating over the severed head of John, still dripping blood. In a few lines, Beardsley captured the essence of the necrophiliac theme which had been Wilde's contribution to the legend. The finished illustrations were something else, however, starting with a titlepage which featured a grinning Satyr admiring his own elegantly drawn penis and testicles. The drawing for "The Toilette of Salome" contained the figure of a beautiful young serving boy seated on a hassock with his hands buried in his dainty pubic patch. He is looking across not at Salome, who, judging by her expression and the position of her hand, is similarly engaged, but at another naked page boy standing to her side.

Lane objected to these details, and Beardsley removed them for the printed version, but such was his skill at evoking an embracing aura of sexuality that one has to study the original and altered drawings side by side to see what touches are missing.* One of the drawings, "Enter Herodias," had contained a handsome naked youth whose genitals Lane demanded be concealed. Beardsley complied by adding a fig leaf so prominent and so cunningly attached that it served the purpose of attracting the eye to the forbidden member it was intended to shield.

On the strength of his eleven drawings for *Salome*, Beardsley was offered the art editorship of a new magazine, *The Yellow Book*, which was intended to provide a vehicle for the English Aesthetic Movement. Its career was cut short by angry mobs which, aroused by Oscar Wilde's trial, stormed its editorial offices in 1895. Wilde had, in fact, never contributed so much as a word to *The Yellow Book*, but such was his notoriety that anyone associated with him, as Beardsley had been with *Salome*, was assumed to be a homosexual. Most of Beardsley's critics make the same assumption, basing it on the supporting evidence of his artistic output. Judged on this basis, however, he would also have to be charged with transvestism, flagellation, incorrigible fetishism, and a spectator's passion for lesbianism. There is no question, however, that no one in the West-

* Brigid Brophy, in a recent biography of Beardsley, called him "the most intensely and electrically erotic artist in the world" and noted that his sexuality almost perfectly corresponds to what Freud would later define as "polymorphous perversity." [36]

ern tradition of art has more lovingly, painstakingly depicted the human penis.

The high point of Beardsley's phallic art consists of the illustrations he drew for a privately printed version of Aristophanes's *Lysistrata* in 1896. Freed from a publisher's anxious eye, he gave to purchasers of the limited edition a high-spirited, amusing view of the equipment and gymnastics of sex such as had not been drawn by anyone since the anonymous painters of classical Greek vases. Through no accident, he borrowed their technique; save for details such as hair, feathers, and the odd bit of lace, the drawings consist of an unbroken, uncluttered line against an empty background. The subjects, however, are very much his own. In the "Toilet of Lampito," she is having her bottom powdered by a helpful little Cupid—except that, for all his arrows and wings, he is considerably older than most *putti* and, with the hand not occupied at the task, is caressing his erection. "The Lacedaemonian Ambassadors," which had been a favorite with Athenian audiences, defies description: three naked men each displaying an enormous erection, the one on the smallest of them so gigantic that he must support it with his outstretched arms. The looks on their faces, the details of hair, the scrupulous delineation of the organs themselves, all different but quite appropriate to their possessors, make the drawing at once gloriously funny and painful with sexual frustration.

"I have just completed a set of illustrations for *Lysistrata*," Beardsley wrote to his friend and patron André Raffalovich. "I think they are in a way the best thing I have done." [37] They were, and equally accomplished are a series of drawings for a projected new edition of Juvenal's *Sixth Satire*. Beardsley was completing this project, as well as a set of illustrations for *Volpone*, when, as had been long expected, death overtook him at the age of twenty-five.

Although Rops's career spanned more than four decades while Beardsley's was crowded into five years, the two men died within six months of each other in 1898. As other artists before them, both had been obliged to divide their creative energy between the established artistic world and the underground of shady dealers, publishers, and collectors with "advanced tastes." In the decades after their death, this distinction was to be blurred and eventually erased—not without a struggle, to be sure. The first serious challenge to it was issued, appropriately, in Vienna, and by Gustav Klimt, a painter whose work habits were described as follows by a contemporary: ". . . he was surrounded by enigmatic named women who, while he stood silently at his easel, wandered up and down his studio, lazing and stretching and luxuriating through the days—yet always ready, at the artist's signal, to freeze obediently into a pose, a movement that had caught his eye. . . ." [38]

Despite this layman's imagined view of bohemian paradise, Klimt was neither a lecher nor a firebrand. On the contrary, his early career had been that of a dutiful academician. At twenty-six he had been presented with a gold medal from Kaiser Franz Josef. His "Schubert at the Piano" had been hailed by critics as "the most beautiful picture ever painted by an Austrian" [39] and earned him the honor of executing the ceiling of the main hall of the University of Vienna. There were to be three tableaux, entitled "Medicine," "Philosophy," and "Jurisprudence," and what the trustees had in mind most probably was a paprika-scented version of Raphael's Vatican *stanze*. What they got, for "Medicine," was a heroically scaled figure of Hygeia holding out the cup of healing while a snake coiled suggestively around her body and, behind and around her, nude figures engaged in various strenuous and explicit activities representing love, ecstasy, procreation, motherhood, illness, and death. This time, instead of a medal, Klimt received a petition signed by eighty-seven of the university's professors denouncing the work as unacceptable.* In one of his rare public statements Klimt replied by taking a parting bite out of the hand that had been feeding him: "Enough of censorship . . . I want to get free. I want to get out of all these unrefreshing absurdities that hinder my work, and get back to freedom. I refuse all state help. I renounce everything." [40]

The unveiling of "Medicine" took place in 1900. For the next eighteen years Klimt pursued a preoccupation with the darker side of sexuality. His version of the "Danaë" is a nude with long red hair, her body curled in fetal position, her eyes closed and lips parted. One hand grasps her breast while the other is between her legs, the better to guide Jupiter in his manifestation as a shower of gold. His "Water Snakes" presents four nude girls with long, flowing hair speckled with stars, their bodies and limbs evoking a pow-

---

* Nevertheless, Klimt completed the other two subjects. All of them were destroyed by the Nazis in 1945.

erful mixture of sensuality and death. The work drew criticism even among advanced circles because Klimt, in defiance of tradition, had made no effort to hide his subjects' pubic hair.

Egon Schiele, Klimt's best-known pupil and protégé, shared his teacher's obsession with sex as the central moving force of life. But unlike Klimt, who even at his most fanciful never lost his high sense of style, Schiele remained, during a career cut short by influenza in 1918, in the continuous grip of neurotic tension. Most of his surviving work—a number of his drawings were burned in 1912, and he himself thrown into prison as a pornographer—consists of images of men and women, singly or in pairs, in agonizingly twisted positions. In "Friendship," a nude man nervously clutches at the breasts of a nude girl lying beside him. A "Self-Portrait" shows the artist naked from the waist and holding an exaggerated erection. In "Reclining Girl in a Blue Dress," the model's legs are spread wide, and her dress is hitched up to the waist to reveal the vivid red lips of her vulva, again indicating desire that will never achieve fulfillment.

One of the casualties of the First World War was the hallowed faith, professed with increasing dogmatism since the Renaissance, in the rationality of man and the virtue of technical progress as the benign engine of change. No positivist interpretation of history as the interplay of national forces could explain, much less justify the mindless carnage of the Somme or Tannenberg. At the same time, Freud's explorations, starting with *The Interpretation of Dreams*, which was published in an edition of 600 copies in 1899, pointed to the conclusion that conscious human behavior might be the product of unknown motivations and that personality itself was no more than a fragile and precarious superstructure erected over the heaving depths of suppressed, irrational wellsprings.

Artistically, this failure of the old and emergence of the new found expression in a loose, shifting coalition of artists and poets, many of whom had served in the trenches of one or the other side. Karl Marx had called for the reappropriation of labor by mankind. Echoing him, André Breton stated in the *First Surrealist Manifesto* of 1924 that "Man's imagination should be free, yet everywhere it is in chains. . . ." [41]

Surrealism rejected social pressure and the rhythms of the machine and strove, instead, to tap those rich sources Freud had identified. As Salvador Dali, one of its most successful practitioners, explains:

> Realism, practical-rational, includes all the sordid mechanisms of logic and all mental prisons. Pleasure includes our world of subconscious desires, dreams, irrationality and imagination. Surrealism attempts to deliver the subconscious from the principle of reality, thus finding a source of splendid and delirious images.[42]

Inevitably most of the images turned out to be erotic. Georges Bataille observes in his *Eroticism*:

> The passage from the normal state to that of erotic desire supposes within us a relative dissolution of the constituted being . . . the term "dissolution" recalling the familiar expression "dissolute" applied to erotic activity. For what is at stake in eroticism is always a dissolution of constituted forms.[43]

The rational, industrial ethic had identified the good with the useful and stigmatized as unhealthy anything that was pleasurable for its own sake. Therefore, surrealism resuscitated the writings of the Marquis de Sade, who had obeyed no other injunction than that of single-mindedly satisfying desire. However strong their intellectual commitment, surrealists also yielded rather easily to the temptation of tweaking the bourgeoisie. In the movement's early days, Max Ernst was involved in an exhibit which created such a scandal that it had to be closed by the police:

> In order to enter the gallery one had to pass through a public lavatory. Inside, the public was provided with hatchets with which, if they wanted to, they could attack the objects and paintings exhibited. At the end of the gallery a young girl, dressed in white, as for her first communion, stood reciting obscene poems.[44]

Professing to appeal to the mind rather than to the senses, surrealist art took everyday objects and diverted them from their customary purposes into ambivalent symbolic roles. At best, which is to say, at its most shocking, the effect could be as startling as René Magritte's "Rape," in which a woman's face has had breasts substituted for eyes and a pubic triangle for a mouth. At the hand of surrealist artists, erotic possibilities multiply, as in André Masson's phallic landscapes, and the entire human body can become an undifferentiated erogenous zone. Dali's "Young Virgin Autosodomized by Her Own Chastity" shows the rear view of a lady wearing nothing but shoes and leaning over a balcony. Her haunches and thighs have fragmented into phallic shapes which could also be interpreted as symbolizing a unicorn's horn, itself an ancient symbol of chastity. Dali's own explanation of the painting—that "Thanks to dismantling or to deformation of the female anatomy, woman can satisfy her profound exhibitionism by detaching various sections of her anatomy and passing them round for people to admire"—will support a range of interpretations.

One of the most single-minded of the surrealists was Hans Bellmer, who fled Nazi Germany in 1938 and died in Paris in 1975 after a lifetime's artistic preoccupation with the manipulation and superimposition of sexual anatomies. Typical of his drawings is a view of a girl kneeling; her body is a phallus, and her breasts are propped up on it as though she were removing a pullover. The vagina shape of her upper torso is made more realistic by abundant hair. Her legs are squeezed into tight stockings, and in between them is the vague shape of another phallus. The shape of her shoes repeats the motif of the vagina. Another drawing, entitled "After the Weekly Closing," shows a realistic picture of the interior of an empty café. The door is locked, and the chairs are stacked along the wall. An almost naked girl is resting her head on a table, while a phallus is trying to penetrate her from behind. It is not clear whether the phallus forms part of her body or that of the chair on which she is sitting. Artists are not expected to explain, but Bellmer offers this commentary in a published volume of his illustrations:

> Up to now we have probably never considered seriously enough to what extent the image of the desired woman is conditioned by the man who desires her. So that in the last analysis there are a whole row of phallus projections, progressing from a detailed picture of the woman to an overall picture of the female species. So that the finger, the arm, the leg of the woman are colored by his masculinity; so that the woman's leg squeezed into a tight stocking, with the thigh protruding, is colored by his masculinity; so that the egg-shaped pair of buttocks from

which the flexible spine gets its tension are colored by his masculinity; so that the two breasts which hang from the elongated
neck or which hang freely from the body are colored by his
masculinity. . . .[45]

No artist of our time, and few before it, explored a wider range
of human experience than Picasso. Eroticism, from the lyrical to
the brutal, runs like a multicolored thread through his long career.
Asked shortly before his death about the difference between art and
eroticism, he replied, "But there is no difference."[46] Indeed, one
recent critic has cited the parallel between the specific sexual
component of Picasso's work and the events of his personal life:

> At times, sexual impulses, particularly those of women, are
> seen as menacing and destructive; in other cases, these forces
> are viewed as almost Rabelaisian jokes that turn man into a
> clumsy, comical creature; and elsewhere, eroticism is celebrated
> as a lyrical, tender experience saturated with the magic of love
> and the miracle of procreation.[47]

One of the subjects to which Picasso returned several times during his lifetime was that of artists simultaneously painting and
making love to their nude models. His last exploration of the theme
was a series of engravings done in 1968, when he was in his eighties.
The title of the series is "Raphael and La Fornarina," after the celebrated portrait of one of the artist's mistresses. Picasso has shown
the painter as a young man dressed—or, more precisely, half dressed
—in resplendent Renaissance clothing, holding a brush in one hand
and a palette in the other, yet able to surround and penetrate the
woman as she looks up to him in admiration. Apart and to the right,
looking on with mixed excitement and wistfulness, Picasso has
added a third, older figure: one of his rare self-portraits.

This has by no means been an exhaustive survey of the depiction of male genitals in Western art, but it does point to the conclusion, verifiable by a stroll through any museum, that artists
have shown far greater interest in painting or sculpting naked
women than naked men. The commonplace explanation offered
for this preference is that most artists have been men—and, perhaps
as important, that most of the patrons who have supported them
have also been men.

This confirms, unnecessarily, the feminist contention that women have been viewed by men as sexual objects. But it fails to give a reason for artists' reticence in showing the attributes of their own sex and the even greater reticence of the art establishment in allowing the public to view them. In 1916 a very handsome bronze by Brancusi, entitled "Princess X," was banned from an exhibition of modern art in Paris because of its deliberate phallic connotations. Fifty years later, when a London gallery offered a show of amusing watercolors of penises by Jim Dine, the police raided the premises and the gallery's owner was fined for committing a public nuisance.

Even members of the avant-garde observe the convention. Commenting on the famous 1968 erotic exhibition staged by the Kronhausens in Sweden, Margaret Walters notes:

> Many artists were clearly proud of their daring in showing the previously unshowable; female genitals fairly leaped off the wall at the Swedish show. Endless naked girls spread their legs, postured for the spectator, masturbated. Their exposed vaginas were sometimes prettily stylized, sometimes shown in detailed anatomical closeups, and sometimes as nightmare images—as a bleeding wound, a devouring insect, a gaping hole."[48]

And the male equivalent? The same critic notes:

> . . . except in a small section devoted to primitive art, which included some phallic male totems, there were hardly any straightforward male sex objects, and when the penis was represented alone, it was almost always metaphorically, intellectually, as in Man Ray's witty silver *Paperweight for Priapus*, put together out of highly polished spheres and cylinders.

The very different treatment of male and female sexual anatomy in films makes the point even more emphatically. Hedy Lamarr's breasts, Gina Lollobrigida's bare backside, Maria Schneider's pubic triangle are recorded as milestones—attractive milestones—along the road to artistic freedom and integrity.* But there has been no corresponding unveiling of the male. Even in the most torrid

* In, respectively, *Ecstasy* (1933); *Fanfan la Tulipe* (1952); and *Last Tango in Paris* (1973).

scenes of *Last Tango in Paris,* Marlon Brando could confidently have worn a jockstrap.*

Reluctance to display the male genitals seems to become particularly acute when the artist is known to have been a woman. Sylvia Sleigh, Eunice Golden, Alice Neel, Connie Greene would all be better known and more fairly represented in museums of contemporary art were it not for their predilection to paint male nudes, penises and all. Gallery owners and curators, almost universally male, may justify this neglect on artistic grounds, but the quality of the work speaks for itself.

In the primitive societies which practiced them, taboos were erected as shields against particularly pervasive sources of anxiety. The contemporary taboo against displaying the penis, especially the erect penis, may well serve precisely the same purpose—on two levels of consciousness. On the deeper of them, it guards against the fear that the male organ, like the carefully guarded central object of some cult, may suffer diminution of majesty and awesomeness by public exposure, particularly if a woman is responsible for that exposure. And more immediately, it removes the risk, which not many men are secure enough willingly to incur, of simple, direct comparison.

* Analogously there are some dozen magazines available on newsstands which fill their pages with close-ups of vaginas so clinically detailed that they could serve medical students as anatomical handbooks. The two magazines which had tried to publish full-frontal male nudes—*Playgirl* and *Viva*—both gave up the practice. And neither of them, nor any other nonpornographic publication, ever ventured as far as to show an erect penis.

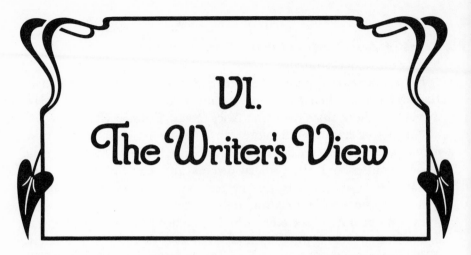

VI.
The Writer's View

Until the recent flinging open of the floodgates, explicit reference to the penis and its function had been, in Western literature at least, almost everywhere proscribed. As high school students quickly discover, however, successive generations of writers learned to circumvent this restriction with metaphor and other wordplay. None succeeded more amusingly or memorably than Boccaccio in his account of how one goes about putting the devil in hell. The tale, told by Dioneo during the third day of the *Decameron*, concerns a beautiful but utterly innocent young girl named Alibech, who wanders off into the desert in search of the best way to serve God. She encounters a hermit named Rustico, who, once he discovers the extent of her innocence, is only too happy to enlighten her. His instructions, which in most English translations are still left in the original Italian (the Modern Library edition notes: "The translators regret that the disuse into which magic has fallen makes it impossible to render the technicalities of that mysterious art into tolerable English"), prove to be at once so efficacious and so rewarding that Rustico, who, we are reminded, subsists on roots and water, turns out to be no match for his young student's newly found religious zeal.*

Poets have conjured imagery which left little to the imagination, as did Thomas Carew, a contemporary of John Donne, in his "A Rapture":

Now in more subtle wreaths I will entwine
My sinewy limbs, my arms and legs, with thine.

* Boccaccio's tale is durable enough to have reappeared, in somewhat modernized dress, as one of the episodes in Terry Southern's *Candy*.

196

Thou like a sea of milk shall lie display'd
Whilst I the smooth calm ocean will invade,
With such a tempest, as when Jove of old
Fell down on Danaë in a stream of gold;
Yet my tall pinnace shall in the Cyprian strait
Ride safe at anchor, and unload her freight:
My rudder with thy bold hand, like a tried
And skilful pilot, thou shalt steer and guide
   My Bark into Love's channel, where it shall
   Dance, as the bounding waves do rise or fall.

One of the rare writers to violate the proscription was John Wilmot, the second Earl of Rochester. His "The Imperfect Enjoyment" starts out conventionally enough:

Naked she lay, clasped in my longing arms,
I filled with love, and she all over charms;
Both equally inspired with eager fire,
Melting through kindness, flaming in desire.
With arms, legs lips close clinging to embrace,
She clips me to her breast, and sucks me to her face.
Her nimble tongue, Love's lesser lightning, played
Within my mouth, and to my thoughts conveyed
Swift orders that I should prepare to throw
The all-dissolving thunderbolt below.

Unfortunately things don't proceed as planned:

But whilst her busy hand would guide that part
Which should convey my soul up to her heart,
In liquid raptures I dissolve all o'er,
Melt into sperm, and spend at every pore
A touch from any part of her had done't:
Her hand, her foot, her very look's a cunt.
Smiling, she chides in a kind, murmuring noise,
And from her body wipes the clammy joys,
When, with a thousand kisses wandering o'er
My panting bosom, "Is there then no more?"

No amount of encouragement on the lady's part seems to help:

This dart of love, whose piercing point, oft tried,
With virgin blood ten thousand maids have dyed;

Which nature still directed with such art
That it through every cunt reached every heart—
Stiffly resolved, 'twould carelessly invade
Woman or man, nor ought its fury stayed:
Wher'er it pierced, a cunt it found or made—
Now languid lies in this unhappy hour,
Shrunk up and sapless like a withered flower.

The remainder of the poem is addressed to the recalcitrant member:

Worst part of me, and hence hated most,
Through all the town a common fucking post,
On whom each whore relieves her tingling cunt
As hogs on gates do rub themselves and grunt,
Mayst thou to ravenous chancres be a prey,
Or in consuming weepings waste away;
May strangury and stone thy days attend;
May'st thou ne'er piss, who dist refuse to spend
When all my joys did on false thee depend.
    And may ten thousand abler pricks agree
    To do the wronged Corinna right for thee.[1]

Although more outspoken than its predecessors, "The Imperfect Enjoyment" still falls within the minor poetic tradition of the rueful recall of sexual failure which originated in Ovid's *Amores**
and was elaborated in the *Satyricon*.[3] But Rochester, whose father had loyally served the royalist cause and who himself became a protégé and companion of Charles II, also addressed himself to the social habits of that monarch's gamy court. One of his satires, "A Ramble in St. James's Park," recounts the goings-on in a favorite haunt of Restoration rakes:

Much wine had passed, with grave discourse,
Of who fucks who, and who does worse
(Such as you usually do hear
From those that diet at the Bear),

---

* Which, in one translation, reads:

I lay without Life's animating Spring
A dull, enervate, worthless, lumpish thing.
. . . .
In vain, alas!, the Nerves were slacken'd still
And I prov'd only potent in my Will.[2]

When I, who still take care to see
Drunkenness relieved by lechery,
Went out into St. James's Park
To cool my head and fire my heart.
But though St. James has th' honor on 't,
'Tis consecrate to prick and cunt.

He notes some of the denizens of the park:

Unto this all-sin-sheltering grove
Whores of the bulk and the alcove,
Great ladies, chambermaids and drudges
The ragpicker, and heiress trudges.
Carmen, divines, great lords, and tailors,
Prentices, poets, pimps and jailers,
Footmen, fine fops do here arrive,
And here they promiscuously swive.

He sees three of his friends, also on the prowl, stop to talk to a woman who turns out to be his own mistress:

In short, without much more ado,
Joyful and pleased, away she flew,
And with these three confounded asses
From park to hackney coach she passes.

Worse than mere treachery, this is a violation of the libertine's code:

Gods! That a thing admired by me
Should fall to so much infamy.
Had she picked out, to rub her arse on,
Some stiff-pricked clown or well-hung parson,
Each job of whose spermatic sluice
Had filled her cunt with wholesome juice,
I, the proceeding should have praised
In hope sh'had quenched a fire I raised.
Such natural freedoms are but just:
There's something generous in mere lust.
But to turn damned abandoned jade
When neither head nor tail persuade;
To be a whore in understanding,
A passive pot for fools to spend in!

In the manner of court favorites, Rochester even hazarded a dart at his royal patron. His "A Satyr on Charles II" reads in part:

> I'th'isle of Britain, long since famous grown
> For breeding the best cunts in Christendom
> There reigns, and oh! long may he reign and thrive,
> The easiest King and best-bred man alive.
>
> . . . .
>
> His scepter and his prick are of a length;
> And she may sway the one who plays with th' other,
> And make him little wiser than his brother.
> Poor prince! thy prick, like thy buffoons at Court,
> Will govern thee because it makes thee sport.
>
> . . . .
>
> This you'd believe, had I but time to tell ye
> The pains it costs to poor, laborious Nelly,
> Whilst she employs hands, fingers, mouth and thighs,
> Ere she can raise the member she enjoys.

"Poor, laborious Nelly" was, as everyone in England knew, the longtime royal favorite Nell Gwyn. One of Rochester's best-known poems is "Signior Dildo." Its occasion was the arrival in England of Mary of Modena, the intended bride of the Duke of York, the king's brother. It begins:

> You ladies of merry England
> Who have been to kiss the Duchess' hand,
> Pray, did you lately observe in the show
> A noble Italian called Signior Dildo?
>
> This signior was one of her Highness's train,
> And helped to conduct her over the main;
> But now she cries out, "To the Duke I will go!
> I have no more need for Signior Dildo."
>
> You'll take him at first for no person of note
> Because he appears in a plain leather coat,
> But when you his virtuous abilities know,
> You'll fall down and worship Signior Dildo.
>
> My lady Southest, heaven prosper her for't!
> First clothed him in satin, then brought him to Court;

But his head in the circle, he scarcely durst show,
So modest a youth was Signior Dildo.

. . . .

The Countess of Falmouth, of whom people tell
Her footmen wear shirts of a guinea an ell,
Might save the expense if she did but know
How lusty a swinger is Signior Dildo.

. . . .

Our dainty fine duchesses have got a trick
To dote on a fool for the sake of his prick:
The fops were undone, did their Graces but know
The discretion and vigor of Signior Dildo.

That pattern of virtue, Her Grace of Cleveland
Has swallowed more pricks than the ocean has sand;
But by rubbing and scrubbing so large it does grow,
It is fit for nothing but Signior Dildo.

And so on for twenty-three stanzas in which the principal ladies of
the court receive individual attention, until:

A rabble of pricks who were welcome before
Now finding the Porter denied 'em the door,
Maliciously waited his coming below
And inhumanly fell on Signior Dildo.

This poem, too, falls into a long-standing tradition. The notion
of an artificial penis, tireless and ever-ready, seems to have preyed
on male minds for centuries. In his *Psychology of Sex*, Havelock
Ellis cites some early examples:

> . . . such instrument is said to be represented in old Baby-
> lonian sculptures, and it is referred to by Ezekiel (Ch. XVI, v.
> 17).* The Lesbian women are said to have used such instru-
> ments made of ivory or gold with silken stuffs and linen.
> Aristophanes, in *Lysistrata*, speaks of the manufacture by the
> Milesian women of a leather artificial penis, or olisbos. In the
> British Museum is a vase representing a *hetaera* holding such

---

* The verse reads: "Thou hast also taken my fair jewels of my gold and of my
silver, which I had given thee, and madest to thyself images of men, and didst
commit whoredom with them."

instruments, which, as found at Pompeii, may be seen in the Museum at Naples. . . . Through the Middle Ages (when from time to time the clergy reprobated the use of such instruments) they continued to be known. . . . Forniti, the Sienese novelist of the sixteenth century, refers in his *Novelle dei Novizi* (7th Day, Novella XXXIX) to "the glass object filled with warm water which nuns use to calm the sting of the flesh and to satisfy themselves as well as they can." [4]

Dildos—probably a corruption of the Italian *diletto*—and godmiches—a French version of the Latin *gaude mihi*, "give me pleasure"—appear in most of the classics of "gallant" literature, such as Brantôme, *L'Escole des Filles*, the British *Cabinet of Love*, and Balzac's *Droll Stories*. A dildo is the hero of a long poem by Thomas Nashe, a contemporary and rival of Shakespeare:

He is a youth almost two handfulls highe,
Streight, round and plumbs, yett having but one eye

. . . .

That bendeth not, nor fouldeth any deale
But stands as stiff, as he were made of steele. [5]

Dildos, usually of massive dimensions, appear almost obligatorily in pornographic writing. In the climactic scene of Harold Robbins's *The Adventurers*, the hero, Dax, who bears more than a passing resemblance to the late playboy-diplomat Porfirio Rubirosa, returns home determined, after some 300 pages of international high living and fancy sex, to relieve the oppression of his people. In this quest, he bursts unannounced into the private chamber of *el Presidente* only to find him naked in bed with Amparo, who is not only *el Presidente*'s daughter but also Dax's wife. And since mere incest is, at this stage of the story, somewhat small beer, there is more: "They were naked on the bed, Amparo's legs wide, *el Presidente* on his knees between them, a huge black dildo strapped around his waist." [6]

That the dildo should be black instead of white or pink is, of course, another instance of Caucasian projection of sexuality onto blacks, but the abiding male preoccupation with the dildo is itself a projection. As Wayland Young notes in *Eros Denied*, "it is a refusal to accept the difference of women, a projection onto them of the need to use and the need to experience what the man has and the woman has not." And he adds, "It is also an excellent emblem of lust itself, of using the body as a thing. . . . Nothing else matters, only the local, concrete, reproducible, purchaseable organ." [7] Dildos and godmiches have, of course, been known in all cultures and at all times, but in numbers small enough to make their very existence worthy of comment. Nor, according to the best evidence garnered by Kinsey and others, are they much favored by women. Women do not, it appears, masturbate by pushing great big pieces of machinery, however cunningly contrived, in and out of themselves.

The taboo-breaking endeavors of the Earl of Rochester and some of his contemporaries * did not set a trend. Save for pornography, the penis did not appear again explicitly in published English writing until 1928, when Oliver Mellors encountered Constance Chatterley:

> He dropped the shirt and stood still, looking towards her. The sun through the low window sent a beam that lit up his thighs and white belly, and the erect phallus rising darkish and hot-looking from the little cloud of vivid gold-red hair. She was startled and afraid.
> "How strange!" she said slowly. "How strange he stands there! So big! and so dark and cocksure! Is he like that?" . . .
> The man looked down in silence at his tense phallus, that did not change. . . . "Cunt, that's what th'art after. Tell Lady Jane tha' wants cunt. John Thomas, an' th' cunt of Lady Jane!" [9]

This chapter will take a look at D. H. Lawrence, John Thomas's creator, and also more recent writers, to see some of the ends which freedom of sexual expression have been made to serve. It will look at how Shakespeare, among others, circumvented the proprieties of his day to entertain and enlighten his audiences. It will trace the remarkable durability of a single theme—the oedipal situation—through much of our literature. And it will attempt to show that, whatever their form or style, writers have unconsciously projected their creations through their own psyches and in the process ended up by saying more than is manifest on the printed page.

---

* Including Sir George Etherege, one of whose lyrics began:

> Dreaming last night on Mrs. Farley,
> My prick was up this morning early. . . .[8]

Consider, as an example, a remarkable short story by Herman Melville entitled "I and My Chimney." It begins:

> I and my chimney, two gray-headed old smokers, reside in the country. We are, I may say, old settlers here; particularly my old chimney, which settles more and more every day. . . .
>
> Within thirty feet of the turf-sided road, my chimney—a huge, corpulent old Harry VIII of a chimney—rises full in front of me and all my possessions. Standing well up a hill-side, my chimney, like Lord Rosse's monster telescope, swung vertical to hit the meridian moon, is the first object to greet the approaching traveler's eye, nor is it the last which the sun salutes. . . .
>
> But it is within doors that the pre-eminence of my chimney is most manifest. When in the rear room, set apart for that object, I stand to receive my guests (who, by the way, call more, I suspect, to see my chimney than me), I then stand, not so much before, as, strictly speaking, behind my chimney, which is, indeed, the true host. Not that I demur. In the presence of my betters, I hope I know my place.[10]

The chimney is described in affectionate detail:

> From the exact middle of the mansion it soars from the cellar, right up through each successive floor, till, four feet square, it breaks water from the ridge-pole of the roof, like an anvil-headed whale, through the crest of a billow. . . .
>
> Large as the chimney appears upon the roof, that is nothing to its spaciousness below. At its base in the cellar, it is precisely twelve feet square; and hence covers precisely one hundred and forty-four superficial feet. What an appropriation of terra firma for a chimney, and what a huge load for this earth! In fact, it was only because I and my chimney formed no part of his ancient burden that that stout peddler Atlas of old was enabled to stand up so bravely under his pack.

For all its great size and massiveness, the chimney has suffered damage over the years:

> The reason for its peculiar appearance above the roof touches upon rather delicate ground. How shall I reveal that, forasmuch as many years ago the original gable roof of the old house had become very leaky, a temporary proprietor hired a band of

woodmen, with their huge, cross-cut saws, and went to sawing the old gable roof off. . . .

All feeling hearts will sympathize with me in what I am now about to add. The surgical operation, above referred to, necessarily brought into the open air a part of the chimney previously under cover, and intended to remain so and, therefore not built of what are called weather-bricks. In consequence, the chimney, though of a vigorous constitution, suffered not a little from so naked an exposure; and, unable to acclimate itself, ere long began to fail—showing blotchy symptoms akin to those in measles.

The narrator's wife is hostile toward the chimney:

In vain my wife—with what probable ulterior intent will, ere long, appear—solemnly warned me, that unless something were done, and speedily, we should be burned to the ground, owing to the holes crumbling through the afore-said blotchy parts, where the chimney joined the roof.

His neighbor is evidently jealous of it:

. . . one day—when I was a little out of my mind, I now think—getting a spade from the garden, I set to work, digging round the foundation, especially at the corners thereof, obscurely prompted by dreams of striking some old, earthen-worn memorial of that by-gone day when, into all this gloom, the light of heaven entered, as the masons laid the foundation-stones, peradventure sweltering under an August sun, or pelted by a March storm. Plying my blunted spade, how vexed was I by that ungracious interruption of a neighbor who, calling to see me upon some business, and being informed that I was below, said I need not be troubled by coming up, but he would go down to me; and so, without ceremony, and without my having been forewarned, suddenly discovered me, digging in my cellar.

"Gold digging, sir?"

"Nay, sir," answered I, starting, "I was merely—ahem!—merely—I say I was merely digging—round my chimney."

"Ah, loosening the soil, to make it grow. Your chimney, sir, you regard as too small, I suppose; needing further development, especially at the top?"

"Sir!," said I, throwing down the spade, "do not be personal. I and my chimney—"

"Personal?"

"Sir, I look upon this chimney less as a pile of masonry than as a personage. It is the king of the house. I am but a suffered and inferior subject."

But the chimney's chief enemy is the wife:

How often has my wife ruefully told me, that my chimney, like the English aristocracy, casts a contracting shade all round it. She avers that endless domestic inconveniences arise—more particularly from the chimney's stubborn central locality. The grand objection with her is, that it stands midway in the place where a fine entrance-hall ought to go. In truth, there is no hall whatever to the house—nothing but a sort of square landing place, as you enter from the wide front door. . . .

And here, respectfully craving her permission, I must say a few words about this enterprising wife of mine. Though in years nearly as old as myself, in spirit she is young as my little sorrel mare, Trigger, that threw me last fall. What is extraordinary, though she comes of a rheumatic family, she is straight as a pine, never has any aches; while for me with sciatica, I am sometimes as crippled up as any old apple tree. . . .

Not insensible of her superior energies, my wife has frequently made me propositions to take upon herself all the responsibilities of my affairs. She is desirous that, domestically, I should abdicate; that, renouncing further rule, like the venerable Charles V, I should retire into some sort of monastery. But indeed, the chimney excepted, I have little authority to lay down. By my wife's ingenious application of the principle that certain things belong of right to female jurisdiction, I find myself, through my easy compliances, insensibly stripped by degrees of one masculine prerogative after another.

Inevitably the conflict is reached:

At last my wife came out with her sweeping proposition—in toto to abolish the chimney.

The narrator's two daughters join the fight on the side of their mother:

Sometimes all three abandon the theory of the secret closet, and return to the genuine ground of attack—the unsightliness of so cumbersome a pile, with comments upon the great addition of room to be gained by its demolition, and the fine effect of the projected grand hall. . . . Not more ruthlessly did the Three Powers away poor Poland, than my wife and daughters would fain partition away my chimney. . . .

Scarce a day I do not find her with her tape-measure, measuring for her grand hall, while Anna holds a yard-stick on one side, and Julia looks approvingly on from the other. Mysterious intimations appear in the nearest village paper, signed "Claude," to the effect that a certain structure, standing on a certain hill, is a sad blemish to an otherwise lovely landscape. Anonymous letters arrive, threatening me with I know not what, unless I remove my chimney. Is it my wife, too, or who, that sets up the neighbors to badgering me on the same subject, and hinting to me that my chimney, like a huge elm, absorbs all moisture from my garden? . . . Assailed on all sides, and in all ways, small peace have I and my chimney.

One day he returns unexpectedly from a trip:

. . . and upon approaching the house, narrowly escaped three brickbats which fell, from high aloft, at my feet. Glancing up, what was my horror to see three savages, in blue jean overalls, in the very act of commencing the long-threatened attack.

And the story ends:

It is now some seven years since I have stirred from home. My city friends all wonder why I don't come to see them, as in former times. They think I am getting sour and unsocial. Some say that I have become a sort of mossy old misanthrope, while all the time the fact is, I am simply standing guard over my mossy old chimney; for it is resolved between me and my chimney, that I and my chimney will never surrender.

It is just possible that Melville is simply describing a marital squabble over an issue of domestic remodeling, but only the most obsessively literal-minded reader will refuse to recognize the story's underlying theme. The narrator's relationship to his chimney—its impressive size, majesty, and importance—is made clear in the first three paragraphs. The objective of his wife—and, by extension, his daughters—is equally clear. *Moby Dick*, as has been exhaustively noted, is replete with phallic allusions and imagery.[11] In "I and My

Chimney," Melville has composed a sustained 13,000-word metaphor of the narcissistic, castrating female and the threatened male.

One of the most frequently cited puns in Shakespeare occurs during the play-within-a-play scene of *Hamlet*. Claudius, Gertrude, and the court have just entered to witness the performance, and the Queen asks Hamlet to sit near her. He refuses and addresses Ophelia:

HAMLET: Lady, shall I lie in your lap?
OPHELIA: No, my lord.
HAMLET: I mean, my head upon your lap?
OPHELIA: Ay, my lord.
HAMLET: Do you think I meant country matters?
OPHELIA: I think nothing, my lord.
HAMLET: That's a fair thought to lie between maids' legs.
OPHELIA: What is, my lord?
HAMLET: Nothing.[12]

The primary meaning of "country" is, of course, geographical—a reference to the reputedly earthy pleasures of the peasantry. The secondary meaning is anatomical, in the tradition of Chaucer, who had considerable fun with "queynt" in *The Canterbury Tales*. This second meaning is further underlined by the double use of "nothing," which, as Professor Thomas Pyles has pointed out, is "unquestionably yonic symbolism, a shape-metaphor intended to call to mind the naught, or 0, which is elsewhere in Shakespeare a symbol of *pudendum muliebre*." [13] *

* As, for instance, in the exchange between the Nurse and Friar Laurence in *Romeo and Juliet*:

NURSE: O! he is even in my mistress's case,
  Just in her case!
FRIAR LAURENCE: O woful sympathy!
  Piteous predicament! Even so lies she,
  Blubbering and weeping, weeping and blubbering.
  Stand up, stand up; stand, an you be a man:
  For Juliet's sake, for her sake, rise and stand;
  Why should you fall into so deep an O? [14]

Or, earlier in the same play, Mercutio's comment:

  . . . 'twould anger him,
  To raise a spirit in his mistress' circle
  Of some strange nature, letting it there stand
  Till she had laid it and conjur'd it down; . . . [15]

Not as commonly noted is the wordplay between Hamlet and Ophelia which takes place later in the same scene:

OPHELIA: You are keen, my lord, you are keen.
HAMLET: It would cost you a groaning to take off my edge.[16]

The meaning of Hamlet's remark becomes clear—and consistent with his previous sexual-verbal attacks on Ophelia—if we read "edge" to mean "erection." Indeed, Shakespeare used the same metaphor in *Cymbeline*, when Imogen apostrophizes her faithless husband:

> . . . and I grieve myself
> To think, when thou shalt be disedg'd by her
> That now thou tirest on, how the memory
> Will then be pang'd by me.[17]

It is again invoked when Cressida, a notorious sharpener of men's sexual appetites, is addressed as a "whetstone." [18] And the whole cluster of images is brought together in the closing couplet of Sonnet 95, which deals with the very palpable perils associated with physical love:

> Take heed, dear heart, of this large privilege;
> The hardest knife ill-used doth lose his edge.[19]

Through an odd oversight, Eric Partridge in his *Shakespeare's Bawdy* does not mention "knife" as a metaphor for penis, although he does list forty-five others, from the commonplace "pike," "yard," "lance," and "tool" to the more fanciful "potato-finger," [20] "holy-thistle," [21] "poperin pear," [22] and "three-inch fool." [23]

Both Partridge and E. A. M. Colman [24] have identified a vast number of Shakespearean expressions for the act of fucking, from the time-honored "making a beast with two backs" [25] to the unusual but graphic "filling a bottle with a tundish." [26] * Breaking them down into groups, Partridge comments that by far the largest number indicate the act as seen from the man's point of view—"terms which state or imply a man's deliberate siege of, or assault upon, a woman's powers of sexual resistance." [27] Among the female-oriented expressions—"dance with one's heels," [28] "put a man in one's belly," [29] "wag one's tail" [30]—he notes "the immemorial hypocrisy, the centuried fiction, that women *give* themselves, or *yield* their bodies to

---

* A tundish is, according to the OED, a "shallow vessel with a tube at the bottom," i.e., a funnel.

men: a fiction extremely insulting to women, for it makes them poor, insentient creatures, the mere puppet-victims of men's lust." [31]

Another of Shakespeare's well-known puns is his invention, in *The Merry Wives of Windsor*, of the "focative" case—the closest he ever ventured to the four-letter expunged word itself. The scene finds Parson Evans questioning young William Page about his knowledge of Latin, as Mistress Quickly listens in and interrupts:

> EVANS: Nominativo, hig, hag, hog; pray you, mark: genitivo, hujus. Well, what is your accusative case?
>
> WILLIAM: Accusativo, hinc.
>
> EVANS: I pray you, have your remembrance, child; accusativo, hung, hang, hog.
>
> QUICKLY: "Hang hog" is Latin for bacon, I warrant you.
>
> EVANS: Leave your prabbles, 'oman. What is the focative case, William?
>
> WILLIAM: O, vocativo, O.
>
> EVANS: Remember, William; focative is caret.
>
> QUICKLY: And that's a good root. [32]

"Caret" is a pun on "carrot," an obvious reference to the penis, as is Mistress Quickly's "good root." There is more sexual punning:

> EVANS: What is your genitive case plural, William?
>
> WILLIAM: Genitive case?
>
> EVANS: Ay.
>
> WILLIAM: Genitive,—horum, harum, horum.
>
> QUICKLY: Vengeance of Jenny's case! fie on her! never name her, child, if she be a whore.
>
> EVANS: For shame, 'oman!
>
> QUICKLY: You do ill to teach the child such words: he teaches him to hick and to hack, which they'll do fast enough of themselves, and to call "horum": fie upon you!

And then the interrogation turns to pronouns:

> EVANS: Show me now, William, some declensions of your pronouns.
>
> WILLIAM: Forsooth, I have forgot.
>
> EVANS: It is qui, quae, quod; if you forget your "quies," your "quaes" and your "quods," you must be preeches.*

---

* "Preeches," according to the glossary in the Modern Library edition of the *Comedies of William Shakespeare*, means "breeched for flogging."

It is necessary to remember, as Professor Colman points out, that the Elizabethan initial *qu* was frequently pronounced as a *k* in the Continental manner—as in the French *quiche* and the Spanish *quiero*. The three words "quies," "quaes," and "quods" thus become "keys," "case," and "cods," and, metaphorically, "penis," "vagina," and "testicles." "Cods," as in codpiece, is self-evident. 'Case" is similarly used elsewhere in Shakespeare and other Elizabethan writings, frequently in contexts of sheathing a sword. The metaphorical use of a key for a penis has an even longer lineage. Chaucer's word for "fuck" was "swyve," which is related to the English "swivel" and the Italian *chiavare*, which means "to turn a key in a lock." [33] In all of them, insertion followed by a circular—a screwing—motion is implied.

But if *qu* is to be pronounced as *k*, then the word "quondam," which appears several times in Shakespeare, deserves a closer look. In *Troilus and Cressida*, for instance, Hector says to Menelaus:

> O, you, my lord? by Mars his gauntlet, thanks,
> Mock not, that I affect th'untraded oath
> Your quondam wife swears still by Venus' glove:
> She's well, but bade me not commend her to you.[34]

The juxtaposition of "gauntlet," "quondam"—which is to say, "condom"—and "Venus' glove" is too much to be a coincidence. Not only does the metaphor fit—like a glove, one might say—but the earliest descriptions of condoms report them as being made of "soft and seamless hides." [35]

Menelaus' response to the speech quoted just above is: "Name her not now, sir; she's a deadly theme." The lady in question, Menelaus's quondam wife, is, of course, Helen, the cause for the tragedy of the Trojan Wars. That is "deadly theme" enough, but in the context to condoms can one not suppose that Shakespeare is alluding as well to another theme, as deadly and far more imminent in the minds of members of his audience—venereal disease?

The quondam-condom pun is developed more fully in *Henry V* when Pistol berates Corporal Nym:

> . . . I thee defy again.
> O hound of Crete, think'st thou my spouse to get?
> No; to the spital go,
> And from the powdering-tub of infamy

> Fetch forth the lazar kite of Cressid's kind,
> Doll Tearsheet she by name, and her espouse:
> I have, and I will hold, the quondam Quickly
> For the only she; and—pauca, there's enough.[36]

The "spital" is a hospital, and the "powdering-tub" was a hot salt-water bath used, ineffectually, in the treatment of venereal disease. Doll Tearsheet, whom the audience had met in *Henry IV*, Part 2, is a pox-infected whore. Pistol is urging Nym to marry her. As for himself, he is safe enough because he is already married to the former (quondam-condom) Mistress Quickly.

It is not likely that Shakespeare, as he was putting speeches into the mouths of his characters, was mindful to provide grist for unborn generations of doctoral candidates. However convoluted these phallic wordplays may sound today, it must be assumed that they were not lost on his audiences. Shakespeare was not only the most gifted but also, by all accounts, one of the most popular playwrights of his day.

There is also to be found in his work evidence of phallic preoccupation on a far more profound level. Freud himself, early in his career, pointed to its presence in the greatest of the Shakespearean plays:

> The play is based upon Hamlet's hesitation in accomplishing the task of revenge assigned to him; the text does not give the cause or the motive of this hesitation, nor have the manifold attempts at interpretation succeeded in doing so! According to the still prevailing conception . . . Hamlet represents the type of man whose active energy is paralyzed by excessive intellectual energy: "Sicklied o'er with the pale cast of thought." According to another conception, the poet has endeavored to portray a morbid, irresolute character, on the verge of neurasthenia. The plot of the drama, however, shows us that Hamlet is by no means intended to appear as a character wholly incapable of action. On two separate occasions we see him assert himself: once in a sudden burst of rage, when he stabs the eavesdropper behind the arras, and on the other occasion when he deliberately, and even craftily, with the complete unscrupulousness of a Prince of the Renaissance, sends the two courtiers to the death which was intended for himself. What is it, then, that inhibits him in accomplishing the task which his father's ghost has laid upon him? [37]

Ernest Jones answered this question in an essay which has become a classic of literary interpretation. He notes that Hamlet is himself bitterly aware of his inability to bring himself to kill Claudius:

> . . . Now, whether it be
> Bestial oblivion, or some craven scruple
> Of thinking too precisely on the event,
> A thought, which, quarter'd, hath but one part wisdom,
> And ever three parts coward, I do not know
> Why yet I live to say "This thing's to do;"
> Sith I have cause and will and strength and means
> To do't.[38]

Using clinical observation as his basis, Jones then points out:

> . . . whenever a person cannot bring himself to do something that every conscious consideration tells him he should do —and which he may have the strongest conscious desire to do— it is always because there is some hidden reason why a part of him doesn't want to do it; this reason he will not own to himself and is only dimly if at all aware of. That is exactly the case with Hamlet. Time and again he works himself up, points out to himself his obvious duty, with the cruellest self-reproaches lashes himself to agonies of remorse—and once more falls away into inaction.[39]

But why? Because Claudius's crime corresponds to what psychoanalysis identifies as the wish common to every male child—to eliminate his father and possess his mother. As Jones writes: "The call of duty to kill his stepfather cannot be obeyed because it links itself with the unconscious call of his nature to kill his mother's husband, whether this is the first or second [husband]; the absolute repression of the former impulse involves the inner prohibition of the latter also." [40] Were Hamlet to punish Claudius for murdering his father and marrying his mother, he would have to punish himself as well, for that is exactly what he himself unconsciously wished to do. Therefore, he delays, and agonizes. Furthermore, the wish in question is unconscious in all of us, and that is why the critics could not say why Hamlet delays.

There is ample evidence, within the play, of both Hamlet's oedipal stirrings and of Gertrude's seductive sensualness toward him. Even Claudius notices that "the Queen his mother lives almost by his looks." [41] The closet scene, which is the play's major confrontation between mother and son, reeks with explicit sexuality.* ("Let the bloat king tempt you again to bed;/Pinch wanton on your cheek; call you his mouse;/And let him, for a pair of reechy kisses,/Or paddling in your neck with his damn'd fingers,/Make you to ravel all this matter out. . . ." [42]

Jones suggests that Hamlet's courtship of Ophelia at least in part "originated not so much in direct attraction for Ophelia as in an unconscious desire to play her off against his mother, just as a disappointed and piqued lover so often has resort to the arms of a more willing rival." Commenting on the part of the play scene which was quoted above, Jones says:

> When . . . he replies to his mother's request to sit by her with the words "No, good mother, here's metal more attractive" and proceeds to lie at Ophelia's feet, we seem to have a direct indication of this attitude; and his coarse familiarity and bandying of ambiguous jests with the woman he has recently so ruthlessly jilted are hardly intelligible unless we bear in mind that they were carried out under the heedful gaze of the Queen. It is as if his unconscious were trying to convey to her the following thought: "You give yourself to other men whom you prefer to me. Let me assure you that I can dispense with your favor and even prefer those of a woman whom I no longer love." His extraordinary outburst of bawdiness on this occasion, so unexpected in a man of obviously fine feeling, points unequivocally to the sexual nature of the underlying turmoil. [43]

As for the play itself, Norman Holland in his *Psychoanalysis and Shakespeare* makes this final observation:

> We in the audience once went through an oedipal crisis, and now we find in Hamlet's echoes of our own. In effect we are projecting our own inner feelings about parents into the play and then "finding" them there, as indeed Hamlet himself does. Perhaps then, as Freud suggested at the outset, this is the secret of the universal appeal of the tragedy; it deals with a universal cluster of impulses, the oedipus complex. But we can add some-

---

* As played in the Laurence Olivier filmed version of *Hamlet*, which leans heavily on the Freud-Jones interpretation, it is more a steamy love scene than a filial conversation.

thing to Freud from modern ego psychology. The play deals
with the universal oedipus complex, but then the play—itself
so much concerned with "play"—provides us out of its very own
being with a defense or adaptation: we in the audience "play"
that the impulses are not those inside us but those we find in
the external reality of the play before us. We do indeed bear
Hamlet to the stage, and there, the play's the thing that catches
the conscience of us all.[44]

The story which gives the Oedipus complex its name was told by
Sophocles in his *Oedipus Rex*: Thebes having been stricken by a
plague, the people ask their king, Oedipus, to deliver them from its
horrors. The oracles say that the plague is punishment for the murder of Laius, Oedipus's predecessor and the late husband of Jocasta.
Oedipus, who is now married to Jocasta, swears to find the culprit
but eventually discovers that he himself is not only the unwitting
murderer of Laius but also his son—and, therefore, the husband of
his own mother. Horror-stricken, he rushes into the palace to discover that Jocasta, who has also learned the truth, has hanged herself. He seizes the golden brooches from her garments and, in what
Sandor Ferenczi first pointed out is an act of symbolic castration,
stabs out his eyeballs.

Early in his elaboration of the unconscious mind and the dynamics
of personality, Freud seized upon the Sophoclean story as central to
his theory of repression: "I have found love of the mother and
jealousy of the father in my own case, too, and now believe it to be
a general phenomenon of early childhood." [45] In oversimplified
terms, as the sexual urge of the young boy increases, he develops an
erotic attachment to his mother and begins to see his father as the
formidable rival for her undivided love and attention. What pre-
vents him from acting out his desire is fear of punishment—and,
specifically, fear of castration—at the hands of the father. As a result
of this anxiety, he represses both his incestuous desire for the mother
and his hostility toward the father. Thus, the complex weakens and
eventually disappears, giving rise in its place to the formation of the
superego.

Whether this renunciation actually takes place—indeed, whether
castration anxiety, the Oedipus complex, and even the id, ego, and
superego actually exist—is questioned in varying degree by non-
Freudian schools of psychology. Evidence from projective experi-

ments and cross-cultural anthropological studies has been advanced, sometimes with more heat than light, to prove and disprove their existence.[46] Some of the most persuasive arguments in favor of the Freudian position come from clinical evidence—case histories of patients who seemed to behave *as if* they suffered from castration fears or unresolved oedipal conflicts. But perhaps the most telling point is, as in the case of explaining Hamlet's behavior, a negative one: No other explanation satisfies the observable facts.

Furthermore, whether it exists or not, something very much like an oedipal triangle seems to bubble up again and again in literature, both before and after Freud gave it a name. In the foreword to *Green Hills of Africa*, Ernest Hemingway warns:

> Unlike many novels, none of the characters or incidents in this book is imaginary. Anyone not finding sufficient love interest is at liberty, while reading it, to insert whatever love interest he or she may have at the time. The writer has attempted to write an absolutely true book to see whether the shape of a country and the pattern of a month's action can, if truly presented, compete with a work of the imagination.[47]

The month's action consists of big-game hunting in East Africa. The principal characters are Hemingway himself, on the trail of a greater kudu, a professional white hunter named Jackson Phillips, who is, throughout the book, referred to as Pop, and Hemingway's second wife—Pauline Pfeiffer—who is never referred to by name, but only as P.O.M.—Poor Old Mama. Her attitude toward the hunter is stated early in the narrative:

> . . . danger was in the hands of Pop, and for Pop she had a complete, clear-seeing, absolutely trusting adoration. Pop was her ideal of how a man should be, brave, gentle, comic, never losing his temper, never bragging, never complaining except in a joke, tolerant, understanding, intelligent, drinking a little too much as a good man should, and, to her eyes, very handsome. "Don't you think Pop's handsome?" . . . "Hell, no. I like him as well as any man I've ever known, but I'm damned if he's handsome." "I think he's lovely looking. But you understand how I feel about him, don't you?" "Sure, I'm fond of the bastard myself." "But *don't* you think he's handsome, really?" "Nope." [48]

The hunt does not go well, and Hemingway decides to try a solitary track. Poor Old Mama solicitously packs his gear and reminds him to take along some clean handkerchiefs. Pop gives him some paternal advice. As Hemingway sets off, "I looked back as we went down the hill and saw the two figures, that tall thick one and the small neat one, each wearing big Stetson hats, silhouetted on the road as they walked back toward camp, then I looked ahead at the dried-up scrubby plain." [49]

The hunt is successful, and Hemingway returns to the camp with his trophy horns:

> Then as we came to where our lights shone on the green tents I shouted and we all commenced to shout and blew the Klaxon and I let the gun off, the flame cutting up into the darkness and it making a great noise. Then we were stopped and out from Pop's tent I saw him coming, thick and heavy in his dressing gown, and then he had his arms around my shoulders and said, "You god damned bull fighter," and I was clapping him on the back.
>
> And I said, "Look at them, Pop."
>
> "I saw them," he said. "The whole back of the car is full of them."
>
> Then I was holding P.O.M. tight, she feeling very small inside the quilted bigness of the dressing gown, and we were saying things to each other.[50]

The conquering hero returns. But this is a Hemingway story, so it is not surprising that another member of the safari party—a rival sibling?—has gone off on his own and brought back a still more imposing kudu.

Green Hills of Africa ends with the writer and his wife having lunch in Haifa and reminiscing about their trip:

> "You know," P.O.M. said, "I can't remember it. I can't remember Mr. J. P.'s face. And he's beautiful. I think about him and I can't see him. It's terrible. He isn't the way he looks in a photograph. In a little while I won't be able to remember him at all. Already I can't see him."
>
> "I can remember him," I said, "I'll write you a piece some time and put him in." [51]

The piece, which Hemingway wrote a year later and about which more will be said, was "The Short Happy Life of Francis Macomber."

The oedipal theme, expressed only slightly less explicitly, also provides the central theme of Ken Kesey's *One Flew over the Cuckoo's Nest*, as Ruth Sullivan has pointed out.[52] Nurse Ratched is the mother figure, a threatening figure this time, against which her sons—the inmates of the asylum—attempt to define their manliness. She is described as being "just like a mother" and "that smiling flour-faced old mother." One of the inmates believes in "that tender little mother crap," another observes that "we are victims of a matriarchy here, my friend," and another says that "man has but one truly effective weapon against that juggernaut of modern matriarchy." The weapon is rape, and the threat it is invoked against is castration. "There's not a man here that isn't afraid he is losing or has already lost his whambam." . . . "We comical little creatures can't even achieve masculinity in the rabbit world, that's how weak and inadequate we are." One of the inmates even makes the analogy to a different kind of diminishing surgical procedure: "Yes, chopping away the brain. Frontalobe castration. I guess if she can't cut below the belt she'll do it above the eyes."

The "Big Daddy" to Nurse Ratched's "Big Mama" is represented by Randall McMurphy. He appears on the sceen "like the logger . . . the swaggering gambler . . . the cowboy out of the TV set. . . ." One of the inmates, Chief Bromden, compares him to his own father: "He's as broad as Papa was tall . . . and he's hard in a different kind of way from Papa." He tries to kindle the inmates' flickering manliness by encouraging manly pursuits such as gambling, deep-sea fishing, sexual play with willing girls.

But Kesey is not so much interested in sex as he is in power: "So I'm saying five bucks to each of you that wants it I can't put a betsy bug up that nurse's butt within a week. . . . Just that. A bee in her butt, a burr in her bloomers. Get her goat." This is a wish not for conquest, but for control. Appropriately the central symbolic act of the novel is the destruction of the asylum's control panel.

In her detailed analysis of the book Ruth Sullivan suggests a possible reason for its enduring popularity as an "underground" classic:

> *Cuckoo's Nest* is gratifying especially to the young then, because while on the one hand it creates an anxiety-ridden phantasy about a destructive mother (and social order), it allays it

by creating a powerful, caring father. It also grants indulgences in certain unconscious needs and wishes to be dependent, to feel unjustly treated . . . and to attack and defeat ambivalently-held authority figures (even McMurphy is killed). . . .

The theme of *Cuckoo's Nest* is not merely the assertion that society will get you. It also realistically affirms that if society gets you, it is because you have complied in both your own and others' destruction. The weak are tyrants, too, subtle and dangerous because they can wake in the strong a sympathetic identification and perhaps guilt.

Oedipal problems and their various possible resolutions underlie many of our most familiar children's fairy tales. Indeed, as Bruno Bettelheim demonstrates convincingly in *The Uses of Enchantment*, this may be their most valuable function:

By dealing with universal human problems, particularly those which preoccupy the child's mind, these stories speak to his budding ego and encourage its development, while at the same time relieving preconscious and unconscious pressures. As these stories unfold, they give conscious credence and body to id pressures and show ways to satisfy those that are in line with ego and superego requirements. . . . They speak about his severe inner pressures in a way that the child unconsciously understands, and—without belittling the most serious inner struggles which growing up entails—offer examples of both temporary and permanent solutions to pressing difficulties.[53]

Thus, in "Jack and the Beanstalk":

. . . the phallic beanstalk permits Jack to engage in oedipal conflict with the ogre—the oedipal father—which he survives and finally wins thanks only to the oedipal mother's taking his side against her husband. But at the same time, Jack relinquishes his reliance on the belief in the power of self-assertion as he cuts down the beanstalk; and this opens the way toward a development of mature masculinity.[54]

In the classic tragedy of Oedipus, the first victim to suffer is not Oedipus, or even Jocasta, but Laius, whose fear that his son will someday replace him causes him to banish Oedipus and thus to set in motion the events that undo them all. "Snow White" describes

how a parent can be destroyed by its jealousy for a child. Bettelheim writes:

> In general, the less a person has been able to resolve his
> oedipal feelings constructively, the greater the danger that he
> may be beset by them again when he becomes a parent. . . .
> Nor does the child's unconsciousness fail to respond to such
> feelings in a parent, if they are part of his relation to his child.
> The fairy story permits the child to comprehend that not only
> is he jealous of his parent, but that the parent may have parallel
> feelings—an insight that can not only help to bridge the gap
> between parent and child but may permit dealing construc-
> tively with difficulties in relating which otherwise would not be
> accessible to resolution.[55]

The basic theme of "Goldilocks and the Three Bears," Bettelheim
suggests, is the child's search for identity: "Through his relations to
his parents and siblings, the child must learn with whom he ought
to identify as he grows up, and who is suitable to become his life's
companion, and with it also his sexual partner."[56] The voyage of
self-discovery begins, he points out, with Goldilocks trying to peek
into the bears' house. "This evokes associations to the child's desire
to find out the sexual secrets of adults in general, and of the parents in particular." Very quickly, she learns that Father's porridge
is "too hot" and his chair "too hard." Male identity or intimacy is
not suitable. So "Goldilocks, like every girl experiencing deep
oedipal disappointment in the father, turns back to the original
relation to the mother." But this is no better. What had once been
a warm relationship is now comfortless—the porridge is too cold.
The mother's chair is too soft—an unwelcome envelopment, once
comforting but now too suffocating. What is left are Baby Bear's
things, and they seem "just right," but then, as she sits in his chair,
the bottom falls to the ground, and she along with it. Remaining a
child forever is no solution either.

The use, conscious or unconscious, of the oedipal situation in fiction, poetry, and drama is too extensive for even cursory summary,
particularly as documentation often requires extensive textual cita-
tion. Under "oedipal conflict" or "oedipus complex," Norman Kiell's
Psychoanalysis, Psychology and Literature, a Bibliography, lists 129
entries, referring to the work of authors such as Sherwood Anderson,
Byron, Dickens, Kafka, Melville, O'Neill, Proust, Coleridge, W. S.

Gilbert, Swinburne, Jane Austen, J. M. Barrie, the Brontës, Dostoyevsky, Gide, Samuel Johnson, Rossetti, Rousseau, and Ruskin.
The list was published in 1963 and is anything but exhaustive.*
Furthermore, it does not include significant isolated allusions which
set a pattern that is then echoed throughout the works, as for instance at the beginning of *Portrait of the Artist as a Young Man*
when young Stephen indulges in a six-year-old's fantasy and is
warned:

> —O Stephen will apologize.
> Dante said;
> —O, if not, the eagles will come
> and pull out his eyes,
> Apologise,
> Apologise,
> Pull out his eyes.[57]

Some critics have looked for the oedipal elements in unlikely
places and found them. Anne Fremantle cites Jacobus de Voragine's
The Golden Legend, an early devotional collection of religious
stories, one for each day of the year.[58] For February 24, it tells the
story of a young man named Reuben, whose wife, Ciborea, dreamed
one night after they had intercourse that she would from this act
bear a son "so evil that he would be the downfall of our race."
When, nine months later, she did beget a male child, the parents,
fearful, yet not willing to kill the child, put him in a little basket
and set it on the Jordan River. Rescued, the child was given the
name Judas, and grew up and in time came to Jerusalem, where he
became a friend of Pontius Pilate. One night Judas was robbing an
orchard of its apples when the owner, who was, in fact, Judas's real
father, surprised him. In the fight which ensued, Judas killed the
older man. Rather than punish him, however, Pontius Pilate
awarded him not only the dead man's garden but his widow as well.
When the truth of what he had done finally struck Judas, he ran
away and sought out Jesus, who was preaching the forgiveness of sins.

---

* The oedipal-incest motif is the subject of many of the articles collected in
Art & Psychoanalysis, edited by William Phillips (New York: 1957), and *Hidden
Patterns,* edited by Leonard and Eleanor Manheim (New York: 1966). An
oedipal reading of Conrad, especially *Heart of Darkness,* appears in *Out of My
System* by Frederick Crews (New York: 1975). D. H. Lawrence is treated in
Oedipus in Nottingham: D. H. Lawrence by Daniel A. Weiss (Seattle: 1962).

What he did later, of course, is better known. Jacobus de Voragine, who either invented or collected this story about the most perfidious of human beings, was born in 1298, long before Freud.

Weston La Barre has proposed that oedipal stirrings are often brought to light in "relaxed social situations which would be comparable to the materials obtainable through the psychoanalytic 'free association' method." [59] What he had in mind are bawdy drinking songs and limericks of the kind which are likely to surface "when the superego is liquidated in ordinary social drinking of a definable sort, when fantasies, wishes and typical anxieties break through the barriers imposed by the psychic censor somewhat." He notes that one aspect of the unresolved Oedipus conflict is a lack of adjustment to authority, often expressed in sexual terms as in the limerick about the monk from Siberia.* Another aspect is the grave fear of castration, which is projected in the numerous limericks, such as the one about the young lady of Baroda,† which deal with phallic injury.

Another writer, George Frumkes, has noted the recurrence of the oedipal theme in opera, where a cue to the roles of the participants is furnished by their voices: bass or baritone for father, soprano and occasionally alto for mother, and tenor for son.[60] And finally, Richard Sterba, possibly writing with just the tip of his tongue in his cheek, offers an example which should be familiar to anyone old enough to have participated in World War II. It is the ubiquitous Kilroy, whose stylized little face peering over a wall appeared, along with the simple statement "Kilroy was here," in the most unimaginable places where some GIs had contrived to crawl, climb, or sneak. Sterba says:

> If the name is cut in two—Kill Roi (Kill the King)—it is obvious that he is the one who killed the king and this is well-known analytic material and territory. . . . In the unconscious the enemy in war is identical with the father figure as the little boy experiences him in the Oedipus phase of his libido devel-

---

* There was a young monk from Siberia
Who of frigging grew wearier and wearier.
At last with a yell, he burst out of his cell
And buggered the Mother Superior.

† There was a young girl of Baroda
Who built a new kind of pagoda
The walls of its halls were hung with the balls
Of all the young fools that bestrode her.

opment. The Kilroy legend confirms the symbolic significance of the enemy as the Oedipal father, and the locality possessed by him as the Oedipal mother. Kilroy's inscription is supposed to be found in the most inaccessible places. It is this inaccessibility of a place which gives it mother significance in the unconscious in accordance with the emotionally frustrating situation of the little boy in the Oedipus phase. Kilroy's presence in all inaccessible places is the expression of a grandiose fulfillment of the Oedipal wish. If Kilroy is the murderer of his father, the oversized nose-penis is his privilege and fruits of his deed.[61]

D. H. Lawrence has always caused a certain amount of discomfort to women critics. Sigrid Undset writes:

> Lawrence is seldom convincing when he tries to force the creatures born of his fancy to realize his own gospel of a new and savage kind of abandonment . . . [He] dreamed of a sexual act in which the individuals die from their old ego and are reborn to a new life, each as a master of his own soul, but united with his mate in profound tenderness, saved from all lust of power involved in sexual feeling, cleansed of all the elements of petty vanity which are a part of all erotics, but with their manly or womanly self-consciousness intensified. It was something of this sort that he wished to believe in. But the people who live in his books are in everlasting revolt against his new religion—irreclaimably timid, bitter and suspicious men and women who are incapable of abandoning themselves to another human being without regretting it and immediately trying to recover themselves.[62]

Writing in 1930, the year of Lawrence's death, V. Sackville-West concluded: "One is never quite sure of what Lawrence meant; one doubts whether Lawrence himself was quite clearly sure; one is certain only that behind Lawrence's huge muddles and mistakes lay a most desperate conviction." [63]

If such uncertainty does exist, the blame for it can hardly be charged to Lawrence himself. His views on one of the sexes are expressed fairly clearly in an essay entitled "Cocksure Women and Hensure Men," published in 1928:

> It is the tragedy of the modern woman. . . . She is cock-

sure, but she is a hen all the time. Frightened of her own henny self, she rushes to mad lengths about votes, or welfare, or sports, or business: she is marvellous, out-manning the man. But, alas, it is all fundamentally disconnected. It is all an attitude, and one day the attitude will become a weird cramp, a pain, and then it will collapse. And, when it has collapsed, and she looks at the eggs she has laid, votes, or miles of typewriting, years of business efficiency—suddenly, because she is a hen and not a cock, all she has done will turn into pure nothingness to her. Suddenly it all falls out of relation to her basic henny self, and she realizes she has lost her life.[64]

Speaking of the other sex, in "A Propos of Lady Chatterley," Lawrence has this to say:

The blood of man and the blood of woman are two eternally different streams, that can never be mingled. Even scientifically we know it. But therefore they are two rivers that encircle the whole of life, and in marriage the circle is complete, and in sex the two rivers touch and renew one another, without ever commingling or confusing. We know it. The phallus is a column of blood that fills the valley of blood of a woman. The great river of male blood touches to its depths the great river of female blood—yet neither breaks the bounds. It is the deepest of all communions, as all the religions, in practise, know. . . . And the phallus is the connecting-link between the two rivers, that establishes the two streams in a oneness, and gives out of their duality a single circuit, forever.[65]

And, farther on in the same essay: "If England is to be regenerated . . . then it will be by the arising of a new blood-contact, a new touch, a new marriage. It will be a phallic rather than a sexual regeneration. For the phallus is only the great old symbol of godly vitality in a man, and of immediate contact."[66]

One may begin to infer from all this that it is Lawrence himself who is far from cocksure—who is, in fact, fearful of the power of women—and that the phallus he brandishes is not so much a mighty weapon as a hopeful talisman. "He wants," wrote Eliseo Vivas, "men once more to approach the fulfillment of their sensual passion in an attitude of reverence for the sacred Dark God, the ithyphallic *membrum virile erectus,* of the first religions." [67]

Among those religions, one which deeply affected Lawrence, and which he wrote about with eloquence and sympathy, was that of the Etruscans: "The Etruscan element is like the grass in the field and the sprouting of corn, in Italy: it will always be so." [68] And elsewhere: "That was a nice thing about the Etruscans, there was a phallic symbol everywhere, so everybody was used to it, and they no doubt offered it small offerings, as the source of inspiration." [69]

During the years when he was living in Italy and working on the three successive versions of what eventually became *Lady Chatterley's Lover*, his letters reveal the turn of his mind. "As for my novel, it's half done, but so improper you wouldn't dare to touch it. . . . It's a declaration of the phallic reality." [70] "Of course the book *isn't* improper, but it *is* phallic. . . . And the phallic reality is what one must fight for!" [71] "It is a nice and tender phallic novel—not a sex novel in the ordinary sense of the word. . . . But anyhow, you know it's quite sincere, and that I sincerely believe in restoring the other, the phallic consciousness, into our lives: because it is the source of all real beauty." [72] *

That *Lady Chatterley's Lover* is a "phallic novel" is undeniable. The title which Lawrence had chosen for one of its earlier versions was *John Thomas and Lady Jane*. As indicated in the passage quoted at the beginning of this section, John Thomas is the name Oliver Mellors uses to address a distinctive part of his body. Had Lawrence retained the title, the book would have had the rare distinction of having, as its eponymous hero, a penis.

But *Lady Chatterley's Lover* is, as Edmund Wilson pointed out in his original review of it in the *New Republic*,[73] also a parable of postwar England. "The cataclysm happened, we are among the ruins . . ." [74] runs the second sentence in the book. It is also very much of a piece with Lawrence's earlier novels, dealing with the intrusion of mechanization, the inability of people to touch each

* The same preoccupation affected Lawrence's other artistic activity: painting. In a letter dating to the same period, he writes: "I stick to what I told you, and put a phallus, a lingam you call it, in each one of my pictures somewhere . . . I do this out of a positive belief, that the phallus is a great sacred image: it represents a deep, deep life which has been denied in us all, and still is denied. Women deny it horribly, with a grinning travesty of sex." This letter, to Lawrence's Buddhist friend E. H. Brewster, was dated February 27, 1927. On June 12, 1929, an exhibition of Lawrence's paintings opened at the Warren Gallery in London. Evidently it contained some of the pictures Lawrence had referred to in his letter because it was closed by the police on July 5.

other, the prevalence of self-destruction. What is different about it, not to mince words, is the fucking. It is described explicitly, of course, which occasioned the original furor over the book. But it is also described in the manner of communiqués in a running account of combat and conquest.

We are, for instance, told almost immediately after being introduced to Constance Chatterley—"A ruddy, country-looking girl with soft brown hair and sturdy body, and slow movements, full of unusual energy" [75]—that as a girl of fifteen she had been sent to Dresden, "for music among other things." There she and her sister, Hilda, had "talked so passionately and sung so lustily" and "had given the gift of themselves, each to the youth with whom she had the most subtle and intimate arguments." [76] But even as she was dispensing this generosity, she was learning that a "woman could take a man without really giving herself away. Certainly she could take him without giving herself into his power. Rather, she could use this sex thing to have power over him. For she only had to hold herself back in sexual intercourse, and let him finish and expend himself without her coming to the crisis: and then she could prolong the connection and achieve her orgasm and her crisis while he was merely her tool." [77]

Constance is married to Sir Clifford Chatterley, a young landowner from the Midlands coal-mining country who has been rendered useless from the waist down by a war wound. He occupies himself by writing short stories—"clever, rather spiteful, and yet, in some mysterious way, meaningless"—and by applying himself to the modernization of his collieries. Life at Wragby Hall, the family seat, consists of long, empty days and even longer evenings of rambling, pseudobright talk with visitors from London and abroad. "Time went on as the clock does, half-past eight instead of half-past seven."

Because he wants an heir to succeed him and cannot himself produce one, Chatterley has made it clear to his wife that he would accept an illegitimate child. At the same time her father notices that she is becoming thin and angular and urges her not to wither into a *demivierge*—"Why don't you get yourself a beau, Connie? Do you all the good in the world." [78] To satisfy both of them, she drifts into an affair with a young and successful Irish playwright named Michaelis who comes to spend a weekend at Wragby Hall. Unfortunately he turns out to have a predisposition to premature ejaculation: "He was the trembling excited sort of lover, whose crisis soon came, and was finished." But Connie knows what to do:

> . . . she soon learnt to hold him, to keep him there inside of her when his crisis was over. And there he was generous and curiously potent; he stayed firm inside her, given to her, while she was still active . . . wildly, passionately active, coming to her own crisis. And as he felt the frenzy of her achieving her own orgasmic satisfaction from his hard, erect passivity, he had a curious sense of pride and satisfaction.[79]

But the satisfaction is evidently short-lived because after a few nights of such calisthenics he turns on her:

> When at last he drew away from her, he said, in a bitter, almost sneering little voice: "You couldn't go off at the same time as a man, could you? You'd have to grind yourself off! You'd have to run the show!"
>
> "What do you mean?" she said.
>
> "You know what I mean. You keep on for hours after I've gone off . . . and I have to hang on with my teeth till you bring yourself off by your own exertions." [80]

One day, in the course of bringing him a message from her husband, Connie happens upon the estate's gamekeeper:

> He was naked to his hips, his velveteen breeches slipping down over his slender loins. And his white slim back was curved over a big bowl of soapy water, in which he ducked his head with a queer, quick little motion, lifting his slender white arms, and pressing the soapy water from his ears, quick, subtle as a weasel playing with water, and utterly alone.

The experience "hit her in the middle of her body." "She saw the clumsy breeches slipping down over the pure, delicate white loins, the bones showing a little, and the sense of aloneness, of a creature purely alone, overwhelmed her." [81]

The gamekeeper, Oliver Mellors, is a collier's son who has managed to escape the mines by joining the army, where, unusual for a man of his class, he earned a commission. Poor health, however, and a sense of restlessness caused him to resign and return home, to a job on the Chatterley estate. After her first visit, Connie takes to returning to the Mellors hut, ostensibly to observe some pheasant hens which he has set out to nest. Finally, the eggs hatch:

> She took the drab little thing between her hands, and there it stood, on its impossible little stalk of legs, its atom of balancing life trembling through its almost weightless feet into Connie's hands. But it lifted its handsome, clean-shaped little head boldly, and looked sharply round, and gave a little "peep." [82]

Connie cries; Mellors consoles her. "He laid his hand on her shoulder and softly, gently, it began to travel down the curve of her crouching loins. . . . 'Shall you come to the hut?' he said, in a quiet, neutral voice." [83]

They make love, or rather he makes love because "She lay still, in a kind of sleep, always in a kind of sleep. The activity, the orgasm, was his, all his." [84]

The next day she comes back to the hut: ". . . he sat down for a moment on the stool, and drew her to him, feeling for her body with his free hand. She heard the catch of his intaken breath as he found her. Under her frail petticoat she was naked." [85] But "when he came into her, with an intensification of relief and consummation that was pure peace to him, still she was waiting. . . . She lay still, feeling his motion within her, his deep-sunk intentness, the sudden quiver of him at the springing of his seed, then slow-subsiding thrust." [86]

Connie stays away from the hut for a few days, but is eventually drawn back. This time:

> . . . as he began to move, in the sudden helpless orgasm, there awoke in her strange thrills rippling inside her. Rippling, rippling, rippling, like a flapping overlapping of soft flames, soft as feathers, running to points of brilliance, exquisite, exquisite and melting her all molten inside. It was like bells rippling up and up to a culmination. She lay unconscious of the wild little cries she uttered at the last.[87]

Back in her own bedroom, however, Connie has second thoughts:

> She must not become a slave. . . . She had a devil of self-will in her breast that could have fought the full soft heaving adoration of her womb, and crushed it. She could even do it now, or she thought so, and she could then take up her passion with her own will.

Ah! Yes, to be passionate like a Bacchante, like a Bacchanal fleeing though the woods, to call on Iacchos, the bright phallus that had no independent personality behind it, but was pure god-servant to women! The man, the individual, let him not dare intrude. He was but a temple servant, the bearer and keeper of the bright phallus, her own.

So, in the flux of a new awakening, the old hard passion flamed in her for a time, and the man dwindled to a contempt-ible object, the mere phallus-bearer, to be torn to pieces when his service was performed.[88]

At their next encounter, she again holds back:

. . . she lay with her hands inert on his striving body, and do what she might, her spirit seemed to look on from the top of her head, and the butting of his haunches seemed ridiculous to her, and the sort of anxiety of his penis to come to its little evacuating crisis seemed farcical. . . . Cold and derisive her queer female mind stood apart, and though she lay perfectly still, her impulse was to heave her loins, and throw the man out, escape his ugly grip, and the butting overriding of his absurd haunches.

Mellors senses something wrong:

"Ay!" he said. "It was no good that time. You wasn't there." [But] as he was drawing away, to rise silently and leave her, she clung to him in terror.

"Don't! Don't go! Don't leave me! Don't be cross with me! Hold me! Hold me fast!" she whispered in blind frenzy, not even knowing what she said, and clinging to him with uncanny force. It was from herself she wanted to be saved, from her own inward anger and resistance.[89]

Mellors is right there:

He took her in his arms again and drew her to him, and suddenly she became small in his arms, small and nestling. It was gone, and she began to melt in a marvellous peace. . . . She quivered again at the potent inexorable entry inside her, so strange and terrible. It might come with a thrust of a sword in her softly opened body, and that would be death. She clung in a sudden anguish of terror. But it came with a strange slow thrust of peace, the dark thrust of peace and a ponderous primordial tenderness, such as made the world in the beginning. . . . She dared to let go everything, all herself, and be gone in a flood.[90]

So Mellors wins. But we learn that he has campaigned over this same terrain before, that he was—and indeed still is—married to an awesome woman named Bertha Coutts:

"Well, I married her, and she wasn't bad. Those other 'pure' women had taken nearly all the balls out of me, but she was all right that way. She wanted me and made no bones about it. . . . But when I had her, she'd never come off when I did. Never! She'd just wait. If I kept back for half an hour, she'd keep back longer. And when I'd come and really finished, then she'd start on her own account, and I had to stop inside her till she brought herself off, wriggling and shouting, she'd clutch with herself down there an' then she'd come off, fair in ecstasy. And then she'd say: 'That was lovely!' Gradually I got sick of it: she got worse. She sort of got harder and harder to bring off, and she'd sort of tear at me down there, as if it was a beak tearing at me. By God, you'd think a woman's soft down there like a fig. But I tell you the old rampers have beaks between their legs and they tear at you with it till you're sick." [91]

Bertha's reward for her vividly described vagina dentata was that Mellors left her when he joined the army and has not seen her since. Connie, however, is a different matter. The very next encounter with her is the occasion for the John Thomas-Lady Jane dialogue previously cited, and for this further exchange:

"John Thomas! John Thomas!" and she quickly kissed the soft penis that was beginning to stir again.

"Ay," said the man, stretching his body almost painfully. "He's got his roots in my soul, that gentleman! An' sometimes I don't know what ter do with him. Ay, he's got a will of his own, an' it's hard to suit him. Yet I wouldn't have him killed."

"No wonder men have always been afraid of him!" she said. "He's rather terrible."

The quiver was going through the man's body. . . . And he was helpless, as the penis in slow, soft undulations filled and surged and rose up, and grew hard, standing there hard and overweening, in its curious towering fashion. The woman too trembled a little as she watched.[92]

It would seem that the point has been made, but Lawrence arranges another engagement between Mellors and Connie. It is a peculiar scene because, for the first and only time in the book, the author abandons his explicit language for some carefully veiled allusions:

> It was a night of sensual passion, in which she was a little startled and almost unwilling: yet pierced again with piercing thrills of sensuality, different, sharper, more terrible than the thrills of tenderness, but at the moment more desirable. Though a little frightened, she let him have his way, and the reckless, shameless sensuality shook her to her foundation, stripped her to the very last, and made a different woman of her. It was not really love. It was not voluptuousness. It was sensuality sharp and searing as fire, burning the soul to tinder.
>
> Burning out the shames, the deepest, oldest shames, in the most secret places. It cost her an effort to let him have his way and his will of her. She had to be a passive, consenting thing, like a slave, a physical slave. . . . In the short summer night she learned so much. She would have thought a woman would have died of shame. Instead of which, the shame died. Shame, which is fear: the deep organic shame, the old, old physical fear which crouches in the bodily roots of us, and can only be chased away by the sensual fire, at last was roused up and routed by the phallic hunt of the man, and she came to the very heart of the jungle of herself. . . . And what a reckless devil the man was! Really like a devil! One had to be strong to bear him. But it took some getting at, the core of the physical jungle, the last and deepest recess of organic shame. The phallos alone could explore it. And how he had pressed it on her.[93]

Despite several clues which Lawrence left elsewhere in the narrative, it was not until thirty-three years after the publication of *Lady Chatterley's Lover* that someone finally pointed out in print that the activity described in this passage is anal intercourse.[94*]

Why Lawrence chose to retreat into discretion in this particular

* Through delicacy or oversight, the passage was not mentioned during the long, exhaustive obscenity trial of the book in London in 1960.

instance—and in a similar scene between Ursula and Birkin in *Women in Love*—is understandable. It would take a few more years before buggery, in its assorted combinations, became acceptable material for serious literary expression. Why he included the scene in the first place has been the subject of considerable critical debate.[95] Some of it makes for hard reading:

> The invasion of the genital by the excremental, the contamination of joy by shame and life by death, was a strategy for the overthrow of the last enemy. We have seen that Lawrence had earlier thought of these polarities as reconcilable only by a third force, his Holy Ghost; the phallus, its representative, will bridge the flow of dissolution and creation, which coming together in the genitalia, also come together in history, at this moment. [96]

All the critics point to the aspect of purification contained in the act. Much is made of "burning out" and of smelting "the heaviest ore of the body into purity." Mark Spilka in *The Love Ethic of D. H. Lawrence* describes it as "a purgation process, and less the norm of love than a release to full, creative life," [97] and Wilson Knight sees Lawrence trying to "blast through . . . degradation to new health." [98]

But if sodomy is the means to purification, one must wonder why Mellors does not feel the need to be purified of *his* shame and fear. Physiology presents no problem because in the scene mentioned above from *Women in Love*, Ursula kneels in front of Birkin and brings him to orgasm by exploring with her fingers at "the back of the loins" to "the quick of the mystery of darkness." In that instance, Lawrence makes his meaning clear by repeating the word "back" several times, by having Ursula say that she thought "there was no source deeper than the phallic source," and by noting that "with perfect finger tips of reality she could touch the reality in him."

If there is an act of purification in the scene, the greater likelihood is that it is Connie's mind which is being purified—cleansed of any remaining vestiges of doubt regarding phallic supremacy. Woman's awareness of the phallic mystery must include a proper awe of man. Or more precisely, the proper awe of man must be driven home by the phallus. Having swept the battlefield, Lawrence, like any conqueror, marks the fact by planting his standard.

In the short story "Fathers and Sons," Ernest Hemingway says of

Nick Adams, who, if not an autobiographical device, is at least the recurring projection for certain subjects: "If he wrote it, he could get rid of it. He had gotten rid of many things by writing them." [99]

That Hemingway was an obsessed writer who often used his craft to relieve his own psychic stresses and tension has been noted by many serious critics of his work. Hemingway himself was aware of this observation and once characteristically refuted it by describing two of those critics as "Professor Carlos Back-up . . . wearing the serious silks of Princeton who 'feeds' my collected works into the Symbol Searcher, which is a cross between a Geiger counter and a pinball machine . . ." and "Professor Philip Youngerdinger . . . wearing the serious silks of N.Y.U.," who uses an "economy-sized death wish indicator, which can also turn up complexes both certified and uncertified at the flick of the dial." [100] Nevertheless, when once asked by an interviewer for the name of his psychiatrist, he replied, "Portable Corona Number 3." [101]

One does not have to read much of what Hemingway confided to Portable Corona Number 3 to sense the pervasive unconscious hostility expressed through anxiety and its defense mechanisms. The anxiety, as will be shown, is largely sexual and not unlike that clinically associated with unresolved childhood fears. The defense mechanisms are what give Hemingway's prose and plots their distinctive style. Time and again, especially when confronted with emotional crisis, characters retreat into ritualistic gestures—the beautiful, evocative, but also repetitive and, in the end, spiritually unsatisfying descriptions of the correct way to catch a trout, pitch a tent, order a meal, fight a war. Without ritual, there is *nada*, as expressed in the prayer at the close of "A Clean Well Lighted Place:" "Our nada who art in nada, nada be thy name thy kingdom nada . . . Hail nothing full of nothing, nothing is with thee." [102]

On the other hand, strict adherence to the proper ritual is what qualifies a man as hero. The code is clear and clearly observed by all of Hemingway's unlikely heroes: the aging welterweight Jack Brennan in "Fifty Grand," who continues to fight despite his opponent's attempts to foul him; Caetano, the mortally gut-wounded gambler in "The Gambler, the Nun and the Radio," who refuses to name his assailants; Manuel Garcia, the old bullfighter in "The Undefeated"; and even Ole Andreson, who, in "The Killers," knows that he has violated the code and therefore makes no attempt to save himself from certain death.

Hemingway sums up the relationship of ritual to code as the "holding of his purity of line through the maximum of exposure." [103] The prescription could be applied to measure the worth of any of the author's stoical heroes. Appropriately, however, it was used to describe the style of Romero, the young bullfighter in *The Sun Also Rises*. Bullfighting always held a special significance for Hemingway. He devoted an entire book to the subject, as well as a number of short stories and articles. News photographs of Papa at Pamplona and other tauromachian shrines did much to generate interest among *nordeamericano* youth in what had been an alien, unfamiliar, and somewhat distasteful spectacle.

On the surface, bullfighting offers the same attractions—violence, danger, death—as other favorite Hemingway pastimes such as war and big-game hunting. But there are even more dangerous civilian occupations—there are more retired matadors than Grand Prix drivers, for instance. Bullfighting had the additional, if not the primary, attraction of being intensely erotic. The bull, as has been shown, is one of the earliest symbols of masculinity and fertility. In going out to fight him, the matador risks injury or death, but the specific part of his body which is most vulnerable is his groin. He is measuring his sexuality against that of the animal, and it is appropriate that the drama should pivot around the horns of the bull and the sword of the man. It is even more appropriate that the successful matador should be presented with the cutoff ears of the fallen bull and that he should in turn offer these trophies of a symbolic castration to the lady of his choice.* Hemingway himself once described his reaction to witnessing a bullfight as "I feel very fine while it is going on and have a feeling of life and death and mortality and immortality, and after it is over I feel very sad but very fine." [104]

These words could as well be used to describe sexual intercourse, except that there is no woman immediately involved in the *corrida*. Rather, a bullfight can be seen as the sexual conflict between two males, the more powerful of which threatens literally as well as symbolically to castrate the younger. In that sense, it is the ritual enactment of the father-son aspect of the oedipal conflict.

Castration, the central oedipal anxiety, held an abiding fascina-

---

* In *The Sun Also Rises*, the bullfighter Romero is the only one who survives sexual encounter with Brett Ashley. She in turn, as she breaks with him, leaves behind in a hotel drawer the ear which he dedicated to her.

tion for Hemingway. It is the explicit subject of the story "God Rest You Merry, Gentlemen" and a recurring theme in many others. Jake Barnes's castration—not, as Hemingway was careful to point out, his emasculation but his physical wound [105]—is central to *The Sun Also Rises*. The closing lines of the novel are:

> "Oh, Jake," Brett said, "we could have had such a damned good time together."
>
> Ahead was a mounted policeman in khaki directing traffic. He raised his baton. The car slowed suddenly pressing Brett against me.
>
> "Yes," I said, "Isn't it pretty to think so?" [106]

The whole thrust of the book requires that Jake's comment be taken as irony. To emphasize this, Hemingway has interposed the figure of the policeman between his principal characters' closing speeches. As one critic notes: "With his khaki clothes and his preventive baton, he stands for the war and the society which made it, for the force which stops the lovers' car, and which robs them of their normal sexual roles." [107] But the raised baton also represents, in the first instance, precisely that which Barnes lacks. If Hemingway had wanted only to stop traffic, the policeman could as well have used a whistle.

The castrating wound appears again in *To Have and Have Not*, when Harry Morgan tries to reassure himself: "To hell with my arm. You lose an arm you lose an arm. There's worse things to lose than an arm. You've got two arms and you've got two of something else. And a man's still a man with one arm or with one of these . . . I got those other two still." [108] Another castrating wound causes the death of Robert Jordan in *For Whom the Bell Tolls:* His leg is broken, and he is left helpless when his horse, pointedly described as a gelding, is hit and falls down on him. In *Across the River and into the Trees*, Renata's gift to Cantwell, which he keeps in his pocket as a talisman and caresses with his bad hand, is a pair of emerald stones. The celebrated story about how Scott Fitzgerald confided to Hemingway that Zelda had accused him of being inadequately endowed, and how Hemingway sought to reassure him, first by a visit to the WC and then by a stroll through the classical statuary galleries of the Louvre, may be an invention.[109] But the fact that Hemingway chose to tell it in the first place says something about his own castration anxiety.

One of the striking castration images appears in the Nick Adams story entitled "Now I Lay Me." Nick has been wounded and is lying in a makeshift hospital behind the Italian lines. Unable to sleep because "if I ever shut my eyes in the dark and let myself go, my soul would go out of my body," [110] he wills himself to think back to the earliest thing he can remember. It is:

> . . . the attic of the house where I was born . . . and, in the attic, jars of snakes and other specimens that my father had collected as a boy and preserved in alcohol, the alcohol sunken in the jars so that the backs of some of the snakes and specimens were exposed and had turned white . . . I remember, after my grandfather died we moved away from that house and to a new house designed and built by my mother. Many things that were not to be moved were burned in the back yard and I remember those jars from the attic being thrown in the fire, and how they popped in the heat and the fire flamed up from the alcohol. I remember the snakes burning in that fire in the back yard. But there were no people in that, only things. I could not remember who burned the things even. . . .[111]

Asked by an interviewer about the presence of symbolism in his writing, Hemingway once replied:

> I suppose there are symbols since critics keep finding them. If you do not mind, I dislike talking about them and being questioned about them. It is hard enough to write books and stories without being asked to explain them as well. Also, it deprives explainers of work. If five or six or more good explainers can keep going why should I interfere with them? [112]

It hardly takes five or six explainers to note that the snakes are emphatically phallic—Hemingway even helps out by specifying that they had turned white. Nor is there any question of what happened to the snakes. As for who is responsible for their destruction, Nick says he cannot remember. The blocking out of painful memories is a familiar psychic defense.

In the next paragraph—the next session with Number 3—Nick does recall:

> About the new house I remember how my mother was always cleaning things out and making a good clearance. One time when my father was away on a hunting trip she made a good

thorough cleaning out in the basement and burned everything that should not have been there. When my father came home and got down from his buggy and hitched the horse the fire was still burning in the road beside the house. . . . "What's this?" he asked.

"I've been cleaning out the basement, dear," my mother said from the porch. She was standing there smiling to meet him. . . . My father raked very carefully in the ashes. He raked out stone axes and stone skinning knives and tools for making arrowheads and pieces of pottery and many arrowheads. They had all been blackened and chipped by the fire.[113]

The mother is remembered as the betrayer. She destroys possessions important to his father, his Indian relics and, before that, the white snakes.

Even his greatest admirers concede that Hemingway is at his weakest when he tries to portray women. They turn out to be either bitches, like Brett or Margot Macomber, or pliable playthings, like Catherine Barkley, Maria, and Renata, who are little more than narcissistic extensions of their men. In "Fathers and Sons," Nick recalls his initiation into love with the Indian girl Trudy:

> Could you say she did first what no one has ever done better and mention plump brown legs, flat belly, hard little breasts, well holding arms, quick searching tongue, the flat eyes, the good taste of mouth, then uncomfortably, tightly, sweetly, moistly, lovely, tightly, achingly, fully, finally, unendingly, never-endingly, never-to-endingly, suddenly ended, the great bird flown like an owl in the twilight only it daylight in the woods and hemlock needles stuck against your belly.[114]

This was the closest the earth came to shaking for Nick Adams or for any other of Hemingway's men. As they grew older, they learned that love of women—erotic love—brought swift consequences of pain and destruction. Venereal disease appears repeatedly as the accomplice of love. Hemingway's attitude toward pregnancy, in his fiction, wavers between dread and hatred. Not inappropriately, one of his collections of stories is entitled *Men Without Women*.

But therein lies hazard as well. Few writers return as frequently, or with as much fascinated disgust, to homosexuality—both kinds of homosexuality. Lesbianism, and its castrating effect on the man, are the subject of "Sea Change" and "Mr. and Mrs. Elliot." It is implicit in Pilar's relationship to Maria. In *A Moveable Feast*, Hemingway ascribes his break with Gertrude Stein to overhearing her during a lesbian quarrel—"It was bad to hear," he says, "and the answers were worse." [115]

In one of the digressions in *Death in the Afternoon* Hemingway rails against "the prissy exhibitionistic, aunt-like, withered old maid moral arrogance of a Gide; the lazy, conceited debauchery of a Wilde who betrayed a generation; the nasty, sentimental pawing of humanity of a Whitman and all the mincing gentry." [116] Many of the stories, such as "Mother of a Queen" and "A Simple Enquiry," seem to have little point other than heaping scorn on "the mincing gentry." In *A Moveable Feast*, Hemingway recalls: "When you were a boy and moved in the company of men, you had to be prepared to kill a man, know how to do it and know that you really would do it not to be interfered with." [117] Presumably the young narrator of "The Light of the World" was prepared because when, at the end of the story, the homosexual cook asked him and his companion, "Which way are you boys going?" he can tell him, "The other way from you." [118]

Hemingway's personal aversion to homosexuality was so well publicized that when Tennessee Williams had lunch with him in Havana in 1959, he reported that the two had enoyed a most affable talk despite the stories he had heard to the effect that "Hemingway usually kicks people like me in the crotch." [119]

The phenomenon of homophobia and its roots have been discussed in a previous chapter of this book. Hemingway himself made a pertinent observation when he described a bullfighter who was too theatrical in demonstrating his courage: "It was as though he were constantly showing the quantity of hair on his chest or the way in which he was built in his more private parts." [120] *

* The sentence inspired one of the most famous fights in recent literary history. In his review of *Death in the Afternoon* which appeared in a June 1933 issue of *New Republic* under the title "Bull in the Afternoon," Max Eastman speculated that Hemingway's aggressive masculinity betrayed something less than "serene" confidence in his own manhood. "Most of us," he says, "suffer at times from that small inward doubt." In Hemingway's case, he suggests, the doubt had led to a "literary style . . . of wearing false hair on the chest."

The chancre must have gnawed because four years later, when Hemingway ran into Eastman in Max Perkins's office at Scribner's, he ripped open his shirt to display a hirsute expanse and then unbuttoned Eastman's shirt to reveal bare naked skin. Still unsatisfied, he pummeled the frailer, older Eastman to the floor.

The rituals, the code, the emasculating female, and the phallo-centric measure of valor all come together in "The Short Happy Life of Francis Macomber," the story which Hemingway promised to write at the end of *Green Hills of Africa*. The plot is familiar enough, if only because "Macomber" is one of the few Hemingway works to have survived, more or less intact, translation into film. The action opens with the Macombers and Robert Wilson, their white hunter, having a preluncheon gimlet—because, as Macomber says, "It's the thing to do" [121]—and pretending that nothing has happened. What did happen is that Macomber, after wounding a lion, panicked and ran while going in to finish it off. "It doesn't have to go any further, does it?" he asks Wilson. "I mean no one will hear about it, will they?" [122]

Wilson replies, "I'm a professional hunter. We never talk about our clients. . . . It's supposed to be bad form to ask us not to talk though." Macomber doesn't know the code. To Wilson, he is "a bloody four-letter man as well as a bloody coward." [123]

Wilson, on the other hand, is well versed in every aspect of the code:

> He, Robert Wilson, carried a double size cot on safari to ac-commodate any windfalls he might receive. He had hunted for a certain clientele, the international, fast, sporting set, where the women did not feel they were getting their money's worth unless they had shared that cot with the white hunter. He despised them when he was away from them although he liked some of them well enough at the time, but he made his living by them; and their standards were his standards as long as they were hiring him.[124]

On the night following Macomber's sorry performance, Wilson gets a chance to use his cot: "Francis Macomber, who had been asleep a little while . . . realized that his wife was not in the other cot in the tent. He lay awake with that knowledge for two hours." [125]

When Margot returns, he asks her where she has been: " 'There wasn't going to be any of that. You promised there wouldn't be.' 'Well, there is now,' she said sweetly." [126]

At breakfast, Wilson asks Macomber whether he slept well. "Did you?" Macomber asks in turn. "Topping," the white hunter re-plies.[127]

The pun is only one of several instances in which Wilson expresses his contempt of Macomber in sexual terms. He repeatedly thinks of him as a "beggar" or a "sod," both of which carry allusions of homosexuality. When Macomber refuses to go back in for the lion, Wilson looks at him and feels "as though he had opened the wrong door in a hotel and seen something shameful." [128] * At the lunch which follows the lion episode, the food served is an eland which Macomber had previously shot. "They're the big cowy things that jump like hares, aren't they?" Margot asks. "They're not dangerous, are they?" "Only if they fall on you," Wilson replies.[130]

It is clear from the story that Wilson is not the first lover Margot has taken, but the baldness of her action, coming on top of his act of cowardice, causes Macomber to change. He goes after buffalo and acquits himself well. Wilson notices the change: ". . . regardless of how it had happened it most certainly had happened. Look at the beggar now, Wilson thought. It's that some of them stay little boys so long, Wilson thought. Sometimes all their lives." [131]

Margot has noted the change, too. " 'You've gotten awfully brave, awfully suddenly,' his wife said contemptuously, but her contempt was not secure. She was very afraid of something." [132]

A few moments after voicing these sentiments, Margot shoots her husband and puts an end to his short, happy life. Virtually every critic—Edmund Wilson, André Maurois, Leslie Fiedler, Carlos Baker, Philip Young—has assumed that she meant to shoot him. The situation is as follows: Macomber has wounded a buffalo and, this time, has gone into the bush to finish him off. The animal charges, but Macomber stands his ground, shooting for the nose but "shooting a touch high each time and hitting the heavy horns, splintering and chipping them like hitting a slate roof." Meanwhile, "Mrs. Macomber, in the car, had shot at the buffalo with the 6.5 Mannlicher as it seemed about to gore Macomber and had hit her husband about two inches up and a little to one side of the base of his skull." [133]

Hemingway is, if nothing else, a man with respect for words. There is nothing in the passage just quoted to suggest that Mrs. Macomber shot at her husband rather than at the buffalo. If she wanted him dead, the simplest action would have been to take no

* Noting these allusions to Macomber's questionable masculinity, one critic even points out that the author gave him the Christian name of Francis, which is "both a masculine and feminine name, with the slightest alteration," and was not uncommonly regarded in the thirties as a sissy's name.[129]

action at all and let the buffalo do the job for her. Nor is there anything in the story to suggest that the reader should at this point question the veracity of the third-person narrative. It is clear that Robert Wilson believes she did it intentionally—"Why didn't you poison him? That is what they do in England," he says to her—but his previous experience with the "international, fast, sporting set" would explain his jumping to that conclusion.

It is not necessary for Margot to have aimed at Macomber's head, even if she was capable of such a well-placed shot. The story makes its point without a final murder. One is reminded of the exchange, in *Death in the Afternoon*, between Hemingway and the "Old Lady" who complained that his stories ended rather mysteriously:

"And is that all of the story? Is there not to be what we called in my youth a wow at the end?"

"Ah, Madame, it is years since I added the wow to the end of a story." [134]

Macomber is killed when a bullet from the 6.5 Mannlicher crashes into his skull, but he is doomed to die because he does not, after all, measure up to the demands of the code, as does Wilson. One does not grow a penis and a fine set of *cojones* overnight, any more than one undoes what has happened over a lifetime:

> He knew about motor cycles—that was his earliest—about motor cars, about duck-shooting, about fishing, trout, salmon and big sea, about sex in books, many books, too many books, about all court games, about dogs, not much about horses, about hanging on to his money, about most of the other things his world dealt in and about his wife not leaving him. [135]

To have died as the victim of a vengeful murderess would have made a final point. To die as the result of a mindless accident is the final, irreducible manifestation of *nada*.

Few serious contemporary writers have found a more congenial home in the once-forbidden thickets explored by D. H. Lawrence than Norman Mailer. Indeed, sex serves as the central metaphor in much of Mailer's work. His literary mission, as he conceives it, is on the heroic side: "The sour truth is that I am imprisoned with a perception which will settle for nothing less than making a revolution in the consciousness of our time." It's a tall order, but nothing short of it will suffice because the oppressor is also conceived on a heroic scale: "What is at stake in the twentieth century is . . . the peril that they will extinguish the animal in us." [136]

The "they," never explicitly identified, emerge as machine technology in its multiple forms and those who contribute to the furtherance of its power. The basic revolutionary strategy, as practiced by Stephen Rojack, the hero of *An American Dream*, is for man to "Trust in the authority of his senses." Other writers, including Lawrence, had preached this brand of neoprimitivism, but Mailer adds to it his own brand of existentialism: "Every moment of one's existence one is growing into more or retreating into less . . . the choice is not to live a little more or to not live a little less; it is to live a little more or to die a little more." [137]

Although he has modified it somewhat in his later work, the fullest rounding out of Mailer's philosophic stance appears in the essay "The White Negro." Its hero is the hipster, who is one of "a new breed of adventurers, urban adventurers who drifted out at night looking for action with a black man's code to fit their facts. The hipster had absorbed the existential synapses of the Negro, and for practical purposes could be considered a white Negro." [138]

Hipdom is a desirable state because "to swing is to be able to learn, and by learning take a step toward making it, toward creating. What is to be created is not nearly so important as the hipster's belief that when he really makes it, he will be able to turn his hand to anything, even to self-discipline." [139] The hipster's rewards are equally desirable:

> But to be with it is to have grace, is to be closer to the secrets of that inner unconscious life which will nourish you if you can hear it, for you are then nearer to that God which every hipster believes is located in the senses of the body, that trapped, mutilated, and nonetheless megalomaniacal God who is It, who is energy, life, sex, force, the Yoga's *prana*, the Reichian's orgone, Lawrence's "blood," Hemingway's "good," The Shavian life-force; "It"; God; not the God of the churches but the unachievable whisper of mystery within the sex, the paradise of limitless energy and perception just beyond the next wave of the next orgasm. [140]

Orgasm is central to the hipster:

> At the bottom, the drama . . . is that he seeks love. Not love as the search for a mate, but love as the search for an orgasm

more apocalyptic than the one which preceded it. Orgasm is his therapy—he knows at the seed of his being that good orgasm opens his possibilities and bad orgasm imprisons him.[141]

As philosophy, or even as reasoned discourse, "The White Negro" is vulnerable to analysis. Thus:

> Hip, as Mailer portrays it, is indeed a "mysticism of the flesh," a romantic glorification of the primordially instinctual. The trouble is that, like most nostalgia for the primitive, Mailer's advocacy of Hip is *phony*. Rape, murder, suicide, orgy, and even orgasm are anything but primitive "instincts." They are in their very nature culturally determined modes of behavior and highly sophisticated forms at that. And, what is more important, they depend for their meaning in Hip on their *negative* quality as rebellious acts against a predominantly square society. There are and could be no hipsters in a primitive African society, nor could hipsterism even become a prevalent mode of conduct. If enough people became hipsters they would of necessity all turn out to be squares.[142]

As an attempt at racial rapprochement, Mailer's essay was also less than a total success. In "The Black Boy Looks at the White Boy," James Baldwin notes: "The Negro jazz musicians, among whom we sometimes found ourselves, who really liked Norman, did not for an instant consider him as being even remotely 'hip.' . . . They thought he was a real sweet ofay cat, but a little frantic." [143]

But the most serious flaw of hipsterism, as far as half of humanity is concerned, is that all the goodies it holds out, including apocalyptic orgasms, are intended for men only. The female's destiny, as prescribed by Mailer, lies elsewhere: "The fact of the matter is that the prime responsibility of a woman is to be on earth long enough to find the best mate possible for herself and conceive children who will improve the species." [144]

Among the technological developments which Mailer considers directly responsible for the sorry state of the world are the diaphragm and the contraceptive pill. With their aid, women are able to evade their prime responsibility. They then are free to become independent and competitive and thus are largely responsible for the tension which exists between the sexes. As Jean Radford notes:

> Militant about the need for an existential conception of

man's life and potentialities, Mailer is blatantly essentialist where women are concerned. Where his male characters are presented with the right and the necessity to choose their destiny, women who attempt to do the same are presented as evil and destructive; *their* salvation, it is implied, lies in a return to *their* natural instincts, *their* biologically determined social roles.[145]

Woman, Mailer claims, is in touch with the mysteries of creation through her womb. It is her link to the future, and the anatomically deprived male can seek only to become a part of the mystery by planting his seed in that womb. This is essentially a fanciful restatement of Micky Spillane's bullet in the lower belly—the apocalyptic fuck she won't forget.

Throughout his writing, Mailer's attitude toward women is closer to Spillane's than that of Tolstoy, Dostoyevsky, and other authors with whom he would probably rather be compared. In *The Naked and the Dead,* for instance, General Cummings thinks of his wife waiting for him at home:

"He must subdue her, absorb her, rip her apart and consume her . . . I'll take you apart, I'll eat you, oh, I'll make you mine, you bitch."[146]

Hollingsworth, in *Barbary Shore,* muses on love:

> . . . he named various parts of her body, and described what he would do to them, how he would tear this and squeeze that, eat here and spit there, butcher rough and slice fine, slash, macerate, pillage, all in an unrecognizable voice which must have issued between clenched teeth until, his appetite satisfied, I could see him squatting beside the carcass, his mouth wiped carefully with the back of his hand. With that, he sighed, as much as to say, "A good piece of ass, by God."[147]

Or Sergius O'Shaughnessy, approaching the movie sex goddess Lulu Meyers in *The Deer Park:*

> Like a squad of worn-out infantrymen who are fixed for the night in a museum, my pleasure was to slash tapestries, poke my finger through nude paintings, and drop marble busts on the floor. Then I could feel her as something I had conquered, could listen to her wounded breathing, and believe that no

matter how she acted at other times, these moments were Lulu, as if her flesh murmured words more real than her lips.[148]

Even in his nonfiction, Mailer cannot resist turning sex into a battlefield. In "Some Children of the Goddess," which is largely a personal assassination of ten contemporary authors, he writes:

> Every novelist who has slept with the Bitch (only poets and writers of short stories have a *Muse*) comes away bragging afterward like a G.I. tumbling out of a whorehouse spree— "Man, I made her moan," goes the cry of the young writer. But the Bitch laughs afterward in her empty bed. "He was so sweet in the beginning," she declares, "but by the end he just went, 'Peep, peep, peep.' " [149] *

Sexual combat is the subject of Mailer's best-known short story, "The Time of Her Time." The title comes from the closing paragraph of *The Deer Park*, in which Sergius O'Shaughnessy asks God whether sex is where philosophy begins, and the deity replies: "Rather think of Sex as Time, and Time as the connection of new circuits." The exact meaning of this exchange has presented some difficulty for interpreters of Mailer's thought, possibly compounded by the fact that the author was, as he relates in *Advertisements for Myself*, under the influence of mescaline when he wrote it.

Sergius is again the hero of the story, now living in a loft in Greenwich Village, where he teaches bullfighting by day and indulges in sexual athletics by night—"there must have been at least fifty girls who spent at least one night in the loft . . . when I woke in the morning, I could hardly wait to get the latest mouse out of my bed and out of my lair." [150] The heroine is Denise Gondelman, a nineteen-year-old Jewish liberal pseudointellectual ("she was gone on Thomas Stearns Eeeee") undergoing psychoanalysis—a three-time loser by the standards of hipsterism.

The two meet at a party, and Sergius is attracted to the girl: "Her college-girl snobbery, the pith for me of eighty-five other honey-pots of the Village aesthetic whose smell I knew all too well, so inflamed the avenger of my crotch, that I wanted to prong her then and

---

* Mailer also has an explanation for why no woman novelist is even worth talking about: ". . . and all the lady writers, bless them. But one cannot speak of a woman having a piece of the Bitch."

there, right on the floor of the party. . . ." [151] He manages to re-
strain himself until they get back to the loft, but the experience
does not live up to expectations:

> She made love as if she were running up an inclined wall so
> steep that to stop for an instant would slide her back to disaster.
> . . . I had been frustrated, had waited, had lost the anger, and
> so been taken by her. That finally got me—all through the talk
> about T. S. Eliot I had been calculating how I would lay waste
> to her little independence, and now she was alone, with me
> astride her, going through her paces, teeth biting the pillow,
> head turned away, using me as the dildoe of a private gallop
> . . . she had fled domination which was liberty for her, and
> the rest of the night was bound to be hell.[152]

The remainder of the story is concerned with Sergius's determined efforts to bring Denise to orgasm. The stakes are high because victory "would add to the panoplies of my ego some peculiar
(but for me, valid) ingestion of her arrogance, her stubbornness and
her will—those necessary ingredients of which I could not yet have
enough for my own ambitions." Defeat, on the other hand, "would
bring me closer to a general depression, a fog bank of dissatisfaction
with myself." [153]

He goes at it like a man with a mission:

> I worked on her like a riveter, knowing her resistances were
> made of steel, I threw her a fuck the equivalent of a fifteen-
> round fight, I wearied her, I brought her back. . . . I sprinted,
> I paced, I lay low, eyes all closed, under sexual water, like a
> submarine listening for the distant sound of her ship's motors,
> hoping to steal up close and trick her rhythms away.

In the end Sergius emerges victorious, but only after a technical
infraction of the Marquess of Queensberry's rules:

> . . . I turned her over suddenly on her belly, my avenger wild
> with the mania of the madman, and giving her no chance,
> holding her prone against the mattress with the strength of
> my weight, I drove into the seat of all stubbornness, tight as a
> vise, and I wounded her, I knew it, she thrashed beneath me
> like a trapped little animal. . . .

Then:

> I turned her once again on her back, and moved by impulse
> to love's first hole . . . I was nothing but a set of aching balls
> and a congested cock, and I rode with her wistfully, looking at
> the contortion of her face and listening to her sobbing sound
> of "Oh, Jesus, I made it, oh Jesus, I did." [154]

Denise is properly grateful—" 'Was it good for you too?' she whispered half awake, having likewise read the works of The Hemingway"—but by morning she has second thoughts and leaves with a
parting shot: " '. . . your whole life is a lie, and you do nothing but
run away from the homosexual that is you.' "

One critic has characterized "The Time of Her Time" as "wild
and funny." [155] It is both, but whether Mailer intended it to be read
as satire is questionable. If so, the joke would have to be on Sergius
and, therefore, on his creator as well. As Jean Radford points out,
"Again and again the critical reader is forced to question the re-
liability of the narrator, but there are no clear signs in the *text*—
in the form of authorial comment, or in the images and symbols—
which denote the author's distance from his narrator's statements." [156] *

In Advertisements for Myself, Mailer promised to write a novel
which would be "the longest ball ever to go up into the accelerated
hurricane of our American letters." His next work of fiction, *An
American Dream*, relates the story of thirty-two hours in the life
of Stephen Rojack, war hero, ex-congressman (D-N.Y.), professor of
existential psychology, television talk-show host, friend of Jack
Kennedy, and author of *The Psychology of the Hangman*. Rojack
is married to but estranged from Deborah Caughlin Mangaravidi
Kelly, who is "a great bitch . . . a lioness of the species: uncondi-
tional surrender was her only raw meat." [158] As the story opens, he

---

* Diana Trilling has offered another interpretation: "Just as in *The Naked
and the Dead* the Army symbolizes the destructiveness of modern society, so in
Time of Her Time woman, the female, represents the fearful social power
against which man must defend himself: woman and society have become
synonymous. The castrating woman is not new in literature any more than the
male phantasy of the castrating woman is new in life; but what Mailer's story
demonstrates better than any piece of contemporary fiction I can bring to mind
is the new impulse of the writer to identify the destructive female force with
the destructive social force: woman *is* society in all its dark, unspecifiable lust
and horror.[157]

visits her; she taunts him with accounts of her current lovers—" 'I can't tell you how shocked they were when I began. One of them said: "Where did you ever learn to root about like that? Didn't know such things went on outside a Mexican whorehouse." ' " He slaps her: ". . . the blow caught her on the side of the ear and knocked her half out of bed. She was up like a bull and like a bull she charged . . . she drove one powerful knee at my groin (she fought like a prep school bully) and missing that, she reached with both hands, tried to find my root and mangle me." [159]

He throttles her to death, then, on his way out of the apartment, barges into the room of her maid:

> The lamp by her bed was on . . . and, nice shock, there was Ruta, Fräulein Ruta from Berlin, lying on top of the covers with her pajama pants down, a copy of a magazine in one hand (a flash of nude photographs in color) and her other hand fingering, all five fingers fingering like a team of maggots at her open heart.

Wordlessly he takes his clothes off: "My bare foot came up from the carpet and I put my five toes where her hand had been, drawing up on the instant out of her a wet spicy wisdom of all the arts and crafts of getting along in the world." He then proceeds to fuck her, alternately using her vagina and anus:

> So that was how I finally made love to her, a minute for one, a minute for the other, a raid on that Devil and a trip back to the Lord . . . like some cat caught on two wires I was leaping back and forth, in separate runs for separate strokes, bringing spoils and secrets up to the Lord from the red mills, bearing messages of defeat back from that sad womb, and then I chose— ah, but there was time to change—I chose her cunt. It was no graveyard now, no warehouse, no, more like a chapel now. . . .

In the end, however, hell wins: ". . . the seed was expiring in the wrong fields. . . . It was perishing in the kitchens of the Devil. Was it a curse on me?" Ruta, however, is properly impressed. "*Der Teufel* is so happy," she says.[160]

Rojack then plays cat-and-mouse games with the policemen sent to investigate the death of his wife, whose body he tosses out a tenth-story window. He meets a beautiful blond soiled-but-pure nightclub singer named Cherry Melanie—so named because, despite much trying, she had never experienced an orgasm through genital intercourse. He corrects this defect, but only after some difficulty: "We reached into some middle ground of a race, we were bicycle riders caught in the move of lap after lap around a track, soon we would be nothing but a rhythm which was nothing but a rhythm which would pump on to a climax I knew would never come. . . ." But Rojack knows what's wrong: ". . . I searched for that corporate rubbery obstruction I detested so much, found it with a finger, pulled it forth, flipped it away from the bed." Immediately, things improved:

> Like diving on a cold winter day back to a warm pool, I was back in her, our wills now met . . . and [I] felt love fly in like some great winged bird, some beating of wings at my back and felt her will dissolve into tears, and some great deep sorrow like roses drowned in the salt of the sea came flooding from her womb and washed into me like a sweet honey of balm for all the bitter sore of my soul . . . some shield broke in me, bliss, and the honey she had given me I could only give back, all sweets to her womb, all come in her cunt. "Son of a bitch," I said, "so that's what it's all about." [161]

There's more to the story—a confrontation with Shago Martin, Cherry's black stud; another confrontation with Barney Oswald Kelly, Rojack's father-in-law and omnipresent *éminence grise* of the political and corporate world; Cherry's death at the hands of a confused friend of Shago's; and Rojack's own hegira to Las Vegas, from where he telephones to Cherry in heaven and is told, " 'It's kind of cool right now, and the girls are swell. Marilyn says to say hello.' " [162]

Clearly, *An American Dream* is an allegory, an extended metaphoric vision of contemporary America as Mailer sees it. But however fanciful—and effective—the images and muscular the prose style, the vision is seen through the prism of Mailer's long-standing sexual attitudes. Forceful anal intercourse may be poeticized into entering "deserted warehouses," but it is also, as Leslie Fiedler has pointed out, an expression of sadistic impulses: "Buggery is the essential aspect of a sexual connection whose aim is annihilation." [163] Rojack is, by his own assessment, a nifty swordsman—the opening of *An American Dream* reads: "I met Jack Kenendy in November, 1946 . . . we went out one night on a double date and it turned out to be a fair evening for me. I seduced a girl who would have been bored by a diamond as big as the Ritz." Yet he needs reassurance even from such lesser game as Ruta, the maid. After his bout with her, "She lay for a minute half in sleep, half in stupor, and her tongue licked idly at my ear. . . . 'Mr. Rojack,' she said at last with gutty fleshy Berlin speech, 'I do not know why you have trouble with your wife. You are absolutely a genius, Mr. Rojack.' " To which he modestly replies: "A doctor is not better than his patient." [164]

As Stanley Gutman points out:

> The theme of the "heroic penis" is central to Mailer. . . . It is as if he is acting out his own neuroses in discussing the male sexual power; he has never progressed beyond a stage in which "the good lay makes all ok," in which a man is a man only if he can satisfy a woman sexually. One has a feeling that Mailer must continually prove his masculinity, as if he is very dubious of it: implications can be seen in escapades in his personal life, such as acting the part of a mobster in his films (*Beyond the Law*), playing the boxer, being champion drunk, or battler, or lover; and in his fiction as a belief in the power of the penis and disgust with homosexuality.[165]

Mailer's stance—the "Jimmy Cagney of literature," as Richard Gilman termed him—[166] has made him the central target of female writers.* It was, therefore, with some anticipation that readers picked up the May 1971 issue of *Harper's* which contained *The Prisoner of Sex*, Mailer's measured reply to his female critics. The champ came out fighting, characterizing his detractors as "a squadron of enraged Amazons, an honor guard of revolutionary vaginas." [167] With well-aimed jabs, he punished Kate Millett for the extensive misquotations and distortions she committed upon D. H. Lawrence and Freud in her *Sexual Politics*.† But it soon became clear that the much-touted main event was going to be a dud. Mailer had little or nothing to add to what was by now his Standard Version. Speaking as a male, he insisted that "The eternal battle with woman sharpens our resistance, develops our strength, enlarges the scope of our cultural achievements" and that "the loss of sex polarity is

---

* Notably Kate Millett in *Sexual Politics,* and Mary Ellmann in *Thinking About Women.*

† A similar but more thorough demolition job had already been performed months earlier by Irving Howe in *The Atlantic* magazine.

part and parcel of the larger disintegration, the reflex of the soul's death, and coincident with the disappearance of great men, great causes, great wars." [168] Conceding that economic discrimination on the basis of sex was unfair, he nevertheless accused what he refers to as Woman's Lib of being the unwitting handmaiden of the evil forces of technology. Rejecting the possibility that sexual characteristics may largely be the result of cultural conditioning, he insisted that "the primary quality of man was an assertion, and on the consequences an isolation, that one had to alienate oneself from nature to become a man . . . be perhaps directly opposed to nature . . . if the calm of the seas is seen as the basic condition of nature, that man was a spirit of unrest who proceeded to become less masculine whenever he ceased to thrive" [169]—a reworking of his old "grow or die" theme. Women, on the other hand, have a womb, and short of surrendering themselves and the species to technology, they are stuck with it. As he has said before, Mailer believes that their highest mission on earth—and just about their only mission—is to make the best possible use of it. He does concede that the task has its heroic aspects:

> Was it too late now to suggest that in the search for the best mate was concealed the bravery of a woman, for to find the best mate . . . was no easy matter but indeed a profound and artistic search for that mysterious fellow of concealed values who would eventually present himself in those twenty-three most special chromosomes able to cut through fashion, tradition and class.[170]

Surveying this unequal apportionment of the world's work, Laura Adams aptly notes: "[Mailer's] idea about the nature of masculinity would be intriguing if it were applied to women as well and called humanism." [171]

But the likelihood of this is slim. Seeking an explanation for Mailer's attitudes toward women and sex, Kate Millett uses the same dime-store Freudianism as Denise Gondelman did in "The Time of Her Time":

> The real abyss which portentous phrases such as "existential dread" were invented to mask is the fear of nonexistence. That or the secret terror of homosexuality; a mixture of sin, fascination, and fear which drives Mailer to his heterosexual posturing.

> To be faggot, damned, leprous—to cease to be virile were either
> to cease to be—or to become the most grotesque form of feminine
> inferiority—queer.[172]

A less superficial psychoanalytic reading was attempted by Andrew
Gordon in "The Naked and the Dead: The Triumph of Impotence."
The article's subtitle suggests the line of the argument:

> The family trinity of son, father and mother . . . is re-
> peated in all of Mailer's fiction. First is the innocent, tormented,
> basically blameless hero, who must prove his masculinity in a
> sordid, anal world. He is reincarnated as Lt. Hearn in *The
> Naked and the Dead*, Mike Lovett in *Barbary Shore*, Sergius in
> *The Deer Park* and *The Time of Her Time*, Rojack in *An
> American Dream*, DJ in *Why Are We in Vietnam?*, and as
> Norman Mailer in *The Steps of the Pentagon*.
>
> Next comes the father or father figure, whom the hero
> must best. He comes in two flavors: either a brutal reactionary
> ogre who wields power ruthlessly, or a kindly, sympathetic, but
> fallible mentor who once held power, but proved incompetent
> in office because of moral scruples, and voluntarily relinquished
> his sceptre. . . . In either guise the father figure is invariably
> impotent or compensating for his sexual inadequacy through
> violence. In fact it would not be overly speculative to state that
> every male in the Mailerian canon, hero or villain, suffers from
> psychic impotence or castration anxiety. . . .
>
> To this family portrait, we can add the indispensable mother-
> figure around whom the entire action usually pivots. The
> standard female in Mailer is aggressive, belittling to men,
> dominating, and castrating to the touch. . . .[173]

Gordon finds the trinity in place and operating in a story entitled
"Maybe Next Year" which Mailer wrote as an eighteen-year-old
junior at Harvard and caused to be reprinted in *Advertisements for
Myself*:

> The boy, acutely conscious of his inferior status, longs for
> power, which involves usurping the father's role and winning
> the affection of the mother. In this instance, however, the
> mother is viewed as fearful. His father is so henpecked that
> the son fears his mother will do to him what she seems to have
> done to his father—that is, emasculate him . . . he regresses to

an earlier, narcissistic stage of development in which fulfillment revolved around his own feces. The fixation intensifies
the dilemma, since his anally compulsive mother has distilled
a fear of all sexuality as "dirty." His inhibition against anality
then is as powerful as that against genital sexuality.

In fact, the two become united in his unconscious as destructive, befouling and potentially uncontrollable forces against
which he must defend himself.[174]

Gordon goes on to catalogue an impressive number of metaphors
and allusions in Mailer's work, a chore which has been performed by
a number of other critics. The astounding number and variety of
olfactory references, largely dealing with excretion and putrefaction,
which imbue Mailer's later fiction are surely unique in literature.

Mailer himself seems aware of this bent because in reply to an
interviewer's question regarding the buggery episodes, he once said:

> The reason I wrote about those things twice deliberately
> was something writers will understand but no critic ever will;
> it was just to say to the critics "Fuck you. I wrote about it once;
> I'll write about it again. What are you going to do about it?
> Say I'm anally oriented? O.K. Say I'm anally oriented. I'll say
> I'm Cassius Clay. Fuck you." [175]

Hostility tuned to such intense pitch betrays underlying anxiety.
In an earlier interview with Paul Krassner, Mailer made other
statements which hint at the nature of his defense mechanisms:

> I hate contraception. . . . There's nothing I abhor more
> than planned parenthood. Planned parenthood is an abomina-
> tion. I'd rather have those fucking Communists over here. . . .
> There's a great many men who think of the cock as The
> Avenger. . . . I would guess that most men who understand
> women at all feel hostility toward them. At their worst, women
> are low sloppy beasts.[176] *

Asked whether he thought of the sex act as pleasure or procreation, Mailer replied:

> As you get older, you begin to grow more and more obsessed

* If these were offhand comments, they still represent Mailer's considered
judgment. As he himself explains, he "worked over" the transcript before its
appearance in *The Realist* and chose to include it in *The Presidential Papers*.

with procreation. You begin to feel used up. Another part of oneself is fast diminishing. There isn't that much of oneself left. I'm not talking now in any crude sense of how much semen is left in the barrel. I'm saying that one's very *being* is being used up. . . .

Sooner or later, every man comes close to his being and realizes that even though he's using the act, the act is using him too. He becomes, as you say, more selective. The reason he becomes more selective is that you can get killed, you literally *can* fuck your head off, you can lose your brains, you can wreck your body, you can use yourself up badly, eternally—I know a little bit of what I'm talking about.[177]

Indeed, he does. In the first paragraph of *Why Are We in Vietnam?*, DJ announces that "there's blood on my dick." Mailer's own is stained with ink.

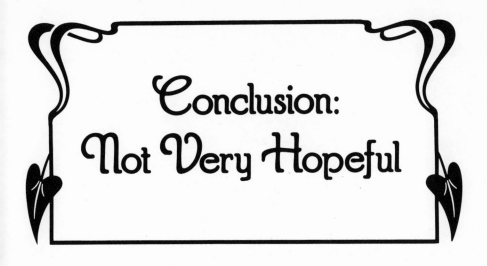

Conclusion:
Not Very Hopeful

There is, then, in contemporary writing, as in contemporary art, intimation that the male's grasp on his own sexuality is something less than totally firm. Moreover, the popularity and critical regard gained by such writers as Lawrence, Hemingway, Mailer, and others who could have been cited would suggest that they have struck a sympathetic chord among readers.

This book has tried to trace some of the consequences of male insecurity. In this final chapter, it will look at three more manifestations of it, the first two admittedly trivial, and then pass on a proposal which might possibly solve the problem once and for all.

The British anthropologist Somerville has described the peculiar costume—the total costume—favored by several groups in the New Hebrides:

> The natives wrap the penis around with many yards of calico, and other materials, winding and folding them until a preposterous bundle of eighteen inches or two feet long and two inches or more in diameter is formed, which is then supported upwards by means of a belt, in the extremity decorated with flowering grasses, etc. The testicles are left naked.[1]

Similar phallic sheaths, or phallocrypts, are common among the peoples of the Pacific, Africa, and the river valleys of South America. Depending on available materials, they may be made of twisted or folded leaves, bamboo, shells, or gourds. Claude Lévi-Strauss, who spent several seasons among the Bororo of central Brazil, described their daily dress: "The men were quite naked except for the little straw corner covering the tip of the penis and kept in place by the foreskin, which is stretched through the opening to form a little roll of flesh on the outside." [2] There is also evidence that the practice has a long history. The anthropologist Leo Frobenius has collected Bantu penile sheaths which bear a striking resemblance to similar artifacts depicted in 9,000-year-old African rock carvings.

Various theories have been proposed for the existence of clothing—modesty, protection, decoration. In *The Psychology of Clothes*, one of the most thoughtful reviews of the subject, J. C. Flugel maintains:

> . . . it has been manifest to all serious students of dress that of all the motives for the wearing of clothes, those connected with the sexual life have an altogether predominant position. . . . Among savage peoples, clothing and decoration start anatomically at or near the genital region, have frequently some definite reference to a sexual occasion (puberty, marriage, etc.). Among civilized peoples, the overtly sexual role of many clothes is too obvious and familiar to need more than a passing mention. . . . Their ultimate purpose, often indeed their overt and conscious purpose, is to add to the sexual attractiveness of their wearers, and to stimulate the sexual interest of admirers of the opposite sex and the envy of rivals of the same sex.[3]

Women have always had an easier time in achieving this dual objective because, as psychologists have noted, there is a tendency for their libido to be more diffused than it is among men. In women the whole body is sexualized; in men sexual feelings are more definitely concentrated on the genital zone. This is true both subjectively and objectively, both for showing the body and for looking at it, and has led to the constant shifting of erogenous zones which has constituted much of feminine fashion through history. As Edmund Bergler notes in *Fashion and the Unconscious*, "Stripped to its essentials, fashion is no more than a series of permutations of seven themes: the breasts, waist, hips, buttocks, legs, arms and length (or circumference) of the body itself."[4]

Men, limited to their single erogenous zone, have responded as best they could. They have decked themselves out with exaggeratedly padded shoulders, still retained in the epaulets of military officers and hotel doormen, or climbed into high heels in order to present a more commanding and virile figure. They have worn tights, padded if necessary, to accentuate their musculature and agility. They have used the skin, fur, feathers, and fangs of animals to attest to their valor. More recently they have begun exposing their bare chests to convey the same message. But only once, with the introduction of the codpiece, did they overcome their insecurity to the extent of calling direct attention to the tool of their manhood.

Originally intended as merely a flap to contain the genitals within the skintight hose then in fashion, the codpiece quickly took on enough padding to resemble a permanent erection and enough color and other decorations to make certain that it would not escape the notice of the most modest feminine eyes—and envious masculine ones as well. It became such an accepted form of adornment that examples, in sumptuous silk, can still be seen in the portraits of such eminent personages as the Emperor Charles V and Baldassare Castiglione, the author of *The Courtier*. But the codpiece fad lasted only some fifty years and was defeated not by religious or moral objections but by ridicule. By Shakespeare's day it had become a theatrical convention, intended to identify a fop or a fool.

Never again would men run the risk of putting their genitals on the line.* But the need to emit a sexual signal remained and, as often happens to suppressed desires, became satisfied through the mechanism of displacement.

Headgear of any shape and size has a strong phallic character. The placement of a royal crown, whether celebrated in a European cathedral or an African chief's village, has powerful symbolic overtones of a marriage between a sovereign and the body politic he will rule. The removal of the hat, as a greeting or as a sign of respect, may well be related to the primitive custom of taking trophies from fallen foes. As such, it may also, as Freud suggested, symbolize castration. Flugel has commented on the odd distinction which requires men to bare their heads and women to cover theirs when entering a church:

> The psychological reason for this distinction is probably that the displacement of exhibitionism from the body on to clothes has gone further with man than with woman. In virtue of this displacement, the wearing of a hat would be regarded as a proud piece of display on the part of the man—a display that contravenes the essential elements of religious humility—whereas

---

* Not long ago, Eldridge Cleaver tried to market a line of trousers with a pouch intended to display the genitals. So far these have not become the fashion.

with woman the corresponding sign of disrespect would be the exposure of the naked head.[5]

In *Modesty in Dress,* James Laver notes the curious parallel between the height of men's hats and the prevailing degree of male domination, as during the Puritan epoch. He writes:

> In the nineteenth century it is possible to plot the rise of the curve of feminine emancipation from the height of men's hats. Absolute male domination of, say, 1850, was certainly accompanied by extremely tall hats. With the advent of the New Woman in the 1880's many men adopted the boater, which might be thought of as a very truncated top-hat. And towards the end of the century men began to wear, so to speak, the very symbol of their bashed-in authority: the trilby.[6]

The observable fact that men have now virtually stopped wearing hats altogether speaks for itself. *

But the most distinct form of displacement is evident in another common article of masculine clothing. The necktie can trace its origin—and its more formal name—to a cloth ribbon worn underneath their open-necked shirts by Croatian mercenaries who served in the armies of Louis XIV. It then became the cambric or linen stock meticulously folded and ironed according to the dictates of Beau Brummell and later still evolved into its present form: a length of cloth which is tied around the neck and allowed to hang loosely down the middle of the chest. It serves no purpose other than to call attention to itself. Significantly it was for a long time—and still is for many men—the only article of attire which could be brightly colored or strikingly patterned. Men who wear the same drab uniform year after year—blue or gray suit, black shoes and socks, white or blue shirt—will lavish tender attention on the selection of a necktie. For many boys, the first wearing of a necktie has become an even more distinct rite of puberty than the first pair of long pants.

Frederic Wakeman's *The Hucksters,* one of the earliest fictionalized accounts of life along Madison Avenue, contains a memorable scene in which the hero, on his way to a very important job interview, stops to spend most of his remaining money on an expensive but

---

* As perhaps do such exceptions as men who wear hard hats, ten-gallon hats, and hats which form part of a uniform.

"sincere" necktie. Then, armed with the self-confidence he needed, he goes on to land the job.

There existed for many years a well-known nightclub in Paris, presided over by a hostess who could compel male guests to get up and sing a song. If they refused, or failed to do so to the audience's satisfaction, she would cut their neckties off with a large pair of scissors. The raucous laughter provoked by the administration of this forfeit left little doubt about the unconscious emotion evoked or about the significance of the necktie itself.

Finally, the custom of wearing a particular necktie which identifies its possessor with some particular group—educational, military, or social, but always exclusively masculine—may simply be a convenient form of communication, but there is one detail of professional costume which is hard to explain in other than phallic terms. Most men, when they dress formally or for business, wear neckties. Men of the cloth do not—and for good measure turn their collars around in order to present to the world an unbroken surface which could not possibly accommodate a necktie.*

The length of men's hair, like the wearing of neckties, may well, in the greater scheme of events, be a relatively trivial matter. But in an article entitled "The Rape of the Lock Revisited," David Kentsmith calls attention to an incident reported by a Buffalo, New York, newspaper in 1970. "A long-haired, 'hippie-looking' young man was walking down the street. Three 'hard-hat' laboring men, in a fit of spontaneous, apparently unprovoked rage and anger, grabbed the young man, threw him to the ground and cut off his long hair." [8] Kentsmith notes that the workmen had never seen the young man before and knew nothing about him. What, then, prompted the aggression? Obviously, it was a response to the stimulus of the long hair. But why? Because, he proposes, it symbolized "dirty, drug-taking hippie," which in turn is a label for "a primitive, a person unresponsive to and uninfluenced by the societal dictates and prohibitions against the expression of his naturalness and primitiveness, especially in sex."

No one asked the young man why he wore his hair long, nor, had

* In this respect, Laver points out that until two generations ago some clergymen did wear a tie, but only a white one, "as if to indicate that they were 'potent but pure.'" [7]

they done so, is it likely that they would have received an illuminating answer. Superficially the current male mode for long hair and beards may be a mute but visible protest against regimentation and social constraint. Long hair on men has, since antiquity, been a sign of freedom. In successive eras, only slaves, serfs, monks, soldiers, convicts, and industrial workers, for whom long hair posed an occupational hazard, were shorn. The term "longhair" itself suggests not only artistic or intellectual pursuits but a certain degree of personal freedom in expression and behavior.

But Havelock Ellis long ago noted: "Of all physical traits, vigor of the hairy system has most frequently perhaps been regarded as the index of vigorous sexuality. In this matter modern medical observation are at one with popular belief. . . ." [9] That there was a connection between the appearance of body hair and sexual maturity did not require the confirming evidence of endocrinologists. Although the evolutionary purpose of such hair is not clear, it seems more than coincidental that it should grow in greatest profusion over those areas, pubic and axillary, where the skin contains scent glands whose secretions need exposure to air in order to develop their full odor. The presence of tufts of hair provides a holding surface for this exposure, which in turn releases a distinctive scent that may have served as a sexual stimulant. At the same time facial hair, by giving its possessor a fiercer appearance, may have helped frighten off rivals in the competition for mates—as it still does among many species of monkeys.

The symbolism in the story of Samson and Delilah is self-evident, but it is hardly unique. At Delos and Delphi, youths offered their first beard to Apollo, and Suetonius relates that the young Nero offered his to Jupiter and marked the occasion with gymnastic contests and the slaying of bullocks. Virility is implicit in the extravagantly bearded statues and reliefs of Mesopotamian kings, as it is in the many representations of Hercules, in Michelangelo's "Moses," and in the naming of such warriors as Harold Fairhair, who unified Norway in the tenth century, and the less successful Clodion the Hirsute, who lost the Frankish crown to Clovis. Until recently the Masai of Kenya believed that their chiefs would lose their power if their beards were cut off. Orthodox Jews still observe the law forbidding a man to shave "the four corners of the face." And the hair-inspired exchange between Hemingway and Max Eastman has been noted earlier.

The North American Indian's war bonnet was a symbolic mane of hair. Symbolic hair is still worn as a badge of manhood by elite regiments: the bearskin busbies of the Brigade of Guards; the cascading black feathers of the Bersaglieri; the horsetail plumes of the Garde Républicaine; the shakos of a dozen military academies and countless drum majors. In Scotland it is even worn, as a sporran, over the appropriate part of the body.

In *The Unconscious Significance of Hair,* the psychoanalyst Charles Berg has assembled a mass of clinical material to demonstrate that the sexual symbolism of hair is universal and has been repressed into the unconscious. He cites dreams in which the cutting or shaving of hair can be clearly related through analysis to sexual fears. He describes and explains widespread customs of ritual head shaving or of cutting hair in special ways. And he proposes that as an exhibitionist object, hair is the only phallus that the conventions of society permit a man to display in public. It is this association, he says, which underlies men's concern over baldness and which accounts for the social unacceptability of uncombed, upstanding hair. Boys are taught that they must comb their hair neatly because uncombed, wild hair symbolically represents the erect penis.[10] *

This may be farther along the Freudian road than many people are willing to wander, but it does provide the basis of an explanation for a current tonsorial phenomenon: the Afro haircut. Undoubtedly ethnic pride and the desire to proclaim that "black is beautiful" have contributed to its popularity. But in a society where attitudes about black virility are deeply rooted, it is impossible to disregard the implicit sexual message which the Afro is intended to convey. Or why would men, including white men whose heritage in no way touches the Dark Continent, affect to wear it or to emulate it to the extent that the consistency of their hair will permit?

The Afro haircut serves as the visible reminder of what most white men, and women, apparently already know. In *Eros Denied,* Wayland Young cites the incredulous comment of an American black in Rome about some society ladies he had met at a party:

---

* At the end of the nineteenth century a French anthropologist named O. Ammon took careful measurements of nearly 4,000 military conscripts and found that the hairier a man was, the greater the diameter of his testicles. However, until a relationship between testicular girth and virility has been established, Dr. Ammon's findings must remain inconclusive.

"They ask you . . . the length of . . . your prick."[11]

Unless they had been brought up in hermetic isolation, the ladies' curiosity was something less than ingenuous. One of the earliest accounts of white travelers in Africa noted that indigenous males were endowed with "large Propagators." In 1623 Richard Jobson, a generally sympathetic observer, reported that Mandingo men were "furnisht with such members as are after a sort burthensome unto them," so large in fact that it was the custom of the tribe not to have intercourse during pregnancy so as not to "destroy what is conceived."[12]

In a learned work entitled *An Account of the Regular Gradation in Man, and in Different Animals and Vegetables; and from the Former to the Latter,* which was published in London in 1799, Dr. Charles White, a member of the Royal Society, categorically states: "That the Penis of an African is larger than that of an European has, I believe, been shewn in every anatomical school in London. Preparations of them are preserved in most anatomical museums; and I have one in mine."[13] Nor was certitude on this subject limited to Anglo-Saxon observers. *The Anthropological Treatises of Johann Friedrich Blumenbach,* published in German in 1795, states: "It is generally said that the penis in the Negro is very large. And this assertion is so far borne out by the remarkable genitory apparatus of an Aethiopian which I have in my anatomical collection."[14]

The corollary notion received its share of attention as well. Black women were "hot constitution'd ladies," driven by a "temper hot and lascivious, making no scruple to prostitute themselves to the Europeans for a very slender profit. . . . If they can come to the place the Man sleeps in, they lay themselves softly down by him, soon wake him, and use all their little Arts to move the darling Passion."[15] *

---

* *In White over Black,* Winthrop Jordan quotes a poem which was popular in 1777:

> Next comes a warmer race, from sable sprung,
> To love each thought, to lust each nerve is strung;
> The Samboe dark, and the Mullatoe brown,
> The Metsize fair, the well-limb'd Quaderoon,
> And jetty Afric, from no spurious sire,
> Warm as her soil, and as her sun—on fire.

But it was the sexuality of the black man, especially the size of his equipment for the purpose, which preyed on white imaginations. Summing up what is still tantamount to folk wisdom, Louis West notes in "The Psychobiology of Racial Violence":

> The clinical experience of psychiatrists and marriage counselors clearly reveals that a large penis does not correlate at all with virility or special satisfaction in coitus, and it is evident from studies of sexual physiology, such as those of Masters and Johnson, that a small penis is a most unlikely basis for sexual incompatibility. In fact, too large, rather than too small, is the much more common complaint of the allegedly maladjusted woman. We know these things, but I hear no sigh of, "Alas, the poor Negro, his penis is too large!" [17]

Almost as firm as the white man's conviction about the size of the black man's penis was the belief that he lusted to use it on a white woman—and the accompanying unspoken fear that she would find it more satisfying than his own. The specter of the slave revolt, which began haunting the South long before the Revolution, was almost invariably expressed in sexual terms. An article in the *London Magazine* in 1757, for instance, describes how the leaders of a slave insurrection in South Carolina were "executed, after confessing the conspiracy, and each of them declaring whose wife, daughter, or sister he had fixed on for his future bedfellow." [18] One can imagine how these declarations were extracted.

Two centuries later, on the occasion of the 1965 march on Selma, local whites unsympathetic to the demonstration's motives attempted to discredit it by publicizing episodes they claim to have witnessed:

> This one particular couple on St. Margaret's lawn were engaged in sexual relations, a white woman (a skinny blond) and a Negro man. After they were through, she wiggled out from beneath him and went over to the man lying on the left of

---

These sooty dames, well vers'd in Venus' school
Make love an art, and boast they kiss by rule.

"If such amiable assessments could find their way into public print," Jordan adds, "one can imagine what tavern bantering must have been like." [16]

them on the lawn and started kissing and caressing his face.
. . . On one occasion I saw a Negro boy and a white girl engage in sexual intercourse on the floor of the church. At this
time the church was packed and the couple did nothing to hide
their actions. While they were engaged in this act of intercourse other boys and girls stood around and watched, laughing and joking.[19]

After thousands of lynchings, hundreds of castrations, the Scottsboro
case, Emmett Till, the specter still walks. *

In a detailed report entitled "Physical Anthropology of the American Negro," William Montague Cobb stated in 1942: "It is said
that the penis of the Negro is larger than that of the White. The
writer's impression from ample observations is that the American
hybrid has not been markedly affected in this respect by his infusion
of white blood, but suitable data are lacking." They still are. Nor
is there comparative evidence of the levels of white and black
sexuality, male or female. If such studies were ever to be constructed
and carried out, they would probably favor the white, at least as
far as males are concerned. Broken homes, dependency, and economic deprivation are more likely to cause passivity and even impotence than to generate extraordinary heterosexual drives.[21] †

Yet the myth prevails and finds reinforcement every time a well-
known, attractive white woman marries a black man—never the
other way around—and when, even in the most liberated, color-blind
social circles, a black man and an attractive white woman—again,
never the other way around—display public signs of a private intimacy.

It has been suggested that blacks may be the innocent victims of

* And not just in Mississippi and Alabama. Writing about contemporary
England, Michael Banton says: "It seems fairly clear that coloured immigrants
and white men in Britain regard each other as sexual competitors." [20] The
failure of the Soviet Union to provide university educations for large numbers of
African students has been due at least in part to their interest, once enrolled,
in dating Russian girls. And the "color problem" which is emerging in some
parts of Israel appears to be accompanied by hostility on the part of the whites
toward sexual attentions to white women by the darker-skinned Oriental Jews.

† The effect on personality of the deprivation of hope and the enforcement
of caste sanctions—conditions which still define the existence of many if not
most blacks in the United States—were chillingly detailed by B. P. Karon in
The Negro Personality (New York: 1958).

the "stranger complex"—the near-universal tendency to look upon anything that is different, unfamiliar, or alien as also being threatening and hostile. It has been said that their single misfortune is to be born, well, black—as in blackmail, blackguard, blacklist, blackball, black words, black deeds, black bile, black magic, black looks, and blackening of character, which is also known as denigration. On a more subtle level, the National Commission on the Causes and Prevention of Violence in 1969 proposed that certain personality types and categories of persons located in particular structural positions in society are uniquely disposed to violent expressions of racism. According to this theory, which views the phenomenon of antiminority group prejudice as an externalization of inner conflict:

> The authoritarian personality is said to be most comfortable with clear-cut systems of authority and status, to be unusually submissive to those above him, and unusually oppressive toward those he perceives as below him. Insecurity about one's own negative characteristics results in the projection onto minority groups of these negative characteristics and blame for one's own undesirable situation.[22]

That projection is involved in the white's perception of blacks, particularly of some aspects of black sexual characteristics, is undeniable. There is no physical basis for that perception. But what is being projected is more than just the maladjustment of an authoritarian personality. True, the passage just cited accurately describes many people who harbor virulently racist views. But there are many others who share these views, yet are comfortable with both their superiors and inferiors.

Why should white men assume and, on the basis of no evidence, perpetuate the belief that black women are passionate, uncontrollably sexed animals? Possibly it was because of their own attraction toward the women, which they gratified even as they realized that their actions were not fully acceptable to society or to themselves. Ah, but if the women were *that* lascivious, a man could hardly be blamed for being overwhelmed. Projection is the defense mechanism whereby desires the satisfaction of which would cause anxiety or guilt are denied and imputed to others. It is not we who are guilty, but they. It is not we who lust, but they.

Projection can also explain the white perception of the black male. Winthrop Jordan, describing race relations after the Civil War, eloquently writes:

> For in advancing as the principal reasons for curbing the free Negro the dangers of intermixture and insurrection, white Americans were expressing—in the language in which such things are expressed—how greatly they feared the unrestrained exercise of their most basic impulses. Neither danger existed in anything like the proportions they saw; the proportions were much more theirs than the Negro's. In this sense, white men were attempting to destroy the living image of primitive aggressions which they said was the Negro's but was really their own. . . . If the gates fell, so did humaneness; they could not fall; indeed there could not be any possibility of their falling, else man was not man and his civilization was not civilized. We, therefore, do not lust and destroy; it is someone else. We are not great black bucks of the fields. But a buck *is* loose, his great horns menacing to gore into us with life and destruction. Chain him, either chain him or expel his black shape from our midst, before we realize that he is ourselves.[23]

And just to make sure that there is no mistake about the buck's potency or his intent, let's be sure and hang between his legs a great, big, oversized black penis.

"At the core of the heart of the race problem," James Weldon Johnson writes, "is the sex problem." [24] This view, which has been expressed by others, was subjected to ingenious experimental test a few years ago by psychologist Gary Schulman at the University of California.[25] Using a variation of Stanley Milgram's now-classic demonstration that normal, ordinary people could be induced to inflict lethal doses of pain on other human beings, Schulman set up a controlled situation in which white male students were placed in a position where they could choose to administer what they believed to be extremely painful electric shocks to a group of volunteers. The test procedure was arranged in such a way that half the subjects knew their "volunteer" was white, and the other half that he was black. Furthermore—and this was the crux of the experiment—some of the subjects were led to believe that the volunteers were living with a partner of the opposite color. (This was accomplished by having an attractive young woman, black or white as required, come into the subject's room and leave a set of keys for the volunteer, along with the message that she would meet him back at the apartment at 10:00 P.M.)

The hypothesis of the experiment was that black men perceived to be living with white women would receive greater punishment—which the white subjects were free to administer as they chose—than the others. This proved to be the case. They were in fact "punished" at a rate almost double that of the white men about whose sexual arrangements nothing had been suggested, and almost three times that of white men perceived to be living with a black woman, who as a group received the least punishment.

In selecting his eighty-four subjects, all freshmen or sophomores at the University of California at Santa Barbara, Schulman used a questionnaire designed to single out "young, educated white males from relatively stable homes whose self-identification and attitudes as typically measured are weighted in a decided liberal direction." To the question of whether progress is civil rights was moving at the right speed, for instance, more than half of those chosen replied either "Too slowly" or "Mostly about right, but some going too slowly." Consequently he was able to conclude:

> Limited though the number of cases is, the data is [sic] consistent with a position that does not limit the potential for racist behavior in the form of physical violence to the bigot, the uneducated, the economically marginal, the southerner or the mentally ill. The fact that a greater willingness to inflict pain upon a black man than a white is found even among the most liberal segment of a subject group that is itself considerably more liberal than the national norm speaks rather forcefully to the issue of the generality of the potential for racist behavior.

And the sexual antagonism implicated in that racist behavior is sad evidence that the male's penile preoccupation bears consequences which at times are less trivial than neckties or haircuts.

A proposal which would forever eliminate this preoccupation has been made by Karen Rotkin in an article entitled "The Phallacy of Our Sexual Norm":

> Though a few women report erotic sensitivity in the vagina, neurological research has failed to find a common source of such sensitivity in the vaginal interior. . . . Since the clitoris is the

center of female sexual response, the phallus is less relevant to female sexuality than is a finger or a tongue, either of which is a more effective stimulator of a clitoris than a penis could possibly be. We can stimulate ourselves or be stimulated by other women as well as men can stimulate us because that unique male offering, the phallus, is of peripheral importance, or may even be irrelevant, to our sexual satisfaction. [26]

This is familiar, well-trod feminist ground. But having gone this far, Rotkin takes a bold step forward:

First, let's imagine a society with a very different notion of heterosexuality. Here it has been found through common practice that a man's right index finger is the most satisfying stimulator of the female's clitoris. Such stimulation is therefore the essential mode of *sexual* (not reproductive) behavior. Sometimes in the course of this practice a man ends up in a position in which his penis is accidentally (or even sometimes intentionally) stimulated, and he achieves a penile orgasm—an enhancement, perhaps, of the sexual act, but of peripheral importance to his digitally-oriented sexuality. The man's real organ of sexuality is his finger, and to wish for penile stimulation is a sign of immaturity. Sometimes people copulate, but this is for the purpose of reproduction, and has nothing to do with sexuality, except for the retarded male who cannot achieve digital orgasm from stimulation by the wondrous clitoris.

It's a lovely idea, well worth trying. But let no one place too high expectations on its success. Sooner or later, men will begin to erect finger-shaped monuments, wear artfully padded gloves, and surreptitiously start to look over at the fellow washing his hands at the next basin.

Reference Notes

Introduction

1. This, at any rate, has become the frequently reprinted account of the discovery. However, Jacques Marsal, who is now a guide at Lascaux and was one of the four boys in the story, told this writer that they were in fact not hunting on that day but prospecting for caves and that, emphatically, they had no dog with them.

2. See A. H. Broderick, *Lascaux: A Commentary* (London: 1949); A. Laming and M. Roussel, *La Grotte de Lascaux* (Paris: 1950); F. Windels, *Lascaux, "Chapelle Sixtine" de la Préhistoire* (Montignac-sur-Vézère, Dordogne: 1948).

3. R. R. Marett, *The Threshold of Religion* (London: 1914), p. 218.

4. For a comprehensive, modern interpretation of the significance of cave paintings, see Annette Laming-Emperaire, *La Signification de l'Art Rupestre Paléolithique* (Paris: 1962), and Andre Leroi-Gourhan, *Treasures of Prehistoric Art* (New York: 1967).

5. Abbé H. Breuil, *Four Hundred Centuries of Cave Art* (Montignac-sur-Vézère, Dordogne: 1952), pp. 134–36.

6. James G. Frazer, *The Golden Bough* (New York: 1944), p. 52.

7. H. Kirchner, "Ein archäologischer Beitrag zur Urgeschichte der Schamanismus," *Anthropos*, vol. 47 (1952), p. 244.

Chapter I

1. Luce Passemard, *Les Statuettes Féminines Paléolithiques dites Vénus Steatopyges* (Nimes: 1938), p. 36.

2. James G. Frazer, *The Golden Bough* (New York: 1944), p. 51.

3. J. G. H. Clarke, *From Savagery to Civilization* (New York: 1953), p. 56.

4. Franz Hancar, "Zum Problem der Venusstatuetten im eurasiatischen

Jungpälaolithikum," *Praehistorische Zeitschrift*, vol. 30–31 (1939–40), p. 85.

5. James Mellaart, *Earliest Civilizations of the Near East* (New York: 1965), p. 92.

6. John E. Pfeiffer, *The Emergence of Society* (New York: 1977), p. 16.

7. The first full-scale formulation of the theory, written in the nineteenth century, appears in J. J. Bachofen's *Myth, Religion and Mother Right*, translated by Ralph Manheim (Princeton: 1967). A more recent version is contained in Elizabeth Gould Davis's *The First Sex* (New York: 1971).

8. *Christian Science Monitor*, June 3, 1969.

9. United Nations, *The Data Base for Discussion on the Interrelations Between the Integration of Women in Development, Their Situation and Population Factors in Africa* (Addis Ababa: 1974).

10. Elise Boulding, *The Underside of History* (Boulder, Colo.: 1976), p. 132.

11. *Ibid.*, p. 120.

12. Elizabeth Colson, "Plateau Tonga," in David M. Schneider and Kathleen Gough, eds., *Matrilineal Kinship* (Berkeley: 1962), p. 36.

13. Jonathan Norton Leonard, *The First Farmers* (New York: 1973), p. 103.

14. V. Gordon Childe, *The Dawn of European Civilization* (London: 1939), p. 113.

15. Boulding, *op. cit.*, p. 146.

16. *Ibid.*, p. 147.

17. George M. Foster, "Sociology of Pottery," in Yehudi Cohen, ed., *Man in Adaptation: The Biosocial Background* (Chicago: 1968), p. 317.

18. Boulding, *op. cit.*, p. 148.

19. A. Gouldner and R. Peterson, *Notes on Technology and the Moral Order* (New York: 1962).

20. W. Stephens, *The Family in Cross-Cultural Perspective* (New York: 1963).

21. Bronislaw Malinowski, *Sex, Culture and Myth* (New York: 1962), p. 249.

22. Apuleius, *The Golden Ass*, trans. by W. Adlington. Book XL.

23. Cited in H. R. Hays, *In the Beginning: Early Man and His Gods* (New York: 1963), p. 259.

24. *Ibid.*, p. 75.

25. *Ibid.*, p. 76.

26. Joseph Campbell, *The Masks of God: Occidental Mythology* (New York: 1964), pp. 21–22.

27. *Ibid.*, p. 80.

28. Job 41:1–11.

29. William King Leonard, *Chronicles Concerning Early Babylonian Kings* (London: 1907), vol. II, pp. 87–91.

30. Otto Rank, *Der Mythus von der Geburt des Helden* (Leipzig: 1922).

31. Robert F. Harper, *The Code of Hammurabi, King of Babylon* (Chicago: 1904).

32. Genesis 1–3.

33. Campbell, *op. cit.*, p. 158.

34. Jane Ellen Harrison, *Prolegomena to the Study of Greek Religion* (Cambridge: 1903), p. 292.

35. W. L. Hildburgh, "Cowrie Shells as Amulets in Europe," *Folk-lore*, vol. 53 (1942), p. 178.

36. W. Ridgeway, "The Origin of the Turkish Crescent," *Journal of the Royal Anthropological Institute*, vol. 38 (1908), p. 248.

37. Cited in James Laver, *Modesty in Dress* (Boston: 1969), p. 3.

38. Genesis 24:2–3.

39. Genesis 47:29.

40. *Encyclopaedia Biblica*, vol. 3, col. 3453.

41. Cited in R. Morris and D. Morris, *Men and Apes* (London: 1966), p. 44.

42. Claire Russell and W. M. S. Russell, *Violence, Monkeys and Man* (London: 1968), p. 127.

43. *Ibid.*, p. 62.

44. A. H. Maslow, *et al.*, "Some Parallels between Sexual and Dominance Behavior of Infra-human Primates and the Fantasies of Patients in Psychotherapy," *Journal of Nervous and Mental Disease*, vol. 131 (1960), p. 202.

45. Detlev W. Ploog and Paul D. MacLean, "Display of Penile Erection in Squirrel Monkey," *Animal Behaviour*, vol. 11 (1963), p. 32.

46. Irenäus Eibl-Eibesfeldt, *Love and Hate* (New York: 1971), p. 29.

47. Wolfgang Wickler, *The Sexual Code* (New York: 1972), p. 53.

48. *Ibid.*, p. 55.

49. *Ibid.*, p. 57.

50. Eibl-Eibesfeldt, *op. cit.*, p. 30.

51. Charles W. Ferguson, *The Male Attitude* (Boston: 1966), p. 102.

52. Cited in Carl Bakal, *The Right to Bear Arms* (New York: 1961), p. 76.

53. *Int. Zeitschrift für Ärztliche Psychoanalyse*, vol. I, no. 5 (1913), p. 494.

54. Cited in Robert Sherrill, *The Saturday Night Special* (New York: 1973), p. 10.

55. Melitta Schmideberg, "On Motoring and Walking," *International Journal of Psychoanalysis*, vol. 18 (1937), p. 42.

56. Theodor Reik, "Men, Women and Houses," *Psychoanalysis*, vol. 1 (1953), p. 24.

57. Joseph D. Noshpitz, "The Meaning of the Car," in *Sexual Behavior and the Law*, ed. by Samuel G. Kling (New York: 1965).

58. Armand M. Nicholi, "The Motorcycle Syndrome," *American Journal of Psychiatry*, vol. 126 (1970), p. 1588.

59. E. H. Kaplan, "Attitudes Toward Automobiles: An Aid to Psychiatric Evaluation and Treatment of Adolescents," *Journal of Hillside Hospital*, vol. 10 (1961), p. 3. J. C. Neavles and G. Winokur, "The Hot-Rod Driver," *Bulletin of the Menninger Clinic*, vol. 21 (1957), p. 28. I. H. Weiland, "The Psychological Significance of Hot-Rods and Automobile Driving to Adolescent Males," *Psychiatric Quarterly, Supplement*, vol. 31 (1957), p. 261. Norman Tabachnick, "Sexual Aspects of the Automobile," *Medical Aspects of Human Sexuality* (September 1973), p. 138. Paul E. Kaunitz and Leon Tec, "Unsuccessful Initiation Rites Among Adolescent Boys," *Journal of Nervous and Mental Diseases*, vol. 140 (1965), p. 175.

60. James W. Hamilton, "The Rear-end Collision: A Specific Form of Acting Out," *Journal of the Hillside Hospital*, vol. 16 (1967), p. 187.

61. Sigmund Freud, *Three Essays on the Theory of Sexuality* (London: 1949), p. 36.

62. Sigmund Freud, *New Introductory Lectures on Psycho-analysis* (London: 1937), p. 139.

63. H. Hartmann, E. Kris, and R. M. Loewenstein, "Notes on the Theory of Aggression," in *The Psychoanalytic Study of the Child*, vol. 3–4 (New York: 1949).

64. P. D. MacLean, "New Findings Relevant to the Evolution of Psychosexual Functions of the Brain," *Journal of Nervous and Mental Disease*, vol. 135 (1962), p. 289.

65. H. M. Halverson, "Infant Sucking and Tensional Behavior," *Journal of Genetic Psychology*, vol. 53 (1938), p. 365.

66. I. V. Levy and I. A. King, "The Effects of Testosterone Propionate in Young Mice," *Anatomical Record*, vol. 117 (1953), p. 562.

67. M. A. Bennett, "Social Hierarchy in Ring Doves. II. The Effects of Treatment with Testosterone Propionate," *Ecology*, vol. 21 (1940), p. 148.

68. W. C. Allee, N. Collias, and C. Z. Lutherman, "Modification of the Social Order Among Flocks of Hens by Injection of Testosterone Propionate," *Physiological Zoology*, vol. 12 (1939), p. 412.

69. H. Persky, K. D. Smith, and G. K. Basu, "Relations of Psychologic Measures of Aggression and Hostility to Testosterone Production in Man," *Psychosomatic Medicine*, vol. 33 (1971), p. 267.

70. Cited in Robert M. Rose, "Testosterone, Aggression and Homosexuality: A Review of the Literature and Implications for Future Re-

search," in Edward J. Sachar, ed., *Topics in Psychoendocrinology* (New York: 1975).

71. Andrew M. Barclay and Ralph Norman Haber, "The Relation of Aggressive and Sexual Motivation," *Journal of Personality*, vol. 33 (1965), p. 462.

72. Y. Jaffe, *et al.*, "Sexual Arousal and Behavioral Aggression," *Journal of Personality and Social Psychology*, vol. 30 (1974), p. 759.

73. Andrew M. Barclay, "Linking Aggressive and Sexual Motives," *Journal of Personality*, vol. 39 (1971), p. 481.

74. S. Feschbach and W. Jaffee, "Effects of Inhibition of Aggression upon Sexual Arousal," cited in Roger N. Johnson, *Aggression in Man and Animals* (Philadelphia: 1972), p. 105.

75. Calvin Hall, "Slang and Dream Symbols," *Psychoanalytic Review*, vol. 51 (1964), p. 38.

76. Susan Griffin, "Rape: The All-American Game," *Ramparts* (September 1971), p. 36.

77. Susan Brownmiller, *Against Our Will: Men, Women and Rape* (New York: 1975), p. 15.

78. Nancy Gager and Cathleen Schurr, *Sexual Assault: Confronting Rape in America* (New York: 1976), p. 280.

79. Edmund Fuller, "Rape—A Tactic in the War of the Sexes," *Wall Street Journal*, October 31, 1975.

80. Duncan Chappell, Robley Geis, and Gilbert Geis, *Forcible Rape: The Crime, the Victim and the Offender* (New York: 1977), p. 9.

81. Brownmiller, *op. cit.*, p. 177.

82. A. Nicholas Groth, Ann Wolbert Burgess, and Lynda Lyttle Holmstrom, "Rape: Power, Anger and Sexuality," *American Journal of Psychiatry*, vol. 134 (1977), p. 1239.

83. A. Nicholas Groth and Ann Wolbert Burgess, "Sexual Dysfunction During Rape," *New England Journal of Medicine* (October 6, 1977), p. 764.

Chapter II

1. *British Medical Journal*, vol. 170 (1968), p. 641.

2. Manson-Bahr, *Manson's Tropical Diseases* (London: 1895), p. 411.

3. P. C. J. van Brero, "Koro, eine eigenthumliche Zwangsvorstellung," *Allg. Z. Psychiat.*, vol. 53 (1897), p. 569.

4. J. A. Slot, "Koro in Central Celebes," *Geneesk. Tijdschr. Ned. Ind.*, vol. 75 (1934), p. 811.

5. P. M. van Wulfften Palthe, "Koro, a Peculiar Anxiety Neurosis," *Geneesk. Tijdschr. Ned. Ind.*, vol. 74 (1934), p. 1713.

6. T. A. Baaschler, "The Influence of Culture on Psychiatric Mani-

festations," *Transcultural Psychiatric Research*, vol. 15 (1963), p. 51.

7. P. M. Yap, "Koro—A Culture-bound Depersonalization Syndrome," *British Journal of Psychiatry*, vol. 111 (1965), p. 43.

8. Fritz Kobler, "Description of an Acute Castration Fear Based on Superstition," *Psychological Review*, vol. 35 (1948), p. 285.

9. The suggestion was made that the proper term be used—in Lewis W. Brandt, "Some Notes on Penis Loss Anxiety," *American Journal of Psychotherapy*, vol. 15 (1961), p. 248—but it has been universally ignored.

10. Ernest Crawley, *The Mystic Rose* (London: 1927), pp. 47–51.

11. *Ibid.*, pp. 58–60.

12. A. C. Kinsey, *et al.*, *Sexual Behavior in the Human Male* (Philadelphia: 1948), p. 366.

13. H. R. Hays, *The Dangerous Sex* (New York: 1964), p. 11.

14. Acts 18:26.

15. I Timothy 2:11–12.

16. Philip Schaff, ed., *A Select Library of the Nicene and Post-Nicene Fathers of the Christian Church* (New York: 1899), ser. 1, vol. IX, p. 104.

17. Cited in G. L. Simonds, *Sex and Superstition* (London: 1966), p. 109.

18. Cited in Katherine M. Rogers, *The Troublesome Helpmate* (Seattle: 1966), p. 11.

19. Wayland Young, *Eros Denied* (New York: 1964), p. 201.

20. *Malleus Maleficarum*, trans. with an Introduction, Bibliography, and Notes by the Reverend Montague Summers (London: 1928).

21. W. H. Trethowan, "The Demonopathology of Impotence," *British Journal of Psychiatry*, vol. 109 (1963), p. 341.

22. Robert Briffault, *The Mothers* (New York: 1927). 3 vols.

23. Leviticus 20:18.

24. Wolfgang Lederer, *The Fear of Women* (New York: 1968), p. 26.

25. Hunter E. Thompson, *Hell's Angels, a Strange and Terrible Saga* (New York: 1967), p. 149.

26. *Ibid.*, p. 37.

27. Hays, *op. cit.*, p. 39.

28. Germaine Greer, *The Female Eunuch* (London: 1971), p. 259.

29. Simonds, *op. cit.*, p. 109.

30. Karen Horney, "The Dread of Women," *International Journal of Psychoanalysis*, vol. 13 (1932), p. 348.

31. Verrier Elwin, "The Vagina Dentata Legend," *British Journal of Medical Psychology*, vol. 19 (1941), p. 439.

32. Stith Thompson, *Tales of the North American Indians* (Boston: 1929).

33. Robert Gessain, "Vagina dentata dans la clinique et la mythologie," *Psychoanalyse*, vol. 3 (1957), p. 247.

34. Lederer, *op. cit.*, p. 44.

35. Jean-Paul Sartre, *Existential Psychoanalysis* (New York: 1962), p. 110.

36. Geza Roheim, *The Riddle of the Sphinx* (London: 1934), p. 230.

37. Sigmund Freud, "The Taboo of Virginity," in *Sexuality and the Psychology of Love* (New York: 1963), p. 70.

38. Simone de Beauvoir, *The Second Sex* (New York: 1953), p. 386.

39. Greer, *op. cit.*, p. 39.

40. William H. Masters and Virginia E. Johnson, *Human Sexual Response* (Boston: 1966), p. 193.

41. In *Daedalus*, vol. 93 (Spring 1964), p. 582.

42. C. G. Jung, "Psychological Aspects of the Mother Archetype," *Collected Works*, vol. 9/1. Bollingen Series XX (New York: 1960), p. 73.

43. Horney, *op. cit.*, p. 351.

44. Alan P. Bell and Martin S. Weinberg, *Homosexualities, A Study of Diversities Among Men and Women* (New York: 1978), p. 85.

45. Joseph Harry and William B. De Vall, *The Social Organization of Gay Males* (New York: 1978), p. 80.

46. Donald Webster Cory, "Homosexuality," in Albert Ellis and Albert Abarbanel, *The Encyclopedia of Sexual Behavior* (New York: 1967), p. 489.

47. Harry and De Vall, *op. cit.*, p. 101.

48. Clifford Allen, "Perversion, Sexual," in Ellis and Abarbanel, *op. cit.*, p. 808.

49. Irving Bieber, *et al.*, *Homosexuality: A Psychoanalytic Study* (New York: 1962).

50. Evelyn Hooker, "An Empirical Study of Some Relations between Sexual Patterns and Gender Identity in Male Homosexuals," in John Money, ed., *Sex Research, New Developments* (New York: 1965), p. 26.

51. Bell and Weinberg, *op. cit.*, p. 328.

52. *Ibid.*, p. 330.

53. Joseph Harry, "On the Validity of Typologies of Gay Males," *Journal of Homosexuality*, vol. 150 (1976), p. 150.

54. Laud Humphreys, *Tearoom Trade, Impersonal Sex in Public Places* (New York: 1970), p. 47.

55. *Ibid.*, p. 108.

56. *Ibid.*, p. 109.

57. Mary Riege Laner and G. W. Levi Kamel, "Media Mating I: Newspaper 'Personals' Ads of Homosexual Men," *Journal of Homosexuality*, vol. 3 (1977), p. 149.

58. Malcolm E. Lumby, "Men Who Advertise for Sex," *Journal of Homosexuality*, vol. 4 (1978), p. 63.

59. Harry and De Vall, *op. cit.*, pp. 3–4.

60. Martin Hoffman, *The Gay World* (New York: 1973), pp. 139–40.

61. Alan Ebert, *The Homosexuals* (New York: 1977), p. 69.

62. Kinsey, *op. cit.*, p. 66.

63. Geoffrey Gorer, *The American People* (New York: 1964), p. 125.

64. Ronald Pearsall, *The Worm in the Bud* (New York: 1969), p. 474.

65. *Ibid.*, p. 474. The story is cited frequently, and generally attributed to Henry Labouchere, the Liberal leader.

66. Gilbert D. Bartell, *Group Sex, an Eyewitness Report on the American Way of Swinging* (New York: 1967), p. 104.

67. *Ibid.*, p. 118.

68. *Ibid.*, p. 146.

69. Wainwright Churchill, *Homosexual Behavior Among Males* (New York: 1971), p. 218.

70. Gorer, *op. cit.*, p. 127.

71. N. McConaghy, "Penile Volume Changes to Moving Pictures of Male and Female Nudes in Heterosexual and Homosexual Males," *Behaviour Research and Therapy*, vol. 5 (1967), p. 43.

72. George Weinberg, *Society and the Sane Homosexual* (New York: 1969).

73. Gorer, *op. cit.*, p. 126.

74. Cited in Vance Packard, *The Sexual Wilderness* (New York: 1970), p. 110.

75. *Ladies' Home Journal* (January 1969), p. 66.

76. Karl Bednarik, *The Male in Crisis* (New York: 1970), p. 99.

77. William H. Masters and Virginia E. Johnson, *Human Sexual Inadequacy* (Boston: 1970), p. 159.

78. Emil A. Gutheil, in *American Handbook of Psychiatry* (New York: 1959), vol. 1, p. 719.

79. Cited in Vern L. Bullough, *The Subordinate Sex* (Chicago: 1973), p. 28.

80. Cited in Ahmed El Senoussi, D. Richard Coleman, and Allan S. Tauber, "Factors in Male Impotence," *Journal of Psychology*, vol. 48, no. 3 (1959), p. 4.

81. Albertus Magnus, *De Secretis Mulierum* (Lyon: 1615), cited in Julia O'Faolain and Lauro Martines, eds., *Not in God's Image* (New York: 1973), p. 124.

82. Benjamin Rush, *Medical Inquiries and Observations upon the Diseases of the Mind* (1812), cited in Ronald G. Walters, *Primers for Prudery* (New York: 1972), p. 33.

83. W. R. Johnson, "Muscular Performance Following Coitus," *Journal of Sex Research*, vol. 4 (1958), p. 247.

84. *New York Times*, December 21, 1974, p. 74.

85. Bronislaw Malinowski, *The Sexual Life of Savages* (New York: 1929), p. 422, cited in Lederer, *op. cit.*, p. 55.

86. Hays, *op. cit.*, p. 99.

87. Mary Jane Sherfey, *The Nature and Evolution of Female Sexuality* (New York: 1972), pp. 124–25.

88. *Ibid.*, pp. 127–28.

89. William A. Acton, *The Functions and Disorders of the Reproductive Organs in Childhood, Youth, Adult Age and Advanced Life Considered in their Physiological, Social and Moral Relations* (Philadelphia: 1871), p. 163.

90. Cited in Nathan G. Hale., Jr., *Freud and the Americans* (New York: 1971), p. 36.

91. George Henry Napheys, *The Transmission of Life, Counsels of the Nature and Hygiene of the Masculine Function* (Philadelphia: 1871), p. 314.

92. H. Newell Martin, *The Human Body* (New York: 1899), p. 663.

93. Alexander Walker, *Intermarriage: or the Mode in Which and the Causes Why Beauty, Health and Intellect Result from Certain Unions and Deformity, Disease and Insanity from Others* (New York: 1839), p. 256.

94. William M. Capp, *The Daughter, Her Health, Education and Wedlock* (Philadelphia: 1891), p. 94.

95. Margaret Cleaves, "Education in Sexual Physiology and Hygiene," *Women's Medical Journal*, vol. XVIII (1908), p. 223.

96. John Cowan, *The Science of a New Life* (New York: 1880), p. 115.

97. Acton, *op. cit.*, p. 225.

98. N. Venel, *Advice to the Nervous and Debilitated of Both Sexes* (London: 1815), p. 15.

99. Ben Barker-Benfield, "The Spermatic Economy: A Nineteenth-Century View of Sexuality," in *The American Family in Social-Historical Perspective*, Michael Gordon, ed. (New York: 1973), p. 342.

100. C. Bigelow, *Sexual Pathology: A Practical and Popular Review of the Principal Diseases of the Reproductive Organs* (Chicago: 1895), p. 83.

101. John S. Haller and Robin M. Haller, *The Physician and Sexuality in Victorian America* (Chicago: 1974), p. 215.

102. Acton, *op. cit.*, p. 147.

103. J. H. Kellogg, *Plain Facts About Sexual Life* (Battle Creek, Mich.: 1877), p. 177.

104. G. Stanley Hall, *Educational Problems*, vol. I (New York: 1924), p. 478.

105. Augustus Kinsley Gardner, "The Physical Decline of American Women," *The Knickerbocker*, vol. 55, no. 1 (January 1860), p. 37.

106. Barker-Benfield, *op. cit.*, p. 348, who gives four medical citations.

107. Cited in Ilza Veith, *Hysteria: The History of a Disease* (Chicago: 1970), p. 216.

108. Charles E. Rosenberg, "Sexuality, Class and Role in 19th Century America," *American Quarterly*, vol. XXV (1973), p. 139.

109. Barker-Benfield, *op. cit.*, p. 354.

110. Ben Barker-Benfield, *The Horrors of the Half-Known Life* (New York: 1976), p. 122.

111. Howard A. Kelly, "Conservatism in Ovariotomy," *Journal of the American Medical Association*, vol. 26 (1896), p. 251.

112. James W. Cokenower, "A Plea for the Conservative Operations on the Ovaries," *Transactions of the Section on Obstetrics and Diseases of Women of the American Medical Association* (1904), p. 291.

113. Ely Van der Warker, "The Fetish of the Ovary," *American Journal of Obstetrics and the Diseases of Women and Children*, vol. 54 (July–December 1906), p. 369.

114. Rollo May, *Love and Will* (New York: 1969), p. 117.

115. Charles Winick, *The New People* (New York: 1968), p. 319.

116. Morton Hunt, *Sexual Behavior in the 1970's* (New York: 1974), pp. 34, 199.

117. *Ibid.*, p. 200.

118. Winick, *op. cit.*, p. 320.

119. All ads appeared in *Screw* magazine, March 8, 1976.

120. R. Loewenstein, "Phallic Passivity in Men," *International Journal of Psychoanalysis*, vol. 16 (1935), p. 334.

121. *Ibid.*, p. 335.

122. Kinsey, *op. cit.*, p. 331.

123. Louis Bragman, "A Case of Autofellatio," *Medical Journal and Record*, vol. 126 (1927), p. 488.

124. E. Kahn and E. Lion, "A Clinical Note on a Self-Fellator," *American Journal of Psychiatry*, vol. 95 (1938), p. 131.

125. Frank Orland, "Factors in Autofellatio Formation," *International Journal of Psychoanalysis*, vol. 52 (1971), p. 289.

126. William H. Masters and Virginia E. Johnson, *Human Sexual Response* (Boston: 1966), p. 191.

127. "A Conversation with Masters and Johnson," *Psychology Today* (July 1969), p. 54.

128. *Medical Aspects of Human Sexuality* (June 1974), p. 170.

129. J. S. Verinis and S. Roll, "Primary and Secondary Male Characteristics: The Hairiness and Large Penis Stereotypes," *Psychological Reports*, vol. 26 (1970), p. 123.

130. *Ibid.*, p. 126.

Chapter III

1. Henry Gray, *Anatomy of the Human Body* (Philadelphia, 1973).

2. *Ibid.*, p. 1310.

3. Paul Delany, "Constantinus Africanus' *De Coitu*: A Translation," *Chaucer Review*, vol. 4 (1969), p. 556.

4. Eckhardt, C. "Untersuchungen über die Erection des Penis beim Hund," *Beitr. Anat. Physiol.*, vol. 3 (1863), p. 123.

5. J. H. Semans and O. R. Langworthy, "Observations on the Neurophysiology of Sexual Function in the Male Cat," *Journal of Urology*, vol. 40 (1938), p. 836.

6. Herbert F. Newman, Jane D. Northrup, and John Devlin, "Mechanism of Human Penile Erection, *Investigative Urology*, vol. 1 (1964), p. 350.

7. Howard D. Weiss, "The Physiology of Human Penile Erection," *Annals of Internal Medicine*, vol. 76 (1972), p. 793.

8. Paul MacLean, "New Findings Relevant to the Evolution of Psychosexual Functions of the Brain," *Journal of Nervous and Mental Disease*, vol. 135 (1962), p. 289.

9. E. Bors and A. E. Commar, "Neurological Disturbances of Sexual Function with Special Reference to 529 Patients with Spinal Cord Injury," *Urological Survey*, vol. 10 (1960), p. 191.

10. Herbert S. Talbot, "The Sexual Function in Paraplegia," *Journal of Urology*, vol. 73 (1955) , p. 91.

11. Howard D. Weiss, "Mechanism of Erection," *Medical Aspects of Human Sexuality* (February 1973), p. 28.

12. A. C. Kinsey, W. B. Pomeroy, and C. E. Martin, *Sexual Behavior in the Human Male* (Philadelphia: 1948), p. 521.

13. Frank A. Beach, William H. Westbrook, and Lynwood C. Clemens, "Comparisons of the Ejaculatory Response in Men and Animals," *Psychosomatic Medicine,* vol. 28 (1966), p. 749.

14. Ian F. Potts, "The Mechanism of Ejaculation," *Medical Journal of Australia* (April 13, 1957), p. 495.

15. W. H. Masters and V. E. Johnson, *Human Sexual Response* (Boston: 1966), p. 191.

16. *Journal of the American Medical Association*, vol. 216, no. 11 (June 14, 1971), p. 1873.

17. Robert Latou Dickinson, *Atlas of Human Sex Anatomy* (Baltimore: 1949) , p. 73.

18. *Ibid.*, p. vi-a.

19. Masters and Johnson, *op. cit.*, p. 192.

20. "A Conversation with Masters and Johnson," *Psychology Today* (July 1969), p. 56.

21. Heinrich Loeb, "Harnrohrencapacität und Tripperspritzen," *München Med. Wschr.*, vol. 46 (1899), p. 1016.

22. Kenneth W. Feldman and David W. Smith, "Fetal Phallic Growth and Penile Standards for Newborn Male Infants," *Journal of Pediatrics*, vol. 86 (1975), p. 395.

23. Apollodorus, *The Library* (Cambridge: 1956), vol. 5, p. 80.

24. *The Perfumed Garden of the Shayh Nefzawi*, trans. by Richard F. Burton (New York: 1963), p. 110.

25. *Penthouse* magazine (May 1976), p. 170.

26. *Hustler* magazine (July 1976), p. 144.

27. Leon Saltzman, M.D., "Interesting Sexual Cases: Premature Ejaculation," *Medical Aspects of Human Sexuality* (June 1972), p. 43.

28. Kinsey, *op. cit.*, pp. 193–217.

29. Karl Abraham, "Ejaculatio Praecox," in *Selected Papers* (London: 1927), p. 280.

30. Wilhelm Stekel, *Impotence in the Male*, vol. 2 (New York: 1927), p. 25.

31. *Ibid.*, p. 26.

32. Bernard Schapiro, "Premature Ejaculation. A Review of 1130 Cases," *Journal of Urology*, vol. 50 (1943), p. 374.

33. Lay Aycock, "The Medical Management of Premature Ejaculation," *Journal of Urology*, vol. 62 (1949), p. 361. See also Frederick Damrau, "Premature Ejaculation: Use of Ethyl Aminobenzoate to Prolong Coitus," *Journal of Urology*, vol. 89 (1963), p. 936.

34. James H. Semans, "Premature Ejaculation: A New Approach," *Southern Medical Journal*, vol. 49 (1956), p. 353.

35. W. H. Masters and V. E. Johnson, *Human Sexual Inadequacy* (Boston: 1970), pp. 92–109.

36. R. Waelder, *Basic Theory of Psychoanalysis* (New York: 1960), p. 94.

37. R. Michels, "Psychoanalysis and the Sex Therapies," presented at the Annual Meeting of the American Psychiatric Association (1975).

38. Louis J. Ripich, "Roundtable: Premature Ejaculation," *Medical Aspects of Human Sexuality* (May 1971), pp. 35–39.

39. I. Goldiamond, "Self-Control Procedures in Personal Behavior Problems," *Psychological Reports*, vol. 17 (1957), p. 851.

40. John C. Lowe and William L. Mikulas, "Use of Written Material in Learning Self-Control of Premature Ejaculation," *Psychological Reports*, vol. 37 (1975), p. 295.

41. Lionel Ovesey and Helen Meyers, "Retarded Ejaculation: Psychodynamics and Psychotherapy," *American Journal of Psychotherapy*, vol. 22 (1968), p. 185.

42. Helen Singer Kaplan, *The New Sex Therapy* (New York: 1974), p. 320.

43. E. D. Frohlich and E. D. Freis, "Clinical Trials of Guanethidine," *Medical Annals, D.C.*, vol. 28 (1959), p. 419. C. T. Dollery, E. M. Smith, and M. D. Milne, "Guanethidine in the Treatment of Hypertension," *Lancet*, vol. 2 (1960), p. 381. R. H. Irvine, K. P. O'Brien, and J. D. K. North, "Methyl Dopa in the Treatment of Hypertension," *Lancet*, vol. 1 (1962), p. 300. H. Singh, "Therapeutic Use of Thioridazine," *American Journal of Psychiatry*, vol. 119 (1963), p. 891. L. Clein, "Thioridazine and Ejaculation," *British Medical Journal*, vol. 2 (1962), p. 547. J. M. Hughes, "Failure to Ejaculate with Chlordiazepoxide," *American Journal of Psychiatry*, vol. 121 (1964), p. 610.

44. Sandor Ferenczi, "The Symbolism and the Bridge," in *Selected Papers* (New York: 1950), vol. 2, pp. 352–56.

45. Edmund Bergler, "Some Special Varieties of Ejaculatory Disturbance Not Hitherto Described," *International Journal of Psychoanalysis*, vol. 16 (1935), p. 84.

46. Otto Fenichel, *The Psychoanalytic Theory of Neuroses* (New York: 1945), p. 172.

47. Masters and Johnson, *Human Sexual Inadequacy*, p. 117.

48. Javad Razani, "Ejaculatory Incompetence Treated by Deconditioning Anxiety," *Journal of Behavior Therapy and Experimental Psychiatry*, vol. 3 (1972), p. 65.

49. Karel Geboes, Omer Steeno, and Pieter De Moor, "Primary Anejaculation: Diagnosis and Therapy," *Fertility and Sterility*, vol. 26 (1975), p. 1109. See also T. M. C. M. Schellen, "Induction of Ejaculation by Electrovibration," *Fertility and Sterility*, vol. 19 (1968), p. 566, and A. J. Sobrero, H. E. Stearns, and J. H. Blair, "Technic for the Induction of Ejaculation in Humans," *Fertility and Sterility*, vol. 16 (1965), p. 765.

50. Stekel, *op. cit.*, p. 107.

51. Ernest Jones, *Papers on Psychoanalysis* (London: 1918), p. 79.

52. Sigmund Freud, *Sexuality and the Psychology of Love* (New York: 1963), p. 63.

53. *Ibid.*, p. 64.

54. Donald W. Hastings, *Impotence and Frigidity* (New York: 1963), p. 83.

55. Bruce G. Belt, "Some Organic Causes of Impotence," *Medical Abstracts of Human Sexuality* (January 1973), p. 152.

56. R. Leriche and A. Morel, "The Syndrome of Thrombotic Obstruction of Aortic Bifurcation," *Annals of Surgery*, vol. 127 (1948), p. 193.

57. John Johnson, *Disorders of Potency in the Male* (New York: 1968).

58. Warren O. Kessler and A. P. McLaughlin, "Agnesis of Penis, Embryology and Management," *Urology*, vol. 1 (1973), p. 226.

59. Kinsey, *op. cit.*, p. 323.

60. J. E. Howard and W. W. Scott, "The Testes," in *Textbook of En-*

docrinology, R. E. Williams, ed. (Philadelphia: 1955), p. 81.

61. D. Stafford-Clark, "The Etiology and Treatment of Impotence," *Practitioner*, vol. 172 (1954) , p. 397.

62. Sigmund Freud, *Complete Works*, vol. 11 (London: 1957), p. 242.

63. Freud, *Sexuality and the Psychology of Love*, p. 64.

64. Karl Abraham, *Selected Papers* (London: 1949), p. 145.

65. Jones, *op. cit.*, p. 93.

66. Stekel, *op. cit.*, p. 111.

67. Freud, *Complete Works*, vol. 11 (London: 1957), p. 240.

68. Jones, *op. cit.*, p. 90.

69. A. Salter, *Conditioned Reflex Therapy* (New York: 1949), p. 268.

70. Alan J. Cooper, "Factors in Male Sexual Inadequacy: A Review," *Journal of Nervous and Mental Disease*, vol. 149 (1969), p. 337. See also, Ahmed El Senoussi, Richard Coleman, and Allan S. Tauber, "Factors in Male Impotence," *Journal of Psychology*, vol. 48 (1959) , p. 3.

71. Masters and Johnson, *Human Sexual Inadequacy*, p. 12.

72. Joseph Wolpe, *The Practice of Behavior Therapy* (New York: 1969), p. 83.

73. Freud, "A Child Is Being Beaten," in *Sexuality and the Psychology of Love*, p. 40.

74. P. G. Denker, "Results of Treatment of Psychoneuroses by the General Practitioner: A Follow-up Study of 500 Cases," *New York State Journal of Medicine*, vol. 46 (1946), p. 2164.

75. H. J. Eysenck, "The Effects of Psychotherapy," in *Handbook of Abnormal Psychology*, H. J. Eysenck, ed. (London: 1960).

76. J. F. Tuthill, "Impotence," *Lancet*, vol. 1 (1955), p. 124.

77. D. Stafford-Clark, "The Etiology and Treatment of Impotence," *Practitioner*, vol. 172 (1954), p. 397.

78. Alan J. Cooper, "Disorders of Sexual Potency in the Male: A Clinical and Statistical Study of Some Factors Related to Short-term Prognosis," *British Journal of Psychiatry*, vol. 115 (1969), p. 709.

79. John Johnson, "Prognosis of Disorders of Sexual Potency in the Male," *Journal of Psychosomatic Research*, vol. 9 (1965) , p. 195.

80. Cited in R. A. Hunter and I. Macalpine, *Three Hundred Years of Psychiatry (1535–1860)* (London: 1963).

81. S. Rachman, "Sexual Disorders and Behavior Therapy," *American Journal of Psychiatry*, vol. 118 (1961), p. 235.

82. *Ibid.*, p. 246.

83. Sarojini Asirdas and H. R. Beech, "The Behavioral Treatment of Sexual Inadequacy," *Journal of Psychosomatic Research*, vol. 19 (1975), p. 375.

84. J. Wolpe, *Psychotherapy by Reciprocal Inhibition* (Stanford: 1958), p. 81.

85. D. Friedman, "The Treatment of Impotence by Brietal Relaxation Therapy," *Behaviour Research Therapy*, vol. 6 (1968), p. 257.

86. G. Kockott, F. Dittmar, and L. Nusselt, "Systematic Desensitization of Erectile Impotence: A Controlled Study," *Archives of Sexual Behavior*, vol. 4 (1975), p. 493. J. M. A. Ansari, "Impotence: Prognosis (A Controlled Study)," *British Journal of Psychiatry*, vol. 128 (1976), p. 194.

87. Tuthill, *op. cit.*, p. 126.

88. Martin Goldberg, "Selective Impotence," *Medical Aspects of Human Sexuality* (October 1972), p. 93.

89. Henry J. Friedman, "An Interpersonal Aspect of Psychogenic Impotence," *American Journal of Psychotherapy*, vol. 27 (1973), p. 421.

90. Masters and Johnson, *Human Sexual Inadequacy*, p. 198.

91. Jhan and June Robbins, *An Analysis of Human Sexual Inadequacy* (New York: 1970). Fred Belliveau and Lin Richter, *Understanding Human Sexual Inadequacy* (New York: 1970). Nat Lehrman, *Masters and Johnson Explained* (Chicago: 1970).

92. Alan J. Cooper, "Treatments of Male Sexual Disorders: The Present Status," *Psychosomatics*, vol. 12 (1971), p. 235.

93. Kockott, *op. cit.*, p. 495.

94. Kinsey, *op. cit.*, pp. 35–101.

95. Marvin Zuckerman, "Physiological Measures of Sexual Arousal in the Human," *Psychological Bulletin*, vol. 75 (1971), p. 297. Marion A. Wenger, James R. Averill, and David D. B. Smith, "Autonomic Activity During Sexual Arousal," *Psychophysiology*, vol. 4 (1968), p. 4.

96. K. Freund, "A Laboratory Method for Diagnosing Predominance in Homo- or Hetero-Erotic Interest in the Male," *Behaviour Research and Therapy*, vol. 1 (1963), p. 85.

97. J. H. J. Bancroft, H. Gwynne Jones, and B. R. Pullan, "A Simple Transducer for Measuring Penile Erection, with Comments on Its Use in the Treatment of Sexual Disorders," *Behaviour Research and Therapy*, vol. 4 (1966), p. 239.

98. James H. Geer, Patricia Morokoff, and Pamela Greenwood, "Sexual Arousal in Women: The Development of a Measurement Device for Vaginal Blood Volume," *Archives of Sexual Behavior*, vol. 3 (1974), p. 559.

99. John Bancroft, "The Application of Psychophysiological Measures to the Assessment and Modification of Sexual Behavior," *Behaviour Research and Therapy*, vol. 9 (1971), p. 119.

100. Cited in Robert S. Ropp, *Sex Energy* (New York: 1969), p. 83.

101. Elizabeth Gould Davis, *The First Sex* (New York: 1971), p. 152.

102. D. R. Laws and H. B. Rubin, "Instructional Control of an Autonomic Sexual Response," *Journal of Applied Behavior Analysis*, vol. 2 (1969), p. 93.

103. Zuckerman, *op. cit.*, p. 309.

104. Donald E. Henson and H. R. Rubin, "Voluntary Control of Eroticism," *Journal of Applied Behavior Analysis*, vol. 4 (1971), p. 37.

105. Raymond C. Rosen, "Suppression of Penile Tumescence by Instrumental Control," *Psychosomatic Medicine*, vol. 35 (1973), p. 509.

106. Raymond C. Rosen, David Shapiro, and Gary E. Schwartz, "Voluntary Control of Penile Tumescence," *Psychosomatic Medicine*, vol. 37 (1975), p. 479.

107. E. R. Csillag, "Modification of Penile Erectile Response," *Journal of Behaviour Therapy and Experimental Psychiatry*, vol. 7 (1976) , p. 27.

108. Thomas G. Benedek, "Aphrodisiacs: Fact and Fable," *Medical Aspects of Human Sexuality* (December 1973), p. 42.

109. Alan Hull Walton, *Aphrodisiacs, from Legend to Prescription* (Westport, Conn.: 1958), p. 26.

110. Act IV, Scene III.

111. Genesis 30:14–17.

112. Benedek, *op. cit.*, p. 49.

113. *Ibid.*

114. D. E. Bruhl and C. H. Leslie, "Afrodex: Double Blind Test in Impotence," *Medical Record and Annals*, vol. 56 (1963), p. 22. C. H. Leslie and D. E. Bruhl, "An Effective Anti-Impotence Agent: Statistical Evaluation of 1,000 Reported Cases," *Memphis and Mid-South Medical Journal*, vol. 38 (1963), p. 379. R. Margolis and C. H. Leslie, "Review of Studies on a Mixture of Nux Vomica, Yohimbine and Methyl Testosterone in the Treatment of Impotence," *Current Therapeutic Research*, vol. 8 (1966), p. 280. Robert Margolis, *et al.*, "Clinical Studies on the Use of Afrodex in the Treatment of Impotence," *Current Therapeutic Research*, vol. 9 (1967), p. 213.

115. Benedek, *op. cit.*, p. 55.

116. Patrick M. McGrady, Jr., *The Youth Doctors* (New York: 1968), p. 40.

117. *Ibid.*, p. 41.

118. Cited in Benedek, *op. cit.*, p. 58.

119. Hugh T. Carmichael and William J. Noonan, "The Effects of Testosterone Propionate in Impotence," *American Journal of Psychiatry*, vol. 97 (1941), p. 919.

120. Act II, Scene III.

121. H. B. Rubin and Donald E. Henson, "Effects of Alcohol on Male Sexual Responding," *Psychopharmacology*, vol. 47 (1976), p. 123. Dan W. Bridell and G. Terence Wilson, "Effects of Alcohol and Expectancy Set on Male Arousal," *Journal of Abnormal Psychology*, vol. 85 (1976), p. 225.

122. G. Terence Wilson and David M. Lawson, "Effects of Alcohol on Sexual Arousal in Women," *Journal of Abnormal Psychology*, vol. 85 (1976), p. 489.

123. Rubin and Henson, *op. cit.*, p. 133.

124. H. J. Anslinger, "Panel Interview: The Drug Revolution," *Playboy* (February, 1969).

125. Cited in Leo E. Hollister, "Drugs and Sexual Behavior in Man," *Life Sciences*, vol. 17 (New York: 1975), p. 665.

126. Cited in Everett H. Ellinwood and Kenneth Rockwell, "Effects of Drug Use on Sexual Behavior," *Medical Aspects of Human Sexuality* (March 1975), p. 26.

127. Robert C. Kolodny, *et al.*, "Depression of Plasma Testosterone with Acute Marihuana Administration," in *The Pharmacology of Marihuana* (New York: 1976), p. 211.

128. See George R. Gay and Charles W. Sheppard, "Sex in the 'Drug Culture,'" *Medical Aspects of Human Sexuality* (October 1972), p. 28. Also George R. Gay, *et al.*, "Drug-Sex Practice in the Haight-Ashbury, or 'The Sensuous Hippie,'" in Merton Sandler and G. L. Gessa, *Sexual Behavior: Pharmacology and Biochemistry* (New York: 1975). Also Leo E. Hollister, "The Mystique of Social Drugs and Sex," in the same volume.

129. *Medical Aspects of Human Sexuality* (October 1972), p. 49.

130. André Barbeau, "L-Dopa Therapy in Parkinson's Disease: A Critical Review of Nine Years' Experience," *Canadian Medical Association Journal*, vol. 101 (1969), p. 791.

131. Malcolm B. Bowers, *et al.*, "Sexual Behavior During L-dopa Treatment for Parkinsonism," *American Journal of Psychiatry*, vol. 127 (1971), p. 127.

132. Albert Sjoerdsma, *et al.*, "Serotonin Now: Clinical Implications of Inhibiting Its Synthesis with Para-chlorophenylalanine," *Annals of Internal Medicine*, vol. 73 (1970), p. 607.

133. G. L. Gessa and Allesandro Tagliamonte, "Role of Brain Monoamines in Male Sexual Behavior," *Life Sciences*, vol. 14 (1974), p. 425. Federico Sicuteri, "Serotonin and Sex in Man," *Pharmacological Research Communications*, vol. 6 (1974), p. 401.

134. Benedek, *op. cit.*, p. 63.

135. Albert Ellis and Albert Abarbanel, eds., *The Encyclopedia of Sexual Behavior* (New York: 1967), p. 150.

136. William L. Furlow, "Surgical Management of Impotence Using the Inflatable Penile Prosthesis," *Mayo Clinic Proceedings*, vol. 51 (1976), p. 325.

137. Ambroise Paré, *The Works of That Famous Chirurgion Ambroise Parey, Translated out of the Latine and Compared with the French by Th. Johnson* (London: 1634), reprint edition by Milford House, Inc. (Boston: 1968), p. 111.

138. N. Bogoras, "Über die volle plastische Wiederherstellung eines zum Koitus fähigen Penis," *Zentralbl. Chir.*, vol. 63 (1936), p. 1271.

139. H. D. Gillies and D. R. Millard, "Congenital Absence of the Penis," *British Journal of Plastic Surgery*, vol. 1 (1948), p. 8.

140. Joel M. Noe, Dale Birdsell, and Donald R. Laub, "The Surgical Construction of Male Genitalia for the Female-to-Male Transsexual," *Plastic and Reconstructive Surgery*, vol. 53 (1974), p. 511.

141. E. Aserinsky and N. Kleitman, "Regularly Occurring Periods of Eye Motility and Concomitant Phenomena During Sleep," *Science*, vol. 118 (1953), p. 273.

142. W. Dement and N. Kleitman, "The Relations of Eye Movements During Sleep to Dream Activity," *Journal of Experimental Psychology*, vol. 53 (1957), p. 339.

143. C. Fisher, J. Gross, and J. Zuch, "Cycle of Penile Erection Synchronous with Dreaming (REM) Sleep," *Archives of General Psychiatry*, vol. 12 (1965), p. 29.

144. *Ibid.*, pp. 38–39.

145. I. Karacan, *et al.*, "The Effect of Sexual Intercourse on Sleep Patterns and Nocturnal Penile Erections," *Psychophysiology*, vol. 7 (1970), p. 338.

146. I. Karacan, "Clinical Value of Nocturnal Erection in the Prognosis and Diagnosis of Impotence," *Medical Abstracts of Human Sexuality* (April 1970), p. 27.

147. I. Karacan, "Erection Cycle During Sleep in Relation to Dream Anxiety," *Archives of General Psychiatry*, vol. 15 (1966), p. 183.

148. I. Karacan, *et al.*, "Sleep-Related Penile Tumescence as a Function of Age," *American Journal of Psychiatry*, vol. 132 (1975), p. 932.

149. *Ibid.*, p. 936.

Chapter IV

1. Blair O. Rogers, *History of External Genital Surgery* (New York: 1969), p. 7.

2. J. Hastings, *Encyclopaedia of Religion and Ethics* (Edinburgh: 1932), vol. 3, p. 676.

3. Exodus 4:25.

4. Joshua 5:2–3.

5. Philippians 3:5; Acts 16:3.

6. Romans 2:29.

7. Theodore James, "Philo on Circumcision," *South African Medical Journal* (August 21, 1976), p. 1409.

8. Ernest Crawley, *The Mystic Rose* (London: 1902), p. 137.

9. Cited in Hastings, *op. cit.*, p. 666.

10. Sigmund Freud, *Analysis of a Phobia in a Five-year-old Boy*, standard edition, vol. X (London: 1909), p. 116.

11. S. Freud, *Moses and Monotheism* (London: 1939), p. 192.

12. S. Freud, *An Autobiographical Study* (New York: 1952), p. 129.

13. S. Freud, *An Outline of Psychoanalysis* (London: 1949), p. 58.

14. G. Roheim, *The Eternal Ones of the Dream* (New York: 1945). Theodor Reik, *Ritual: Psychoanalytic Studies* (New York: 1946). C. D. Daly, "The Psychobiological Origins of Circumcision," *International Journal of Psychoanalysis*, vol. 31 (1950), p. 217.

15. Herman Nunberg, *Problems of Bisexuality as Reflected in Circumcision* (London: 1949).

16. See John C. Touhey, "Penis Envy and Attitudes Toward Castration-like Punishment and Sexual Aggression," *Journal of Research in Personality*, vol. 11 (1977), p. 1. G. S. Blum, "A Study of the Psychoanalytic Theory of Psychosexual Development," *Genetic Psychological Monographs*, vol. 39 (1949), p. 3. R. B. Levin, "An Empirical Test of the Female Castration Complex," *Journal of Abnormal and Social Psychology*, vol. 71 (1966), p. 181. G. C. Rosenwald, *et al.*, "An Action Test of Hypotheses Concerning the Anal Personality," *Journal of Abnormal Psychology*, vol. 71 (1966), p. 304. S. Friedman, "An Empirical Study of the Castration and Oedipus Complexes," *Genetic Psychology Monographs*, vol. 46 (1952), p. 61. B. J. Schwartz, "An Empirical Test of Two Freudian Hypotheses Concerning Castration Anxiety," *Journal of Personality*, vol. 24 (1956), p. 318. I. Sarnoff, "Reaction Formation and Cynicism," *Journal of Personality*, vol. 28 (1960), p. 129.

17. Michio Kitahara, "A Cross-Cultural Test of the Freudian Theory of Circumcision," *International Journal of Psychoanalytic Psychotherapy*, vol. 5 (1976), p. 535.

18. Margaret Mead, *Coming of Age in Samoa* (New York: 1960), p. 118.

19. Edward Norbeck, *et al.*, "The Interpretation of Puberty Rites," *American Anthropologist*, vol. 64 (1962), p. 463.

20. Frank Zimmerman, "Origins and Significance of the Jewish Rite of Circumcision," *Psychoanalytic Review*, vol. 38 (1951), pp. 108–09.

21. *Ibid.*, pp. 109–10.

22. Leviticus 12:2.

23. Bruno Bettelheim, *Symbolic Wounds* (New York: 1962), pp. 42–43.

24. *Ibid.*, p. 19.

25. *Ibid.*, p. 147.

26. Hawa Patel, "The Problem of Routine Circumcision," *Canadian Medical Association Journal*, vol. 95 (1966), p. 576.

27. William Keith C. Morgan, "The Rape of the Phallus," *Journal of the American Medical Association*, vol. 193 (1965), p. 223.

28. P. C. Remondino, *History of Circumcision from the Earliest Times to the Present* (Philadelphia: 1891), p. 256.

29. *Ibid.*, p. 186.

30. Benjamin Spock, *The Common Sense Book of Baby and Child Care* (New York: 1945), p. 18.

31. Douglas Gairdner, "The Fate of the Foreskin, a Study of Circumcision," *British Medical Journal* (December 24, 1949), p. 1433.

32. V. F. Marshall, *et al., Treatment of Cancer and Allied Diseases* (New York: 1963), vol. 7, p. 9.

33. Gairdner, *op. cit.*, p. 1439.

34. David A. Grimes, "Routine Circumcision of the Newborn Infant: A Reappraisal," *American Journal of Obstetrics and Gynecology*, vol. 130 (1978), p. 125.

35. William Keith C. Morgan, "Penile Plunder," *Medical Journal of Australia*, vol. 1 (1967), p. 1102.

36. "Report of the Ad Hoc Task Force on Circumcision," *Pediatrics*, vol. 56 (1975), p. 610.

37. Grimes, *op. cit.*

38. Morgan, "The Rape of the Phallus," p. 124.

39. Grimes, *op. cit.*, p. 127.

40. R. N. Emde, *et al.*, "Stress and Neonatal Sleep," *Psychosomatic Medicine*, vol. 33 (1971), p. 491. T. F. Anders and R. J. Chalemian, "The Effects of Circumcision on Sleep-Awake States in Human Neonates," *Psychosomatic Medicine*, vol. 36 (1974), p. 174.

41. M. P. M. Richards, J. F. Bernal, and Yvonne Brackbill, "Differences: Gender or Circumcision?," *Developmental Psychobiology*, vol. 9 (1976), p. 89.

42. Herbert Basedow, "Subincision and Kindred Rites of the Australian Aborigines," *Journal of the Royal Anthropological Institute*, vol. 57 (1927), p. 123.

43. Ivor H. Jones, "Subincision among Australian Western Desert Aborigines," *British Journal of Medical Psychology*, vol. 42 (1969), p. 188.

44. *Ibid.*, p. 187.

45. Basedow, *op. cit.*, p. 146.

46. *Ibid.*, p. 151.

47. *Ibid.*, p. 153.

48. *Ibid.*, p. 145.

49. M. F. Ashley Montagu, *Coming into Being Among the Australian Aborigines* (London: 1937), p. 302.

50. *Ibid.*, p. 303.

51. Roheim, *op. cit.*, p. 164.

52. *Ibid.*, p. 177.

53. Bettelheim, *op. cit.*, pp. 100–08.

54. J. E. Cawte, *et al.*, "The Meaning of Subincision of the Urethra to Aboriginal Australians," *British Journal of Medical Psychology*, vol. 39 (1966), pp. 245–53.

Chapter V

1. Otto Brendel, "The Scope and Temperament of Erotic Art in the Greco-Roman World," in *Studies in Erotic Art*, Theodore Bowie and Cornelia V. Christenson, eds. (New York: 1970), p. 9.

2. *Ibid.*, p. 15.

3. *Ibid.*, p. 48.

4. G. Rattray Taylor, *Sex in History* (New York: 1954), p. 19.

5. Romans 7:25.

6. Galatians 5:17.

7. I Corinthians 7:1–9.

8. H. H. Milman, *The History of Christianity* (London: 1840).

9. Geoffrey May, *Social Control of Sexual Expression* (New York: 1931), p. 42.

10. Taylor, *op. cit.*, p. 254.

11. C. Horstmann, ed., *Lives of the Women Saints of Our Contrie of England* (London: 1858), p. 148.

12. Sir Frank Stanton, *The Bayeux Tapestry, a Comprehensive Survey* (London: 1957), plate 15.

13. Walter S. Gibson, *Hieronymus Bosch* (New York: 1973), p. 80.

14. Dirk Bax, *Ontcijfering van Jeroen Bosch* (The Hague: 1948).

15. For other studies of the "Garden of Earthly Delights," see Ch. de Tolnay, *Hieronymus Bosch* (London: 1966); J. Combe, *Jerome Bosch* (Paris: 1957); A. Spychalska-Boczkowska, "Materials for the Iconography of Hieronimus Bosch's Triptich the Garden of Delights," *Studia Muzealne* (1966), p. 49; and W. Fraenger, *The Millennium of Hieronymus Bosch* (Chicago: 1951).

16. Richard Lewinsohn, *A History of Sexual Customs* (New York: 1958), p. 151.

17. Jacob Burckhardt, *The Civilization of the Renaissance in Italy* (Oxford: 1944), p. 81.

18. See Edgar Wind, *Pagan Mysteries of the Renaissance* (New Haven: 1958).

19. Leo Steinberg, "The Metaphors of Love and Birth in Michelangelo's *Pietàs*," in *Studies in Erotic Art* (New York: 1970), p. 231.

20. *Ibid.*, p. 248.

21. Cited in Frederick Hartt, *Giulio Romano*, vol. 1 (New Haven: 1958), p. 280.

22. Wayland Young, *Eros Denied* (New York: 1964), p. 103.

23. *Ibid.*, p. 100.

24. Hartt, *op. cit.*, p. 276.

25. A complete bibliographic history of the "Modi" is included in Peter Webb, *The Erotic Arts* (New York: 1975), p. 354.

26. Cited in Robert Melville, *Erotic Art of the West* (New York: 1973), p. 24.

27. Kurt von Meier, *The Forbidden Erotica of Thomas Rowlandson* (Los Angeles: 1967), p. 14.

28. Cited in Pierre Cabanne, *La Psychologie de l'Erotisme* (Paris: 1971), p. 40.

29. *The Journals of Eugene Delacroix*, translated from the French by Walter Pach (New York: 1948), April 20, 1824.

30. *The Goncourt Journal* (New York: 1946), March 6, 1868.

31. Victor Arwas, *Félicien Rops* (New York: 1972), p. 2.

32. *Ibid.*, p. 3.

33. *Ibid.*, p. 5.

34. *Ibid.*

35. Charles Brison, *Pornocrates, an Introduction to the Life and Works of Félicien Rops* (London: 1969), p. 47.

36. Brigid Brophy, *Black and White, a Portrait of Aubrey Beardsley* (London: 1968), p. 36.

37. *The Letters of Aubrey Beardsley*, Henry Moss, J. L. Duncan, and W. G. Good, eds. (Teaneck, N.J.: 1970), p. 150.

38. Cited in Melville, *op. cit.*, p. 28.

39. Allesandra Comini, *Gustav Klimt* (New York: 1975), p. 7.

40. *Ibid.*, p. 8.

41. André Breton, *Manifestes du Surréalisme* (Paris: n.d.), p. 6.

42. Salvador Dali, *Conquest of the Irrational* (New York: 1935), pp. 14–15.

43. Georges Bataille, *Eroticism* (New York: 1958), p. 7.

44. David Gascoyne, *A Short Survey of Surrealism* (London: 1935), p. 33.

45. Hans Bellmer, *Die Puppe*, quoted in Volker Kohmen, *Eroticism in Contemporary Art* (London: 1972), p. 62.

46. Roland Penrose, *Picasso: His Life and Work* (London: 1971), p. 465.

47. Robert Rosenblum, "Picasso and the Anatomy of Eroticism," in *Studies in Erotic Art* (New York: 1970), p. 345.

48. Margaret Walters, *The Nude Male* (New York: 1978), p. 269.

Chapter VI

1. These and subsequent quotations from Rochester's works are taken from *The Complete Poems of John Wilmot, Earl of Rochester*, David M. Vieth, ed. (New Haven and London: 1968).

2. Riched E. Quaintance, "French Sources of the Restoration 'Imperfect Enjoyment' Poem," *Philological Quarterly*, vol. 52 (1963), p. 190.

3. *Ovid's Epistles: with his Amours*, Tonson-Dryden edition (London: 1776).

4. Havelock Ellis, *The Psychology of Sex* (New York: 1936), vol. 3, p. 169.

5. "The Choise of Valentines, or the Merie Ballad of Nashe his dildo," in the *Works of Thomas Nashe*, Ronald B. McKerrow, ed., vol III (New York: 1966), p. 285.

6. Harold Robbins, *The Adventurers* (New York: 1976), p. 771.

7. Wayland Young, *Eros Denied* (New York: 1954), p. 326.

8. *The Poems of Etherege*, J. Thorne, ed. (Princeton: 1963), p. 35.

9. D. H. Lawrence, *Lady Chatterley's Lover* (New York: 1959), pp. 251–52.

10. Herman Melville, "I and My Chimney," in *Selected Writings of Herman Melville*, Modern Library (New York: 1952), pp. 373–408.

11. Robert Shulman, "The Serious Functions of Melville's Phallic Jokes," *American Literature*, vol. 33 (1961), p. 179. Perry Miller, *The Raven and the Whale* (New York: 1956), p. 39. Howard P. Vincent, *The Trying-Out of Moby Dick* (New York: 1956), p. 313.

12. *Hamlet*, Act III, Scene II.

13. Thomas Pyles, "Ophelia's 'Nothing,'" *Modern Language Notes*, vol. 44 (1949), p. 322.

14. *Romeo and Juliet*, Act III, Scene III.

15. *Ibid.*, Act II, Scene I.

16. *Hamlet*, Act III, Scene II.

17. *Cymbeline*, Act III, Scene IV.

18. *Troilus and Cressida*, Act V, Scene II.

19. Sonnet 95.

20. *Troilus and Cressida*, Act V, Scene II.

21. *Much Ado About Nothing*, Act III, Scene IV.

22. *Romeo and Juliet*, Act II, Scene I. The reference is to a kind of pear (from Poperinge, Belgium) thought to resemble the penis and scrotum.

23. *The Taming of the Shrew*, Act IV, Scene I.

24. E. A. M. Colman, *The Dramatic Use of Bawdy in Shakespeare* (London: 1974).

25. *Othello*, Act I, Scene I.

26. *Measure for Measure*, Act III, Scene II.

27. Eric Partridge, *Shakespeare's Bawdy* (New York: 1948), p. 30.

28. *Much Ado About Nothing*, Act III, Scene IV.

29. *As You Like It*, Act III, Scene II.

30. *Titus Andronicus*, Act V, Scene II.

31. Partridge, *op. cit.*, p. 32.

32. *The Merry Wives of Windsor*, Act IV, Scene I.

33. Thomas W. Ross, *Chaucer's Bawdy* (New York: 1972), p. 17.

34. *Troilus and Cressida*, Act IV, Scene V.

35. Cited in Martin Green, *The Labyrinth of Shakespeare's Sonnets* (London: 1974), p. 23.

36. *Henry V*, Act II, Scene I.

37. Sigmund Freud, *The Interpretation of Dreams* (New York: 1938), pp. 309–10.

38. *Hamlet*, Act IV, Scene IV.

39. Ernest Jones, *Hamlet and Oedipus* (London: 1949), p. 53.

40. *Ibid.*, p. 90.

41. *Hamlet*, Act IV, Scene VII.

42. *Ibid.*, Act III, Scene IV.

43. Jones, *op. cit.*, pp. 81–82.

44. Norman N. Holland, *Psychoanalysis and Shakespeare* (New York: 1976), pp. 205–06.

45. Letter dated October 15, 1897, cited in Holland, *op. cit.*, p. 59.

46. Representative of the pro school is Patrick Mullahy, *Oedipus: Myth and Complex* (New York: 1948).

47. Ernest Hemingway, *Green Hills of Africa* (New York: 1935).

48. *Ibid.*, p. 64.

49. *Ibid.*, p. 214.

50. *Ibid.*, p. 290.

51. *Ibid.*, p. 295.

52. Ruth Sullivan, "Big Mama, Big Papa and Little Sons in Ken Kesey's 'One Flew over the Cuckoo's Nest,'" *Literature and Psychology*, vol. 24 (1976), p. 34.

53. Bruno Bettelheim, *The Uses of Enchantment* (New York: 1977), p. 6.

54. *Ibid.*, p. 187.

55. *Ibid.*, p. 195.

56. *Ibid.*, p. 220.

57. James Joyce, *Portrait of the Artist as a Young Man* (New York: 1964), p. 8.

58. Anne Fremantle, "The Oedipal Legend in Christian Hagiology," *Psychoanalytic Quarterly*, vol. 19 (1950), p. 408.

59. Weston La Barre, "The Psychopathology of Drinking Songs," *Psychiatry*, vol. 2 (1959), p. 203.

60. George Frumkes, "The Oedipus Theme in Stories of the Opera," *Journal of Hillside Hospital*, vol. 4 (1955), p. 14.

61. Richard Sterba, "Kilroy Was Here," *American Imago*, vol. 5 (1948), p. 173.

62. Sigrid Undset, "D. H. Lawrence," in *The Achievement of D. H.*

Lawrence, Frederick J. Hoffman and Harry T. Moore, eds. (Norman, Okla.: 1953), p. 54.

63. Cited in *Critics on D. H. Lawrence,* W. T. Andrews, ed. (London: 1971), p. 36.

64. D. H. Lawrence, *Sex, Literature and Censorship,* Harry T. Moore, ed. (New York: 1953), pp. 49–50.

65. *Ibid.,* p. 110.

66. *Ibid.,* p. 114.

67. Eliseo Vivas, *The Failure and the Triumph of Art* (Evanston, Ill.: 1960), p. 58.

68. Cited in Frank Kermode, *D. H. Lawrence* (New York: 1973), p. 125.

69. D. H. Lawrence, "Making Love to Music," in *Sex, Literature and Censorship,* p. 45.

70. *The Collected Letters of D. H. Lawrence,* ed., with an introduction by Harry T. Moore (New York: 1962), p. 1028.

71. *Ibid.,* p. 1042.

72. *Ibid.,* p. 1046.

73. Edmund Wilson, "Signs of Life: Lady Chatterley's Lover," *New Republic,* vol. 59 (July 3, 1929), p. 184.

74. D. H. Lawrence, *Lady Chatterley's Lover* (New York: n.d.), p. 1.

75. *Ibid.,* p. 2.

76. *Ibid.,* p. 3.

77. *Ibid.,* p. 4.

78. *Ibid.,* p. 20.

79. *Ibid.,* p. 31.

80. *Ibid.,* p. 61.

81. *Ibid.,* p. 75.

82. *Ibid.,* pp. 134–35.

83. *Ibid.,* pp. 135–36.

84. *Ibid.,* p. 136.

85. *Ibid.,* p. 147.

86. *Ibid.,* p. 148.

87. *Ibid.,* p. 157.

88. *Ibid.,* pp. 160–61.

89. *Ibid.,* pp. 205–06.

90. *Ibid.,* p. 207.

91. *Ibid.,* pp. 241–42.

92. *Ibid.,* p. 252.

93. *Ibid.,* pp. 297–98.

94. G. Wilson Knight, "Lawrence, Joyce and Powys," in *Essays in Criticism,* vol XI (1961), p. 403. J. Sparrow, "Regina vs. Penguin Books," *Encounter,* vol. 101 (1962), pp. 35–43.

95. See, for instance, Frank Kermode, "Spenser and the Allegorists," in *Shakespeare, Spenser, Donne: Renaissance Essays* (New York: 1971). Mark Spilka, "Lawrence Up-Tight," *Novel*, vol. IV (1971), pp. 252–67. Ford, Kermode, Clarke, Spilka, "Critical Exchange," *Novel*, vol. V (1971), pp. 54–70. Colin Clarke, *River of Dissolution* (New York: 1969). H. M. Daleski, *The Forked Flame* (Evanston, Ill.: 1965), as well as the sources cited below.

96. Frank Kermode, *D. H. Lawrence* (New York: 1973), p. 141.

97. Mark Spilka, *The Love Ethic of D. H. Lawrence* (Bloomington, Ind.: 1955), p. 119.

98. Knight, *op. cit.*, p. 408.

99. Ernest Hemingway, *The Short Stories of Ernest Hemingway* (New York: 1953), p. 491.

100. Cited in Lisbeth J. Sachs and Bernard H. Stern, "The Little Pre-oedipal Boy in Papa Hemingway and How He Created His Artistry," in *Essays in American Language and Literature*, Costerus, ed., vol. 1 (1971), p. 222.

101. Philip Young, *Ernest Hemingway* (New York: 1952), p. 136.

102. Hemingway, *op. cit.*, p. 383.

103. Ernest Hemingway, *The Sun Also Rises* (New York: 1970), p. 168.

104. Richard Drinnon, "In the American Heartland," *Psychoanalytic Review*, vol. 52 (1965), p. 23.

105. George Plimpton, "An Interview with Hemingway," in *Hemingway and His Critics*, Carlos Baker, ed. (New York: 1961), p. 29.

106. Hemingway, *The Sun Also Rises*, p. 247.

107. Mark Spilka, "The Death of Love in 'The Sun Also Rises,'" in *Hemingway, a Collection of Critical Essays*, Robert P. Weeks, ed. (New York: 1972), p. 137.

108. Ernest Hemingway, *To Have and Have Not* (New York: 1937), p. 103.

109. Ernest Hemingway, *A Moveable Feast* (New York: 1964), pp. 187–93.

110. Hemingway, *Short Stories*, p. 363.

111. *Ibid.*, p. 365.

112. Plimpton, *op. cit.*, p. 29.

113. Hemingway, *Short Stories*, p. 366.

114. *Ibid.*, p. 497.

115. Hemingway, *A Moveable Feast*, p. 119.

116. Ernest Hemingway, *Death in the Afternoon* (New York: 1960), p. 205.

117. Hemingway, *A Moveable Feast*, p. 18.

118. Hemingway, *Short Stories*, p. 391.

119. Cited in Scott Donaldson, *By Force of Will: The Life and Art of Ernest Hemingway* (New York: 1977), p. 185.

120. Cited in Drinnon, *op. cit.*, p. 26.

121. Ernest Hemingway, *Short Stories* (New York: 1967), p. 3.

122. *Ibid.*, p. 6.

123. *Ibid.*

124. *Ibid.*, p. 26.

125. *Ibid.*, p. 22.

126. *Ibid.*, p. 23.

127. *Ibid.*

128. *Ibid.*, p. 17.

129. Robert W. Lewis, Jr., *Hemingway on Love* (Austin: 1965), p. 83.

130. Hemingway, *Short Stories* (New York: 1967), p. 9.

131. *Ibid.*, p. 33.

132. *Ibid.*, p. 34.

133. *Ibid.*, p. 36.

134. Hemingway, *Death in the Afternoon*, p. 87.

135. Hemingway, *Short Stories* (New York: 1967), p. 21.

136. Norman Mailer, *Advertisements for Myself* (New York: 1959), p. 17.

137. *Ibid.*, p. 385.

138. *Ibid.*, p. 341.

139. *Ibid.*, p. 351.

140. *Ibid.*

141. *Ibid.*, p. 347.

142. George Alfred Schrader, "Norman Mailer and the Despair of Defiance," in *Norman Mailer, a Collection of Critical Essays*, Leo Braudy, ed. (Englewood Cliffs, N.J.: 1972), p. 88.

143. James Baldwin, "The Black Boy Looks at the White Boy," *Esquire* magazine (May 1961), pp. 102–06.

144. Norman Mailer, *Presidential Papers* (London: 1964), p. 143.

145. Jean Radford, *Norman Mailer, a Critical Study* (New York: 1975), p. 146.

146. Norman Mailer, *The Naked and the Dead* (New York: 1948), p. 325.

147. Norman Mailer, *Barbary Shore* (New York: 1951), p. 146.

148. Norman Mailer, *The Deer Park* (New York: 1951), p. 140.

149. Norman Mailer, *Cannibals and Christians* (New York: 1966), p. 107.

150. Mailer, *Advertisements for Myself*, p. 486.

151. *Ibid.*, p. 488.

152. *Ibid.*, pp. 489–90.

153. *Ibid.*, p. 497.

154. *Ibid.*, pp. 501–02.

155. Philip Bunfithis, *Norman Mailer* (New York: 1978), p. 61.

156. Radford, *op. cit.*, p. 143.

157. Diana Trilling, "The Image of Women in Contemporary Literature," in *The Woman in America*, Jay Lifton, ed. (Boston: 1964), p. 63.

158. Norman Mailer, *An American Dream* (New York: 1964), p. 16.

159. *Ibid.*, p. 35.

160. *Ibid.*, pp. 44–52.

161. *Ibid.*, pp. 121–22.

162. *Ibid.*, p. 252.

163. Leslie Fiedler, "Master of Dreams," *Partisan Review* (Summer 1967), p. 354.

164. Mailer, *An American Dream*, p. 49.

165. Stanley T. Gutman, *Mankind in Barbary: The Individual and Society in the Novels of Norman Mailer* (Hanover, N.H.: 1975), p. 110.

166. Richard Gilman, "What Mailer Has Done," in Brandy, *op. cit.*, p. 161.

167. Norman Mailer, *The Prisoner of Sex* (New York: 1971), p. 31.

168. *Ibid.*, p. 125.

169. *Ibid.*, p. 132.

170. *Ibid.*, p. 231.

171. Laura Adams, *Existential Battles, the Growth of Norman Mailer* (Athens, Ohio: 1976), p. 167.

172. Kate Millett, *Sexual Politics* (New York: 1971), p. 434.

173. Andrew Gordon, "*The Naked and the Dead:* The Triumph of Impotence," *Literature and Psychology*, vol. 19 (1975), pp. 3–13.

174. *Ibid.*, pp. 5–6.

175. Paul Carroll, "*Playboy* Interview," in *Norman Mailer, the Man and His Work*, Robert F. Lucid, ed. (Boston: 1971), p. 290.

176. Norman Mailer, *The Presidential Papers* (New York: 1964), pp. 143–44.

177. *Ibid.*, p. 157.

Chapter VII

1. Cited in Bernard Rudofsky, *The Unfashionable Human Body* (New York: 1971), p. 58

2. Claude Lévi-Strauss, *Tristes Tropiques* (New York: 1977), p. 237.

3. J. C. Flugel, *The Psychology of Clothes* (London: 1971) , p. 26.

4. Edmund Bergler, *Fashion and the Unconscious* (New York: 1953), p. 221.

5. Flugel, *op. cit.*, p. 104.

6. James Laver, *Modesty in Dress* (Boston: 1969), p. 122.

7. *Ibid.*, p. 124.

8. David K. Kentsmith, "The Rape of the Lock Revisited," *Psychiatric Quarterly*, vol. 47 (1973), p. 571.

9. Havelock Ellis, *Studies in the Psychology of Sex*, vol. 4 (New York: 1936), p. 174.

10. Charles Berg, *The Unconscious Significance of Hair* (New York: 1959).

11. Wayland Young, *Eros Denied* (New York: 1964), p. 322.

12. Cited in Winthrop D. Jordan, *White over Black* (Chapel Hill, N.C.: 1968), p. 34.

13. *Ibid.*, p. 501.

14. *Ibid.*, p. 159.

15. *Ibid.*, p. 35.

16. *Ibid.*, p. 150.

17. Louis Jolyon West, "The Psychobiology of Racial Violence," *Archives of General Psychiatry*, vol. 16 (1967), p. 648.

18. Jordan, *op. cit.*, p. 153.

19. Cited in Charles Herbert Stember, *Sexual Racism* (New York: 1976), p. 18.

20. Michael Banton, *White and Coloured* (New Brunswick, N.J.: 1960), p. 31.

21. William Montague Cobb, "Physical Anthropology of the American Negro," *American Journal of Physical Anthropology*, vol. 29 (1942), p. 158.

22. Cited in Gary I. Schulman, "Race, Sex and Violence: A Laboratory Test of the Sexual Threat of the Black Male Hypothesis," *American Journal of Sociology*, vol. 79 (1974), p. 1260.

23. Jordan, *op. cit.*, p. 579.

24. Cited in Stember, *op. cit.*, p. ix.

25. Schulman, *op. cit.*

26. Karen F. Rotkin, "The Phallacy of Our Sexual Norm," *RT: A Journal of Radical Therapy*, vol. 3, no. 1 (September, 1972).

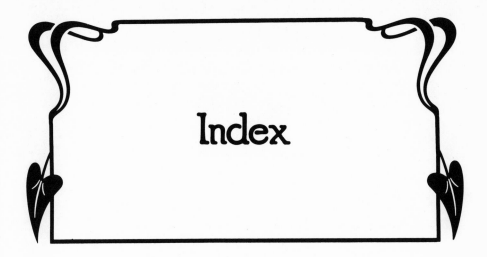

Index